# Jews in Medicine

# JEWS IN MEDICINE

Contributions to Health and Healing
Through the Ages

RONALD L. EISENBERG, MD, JD, DSJS

URIM PUBLICATIONS
Jerusalem • New York

Jews in Medicine:
Contributions to Health and Healing Through the Ages
Ronald L. Eisenberg

Copyright © 2019 Ronald L. Eisenberg

All rights reserved

No part of this book may be used
or reproduced in any manner whatsoever without
written permission from the copyright owner,
except in the case of brief quotations
embodied in reviews and articles.

Typeset by Ariel Walden

Printed in Israel

First Edition

ISBN 978-965-524-300-0

Urim Publications
P.O. Box 52287
Jerusalem 9152102 Israel

**www.UrimPublications.com**

Library of Congress Cataloging-in-Publication Data

Names: Eisenberg, Ronald L., author.
Title: Jews in medicine : contributions to health and healing through the ages /
    Ronald L. Eisenberg.
Description: First edition. | Jerusalem ; New York : Urim Publications, [2019] |
    Includes bibliographical references and index.
Identifiers: LCCN 2018051833 | ISBN 9789655243000 (hardback : alk. paper)
Subjects: | MESH: Physicians—history | Jews—history | Religion and Medicine |
    Judaism—history | Biography
Classification: LCC R694 | NLM WZ 150 | DDC 610.69/5089924—dc23
LC record available at https://lccn.loc.gov/2018051833

# Contents

# Contents

## Modern Era

## Jewish Hospitals in the United States

## The Age of Specialization - Basic Sciences

## The Age of Specialization - Clinical Medicine 265

Contents                                                                    17

# Preface

COMBINING MY PASSION FOR medicine and Jewish studies, *Jews in Medicine* highlights the extraordinary contributions made by Jewish physicians over the ages. The book begins with a traditional Jewish view of medicine based on the Bible and Talmud. Then it focuses on the relationship of Jews and medicine in Islamic and Christian lands, offering a short description of Jewish history of the period followed by accounts of individual Jewish physicians and their major contributions, divided into the regions in which they lived. Turning to the 16th to 18th centuries, the next section details the consequences of the expulsion from Spain, as Jewish physicians moved throughout Europe. This leads into a discussion of the Jewish contributions to medicine in the modern era (19th and 20th centuries), an age that was marked by the development of specialization, broadly categorized into basic sciences and clinical medicine. There is also a section on the rise and fall of Jewish hospitals in the United States. The book ends with a description of Jewish physicians (often non-practicing) who were leaders in the Zionist movement, and those who contributed to the development of medicine in the State of Israel.

Most chapters begin with a general introduction, followed by a series of individual entries on important physicians that provide a brief biography and discussion of their major discoveries and writings. Whenever appropriate, the book includes the relationship of individual physicians with the broader Jewish community. As is customary with postage stamps in both the United States and Israel which do not include personalities who are still alive, no living Jewish physicians have been included in this book, with the exception of winners of the Nobel or Lasker Prizes.

It obviously is impossible to include every Jewish physician who has made meaningful contributions to the development of medicine. There are countless others, such as my father Dr. Milton Eisenberg, who contributed enormously to the welfare of their communities.

Written in a non-technical style and requiring no specialized medical or Jewish knowledge, *Jews in Medicine* is designed for general readers interested in the fascinating history and scope of Jewish contributions to medicine.

*Acknowledgements*

AT URIM, I WANT to thank Pearl Friedman for her brilliant editing and painstaking attention to detail, and publisher Tzvi Mauer for his continued support and advice. I am grateful to both of them for urging me to add photographs of many of the physicians cited. Thanks also to the History of Medicine collection of the National Library of Medicine and to Wikimedia for their vast repositories of free images, as well as to the numerous medical and university archives that freely offered high-resolution images and permission to use their copyrighted material. I greatly appreciate those families of physicians who sent me images of their departed loved ones, as well as the living Nobel Prize winners who graciously supplied images for the book. Finally, as always, I want to thank my wife, Zina Schiff, for her insights and enthusiasm throughout the entire process.

To Zina, Avlana, and Cherina,
who are proof that love and laughter
are the best medicine,

In memory of my father,
Dr. Milton Eisenberg,
an unsung Jewish medical hero,

and

In memory of my mentor,
Dr. Alexander Margulis.

# JEWISH VIEW OF HEALTH

~: ~

In Jewish thought, the concept of "health" entails both physical and emotional/spiritual well-being – health of both the body and the soul. This "holistic" view is evident in the word *shleimut* (completeness), one of the Hebrew terms for health. Another word for health is *beri'ut* (from the root "to create"), which identifies health with creating one's life as a work of art. This implies that one can have a disability, such as an amputation or deafness, and yet be considered healthy in terms of productivity and the ability to contribute to society. Even the word for physician (*rofeh*) comes from a root meaning "to ease," indicating that the doctor treating a "disease" is effectively removing some impediment that is preventing the patient from proceeding further in the creation of a whole and fulfilling life.

Judaism teaches that each person is responsible for taking those steps necessary to preserve health and for seeking qualified medical care when needed. The Bible commands Jews to "take good care of yourself" (Deut. 4:9), requiring that they not endanger themselves through lifestyle choices. Because the body is viewed as a vessel for the soul and the instrument through which one worships God and carries out the Divine will, taking proper care of the body is a *mitzvah*, for only a healthy body is capable of sustaining a holy soul. As the "caretaker" of a body on loan from God, it is incumbent on each person to keep the Divine vessel clean (Lev. R. 34:3). The Talmud stressed the need for personal hygiene, recommending that the hands, legs, and face be washed every day. According to R. Samuel, washing the eyes with cold water in the morning and bathing the hands and feet in warm water at night is better than any medicine for the eye. R. Nathan said that an evil spirit rests on the hands at night and can only be removed by washing the hands three times (Shab. 108b–109a). Indeed, the Talmud states that a Jew may not live in a town without a bathhouse

(BK 46a). Similarly, a Jew is forbidden to mark his body by tattoos and prohibited from the ancient pagan mourning custom of mutilating the flesh (Lev. 19:28).

Once when Hillel was leaving his disciples, they said to him: "Master, where are you going?" He replied: "to do a pious deed." They asked: "What may that be?" He replied: "To take a bath." They asked: "Is that a pious deed?" He replied: "Yes. If in the theaters and circuses, the images of the king must be kept clean by the man to whom they have been entrusted, how much more is it a duty of man to care for the body, since man has been created in the divine image and likeness" (Lev. R. 34:3).

In addition to the stress on hygiene and preventative measures to preserve health, a major biblical innovation was the introduction of a weekly day of rest. No earlier or contemporaneous civilization in Babylonia, Egypt, Greece, or Rome had an institution like the Sabbath, "a seventh day [when] you shall cease from labor" (Exod. 34:21), which was also required "during plowing and harvest time" – periods of the year when there was urgent pressure in the fields and the Israelites would naturally feel that their livelihood demanded continuous work without a break. The requirement to refrain from work was emphasized in connection with the manna, which nourished the Israelites during their years of wandering in the wilderness. On the sixth day, twice as much manna appeared because none was provided on the seventh day when gathering would have constituted work. The severe consequences of violating that prohibition against work on the Sabbath was graphically illustrated by the tale of a man who was sentenced to death by stoning for gathering sticks on the Sabbath (Num. 15:32–36).

## ROLE OF THE PHYSICIAN

Based solely on the literal meaning of the biblical text, it is unclear whether human beings are even permitted to treat illness. Sickness is often described as a Divine punishment for sin – either as a specific statement ("King X did . . . and he became sick") or in nonspecific terms ("If you do . . ., you will be punished by a certain sickness"). Agreeing with the frequent biblical description of sickness as Divine punishment for sin, the Talmud says: "If a man sees that painful sufferings visit him, let him examine his conduct. If he examines and finds nothing [objectionable], let him attribute it to neglect of Torah study." If he still finds nothing, the conclusion must be that these are "chastenings of love" (Ber. 5a). Thus, medical care could be interpreted as a human attempt to intervene in Divine actions, a rejection of God's prerogative. Jeremiah (17:14) exclaims, "Heal me, O Lord, and I shall be healed," and the eighth benediction in the *Amidah* describes God as "Who heals the sick of His people Israel" – implying that only God cures those who are to get well and suggesting that humans should not interfere. One Talmudic-era tract (ARN 36:5) states that the physician is counted among the seven professions whose members have no share in eternal bliss, because he is the accomplice of the patient who should leave his destiny to the decree of the Lord.

Nevertheless, for the majority of Talmudic Rabbis, seeing a doctor when sick was self-evident: "If you are in pain, go to a physician!" (BK 46b). The Talmud suggests various proof texts permitting the physician to attempt to heal. The most quoted citation refers to the situation in which one person strikes and injures another; the first is required to ensure that his victim is "thoroughly healed" (*rapo y'rapei*; Exod. 21:19). A later verse notes that if a person loses something that you know is his, "you shall restore [the lost property] to him" (Deut. 22:2). Maimonides interpreted this phrase as referring to one's health, implying that it is permissible to provide medical care. Commenting on the well-known phrase, "Love your neighbor as yourself" (Lev. 19:18), the Rabbis argued that this even permits curative measures that require inflicting a wound in the process. The rabbinic concept of *pikuach nefesh* associates medical care with the religious requirement of saving a life, implying that the delivery of medical care is legally required. Even desecrating the Sabbath is permitted for *pikuach nefesh*, in keeping with the rabbinic interpretation of the verse, "You shall keep My laws and My rules, by the pursuit of which man shall *live*" (Lev. 18:5), as meaning that violating one Sabbath to save a person's life is more than outweighed by permitting him to observe many others in the future (Yoma 85b). To help save a life, it is permitted to consume forbidden foods and even eat on Yom Kippur (Pes. 25a). The only laws that cannot be violated to preserve a life are those prohibiting murder, idolatry, and sexual immorality (Yoma 85b; Sanh. 74a).

Similarly, one is obliged to "not stand idly by the blood of your neighbor" (Lev. 19:16). The Talmud concludes that human beings and God are partners, not antagonists, in aiding the sick, each playing an important role in the process of health care. R. Akiva noted that just as a farmer works the soil rather than leaving the growing of crops solely to God, so physicians are required to treat the sick – in order to "cultivate" health (Mid. Sam. 52a).

The Talmud observes that "no Jew may live in a town without a physician," and if a Jew feels ill he must immediately consult a doctor (BK 46a). However, it also notes that one should "not dwell in a town where the leader of the community is a physician" (Pes. 113a), either because as a doctor he would be too busy to give proper attention to communal matters or because his civic activities would preclude him from devoting enough time to care for his patients. In addition, the Rabbis counseled that a physician "coming from afar has a blind eye," meaning that he is little concerned about the fate of his patient, whom he does not understand as well as a local doctor does (BK 85a). Nevertheless, "Every sickness has its remedy, provided the physician makes the proper diagnosis and then prescribes the correct medicines" (Tanh. Yitro 8).

Biblical treatments for a variety of ailments included washing; bathing in therapeutic waters for skin disease; the application of oils, balsams, and bandages for wounds and fractures; and a variety of specific medications such as myrrh, cassia, galbanum, niter, and sweet cinnamon. In the story of Rachel and Leah, the mandrake was thought to be an aphrodisiac (Gen. 30:14–16). The prophets Elijah and Elisha are each reported as having performed the modern method of mouth-to-mouth artificial respiration to revive young boys (1 Kings 17:22; 2 Kings 4:35).

The Bible rejects all magical rites and ritual incantations to treat diseases and injuries, with the single exception of the *nechustan* (copper serpent). As punishment for their rebellion in the wilderness, God sent fiery serpents to bite the people who had complained to Moses. When the people repented, God heeded their prayers and ordered Moses to make a serpent and place it on a pole, so that anyone who had been bitten could look at it and recover (Num. 21:6–10). Although God did not specify the material to be used, Rashi concludes that Moses chose copper (*nechoshet*), because in Hebrew it contains the letters of *nachash* (serpent), which was attacking the sinners. This copper serpent eventually became an object of idol worship in the Temple, until it was destroyed by King Hezekiah in the 8th century BCE (2 Kings 18:4), an action that was praised by the Rabbis (Ber. 10b). This righteous monarch, who ruled the Kingdom of Judah for 29 years, also is credited by the Talmud for hiding the "Book of Remedies" (Pes. 4:10). A work of unknown origin, it has been attributed variously to King Solomon, Noah or one of his sons, or to the time of Moses and the years of wandering in the desert. According to the last of these theories, the *Book of Remedies* is a compilation of natural tonics, describing the healing properties of plants, herbs, and other substances found in nature. In Hezekiah's time, the people had come to rely on these cures instead of turning to God, leading the king to hide the book lest the Israelites be led toward idolatry, as well as to force the people to recognize that God was the source of healing.

According to Maimonides, the physician should also see the patient when well, not only when ill, so as to be aware of the patient's normal state, such as a higher-than-normal temperature when healthy. Drugs should be employed only as a final remedy; in mild cases, the physician should first try to find a natural cure so that the body can heal itself. Maimonides argued that using drugs in mild cases may be counterproductive. If a mistake is made, the therapy may prove to be contrary to the course of nature, impeding cure while aggravating pain. Even if the correct drug is given, the inner nature of the patient learns lazy ways rather than exerting itself to heal in the absence of external help. Maimonides also maintained that the physician should not merely treat the disease but rather the person suffering from it, for successfully treating the disease often does not mean that one has cured the patient.

According to Ben Sira, "Honor the doctor for his services, for the Lord created him. His skill comes from the Most High, and he is rewarded by kings. The doctor's knowledge gives him high standing and wins him the admiration of the great. The Lord has created medicines from the earth, and a sensible man will not disparage them. . . . The Lord has imparted knowledge to men, so that by their use of His marvels God may win praise; by using them the doctor relieves pain and from them the pharmacist concocts his mixture. There is no end to the works of the Lord, who spreads health over the whole world" (38:1–8). Should a doctor be paid for providing medical services? As the Talmud observes, "A physician who heals for nothing is worth nothing" (BK 85a).

In essence, the Jewish view is that physicians are agents or partners of God. Although given permission to treat patients, physicians should never feel that their power and skill alone have resulted in a cure. The major duty of the physician is to educate their patients in ways to prevent illness and attain health. They must serve as role models for their patients, for as expressed in the ethical will of Judah ibn Tibbon to his physician son, a doctor cannot expect the patient to listen unless he himself practices what he advises others.

## RITUAL PURITY AND IMPURITY

A major set of biblical laws relates to ritual purity and impurity. After the erection of the Tabernacle, the Israelites were required to free their camp of all ritual contamination (*tumah*) so that the Divine Presence (*Shechinah*) could dwell within it. Although strictly speaking these laws applied only in reference to the Sanctuary and the holy objects connected with it, some have argued that these laws were "hygienic," designed to prevent the spread of infection among the community. They consider the prescribed purification (by water or fire) as a process of "disinfection." However, no prayer or formula was recited, and the sacrifice (which invariably took place *after* purification) was only a formal indication that the person was eligible to return to the camp. Those who hold the other point of view maintain that the laws of purity and impurity were levitical (purely religious) and unrelated to sanitary concerns. They point to multiple biblical passages stressing that these laws were designed to direct the people to holiness and to guard them against anything that was defiling or would prevent them from participating in activities related to the Sanctuary. Neverthe-less, these laws involved sanitary regulations and quarantines to prevent epidemics and the spread of disease.

Among those things that could cause ritual impurity were the carcasses of animals (Lev. 11:24); the carcasses of certain creeping creatures (weasel, mouse, great lizard, gecko, land-crocodile, lizard, sand-lizard, and chame-leon), which were also prohibited as food (Lev. 11:29–30); and food and drink in an earthen vessel into which one of these dead creatures or their droppings had fallen (Lev. 11:34). The most potent source of ritual impu-rity was a dead human body (Num. 19:11). It conveyed ritual uncleanness to anyone or anything that entered or remained within the same tent or under the same roof as a corpse (including household utensils and wearing apparel), even if the person had no direct contact with it. A person who had contact with an individual who had become ritually unclean became himself ritually impure and could even transmit this state to food and drink. Another important source of ritual uncleanness was contact with a menstruating woman (*niddah*). During her period of separation, anyone who touched her, her bedding, or anywhere she sat would become ritu-ally impure.

A man who had a chronic discharge from his sex organ (*zav*) and a woman suffering from non-menstrual bleeding or a genital discharge (*za-vah*) were said to suffer from a "flux" and were deemed ritually unclean (Lev. 15:2–18; 25–28). A male who had an involuntary seminal emission could immerse himself immediately and become ritually pure the evening following the immersion. Semen itself was considered unclean and could make any garment or skin it touched ritually impure (Lev. 15:16–18).

Following childbirth, a woman was deemed ritually unclean (Lev. 12:2–8), presumably due to the physical secretions related to the birth process. Her period of impurity depended on the gender of her offspring. Accord-ing to biblical law, a woman who gave birth to a son was ritually impure for seven days (like a menstruating woman); however, following the birth of a girl, the mother was a *niddah* for fourteen days.

A person afflicted with "*tzara'at*" (*metzora*) was deemed ritually unclean.

Although this term is often translated as "leprosy," the signs described in the Torah and the reversibility of this skin condition make it doubtful that it refers to that incurable disease. To be made recognizable so that people could keep away from him, the *metzora* had to rend his clothes, allow the hair of his head to go loose, cover his upper lip, and cry "unclean, unclean" (Lev. 13:45). It was forbidden for affected individuals to cut out or cauterize the physical signs of *tzara'at* in order to change their appearance. The Rabbis regarded *tzara'at* as a Divine punishment for slander or tale-bearing (*lashon ha-ra*; lit. "evil speech"), indicating that such a person is a "moral leper" who must be excluded from the camp of Israel. The prime biblical example is Miriam, who developed *tzara'at* after she "spoke against Moses because of the Cushite woman whom he had married" (Num. 12:1).

*Tzara'at* also could contaminate garments through contact with an afflicted individual or his sores (Lev.13:47–59). Some explain the spots on the garments as related to mildew or a parasitic infection. In addition, *tzara'at* could affect a house, which might require partial or even complete demolition (Lev.14:33–53). This condition was most likely due to a fungus similar to the cause of dry rot, though some have suggested that it represented parasitic insects or a collection of nitrous material that had formed in the walls.

For all of these cases of ritual impurity, all afflicted individuals had to thoroughly clean themselves with water before being allowed back into the camp (Lev. 15:2–13; Num. 19:16).

When the Israelite army went to war, its encampment was to be completely different from that of any other nation. Because Israel's success was in the hands of God, the camp must be a place of purity, free from dirt and waste, as befitting the Divine Presence. One mechanism for ensuring the cleanliness and sanctity of the camp was the command to reserve a place outside the camp where the troops could go to relieve themselves, so that God would not "see an unseemly thing among you and turn away from you" (Deut. 23:13). Each soldier was commanded to provide himself with a shovel or paddle in addition to his weapons, so that he could dig up the earth and cover his excrement (Deut. 23:15).

## KASHRUT

There is disagreement whether the Jewish dietary laws (*kashrut*) have any health-related basis. The underlying biblical rationale is the verse, "*Sanctify yourself and be holy, for I am holy*" (Lev. 11:44). This demand has two aspects: (a) the positive aspect of imitating God by manifesting such Divine traits as being merciful, loving, and long-suffering; and (b) the negative aspect of withdrawing from things that are impure and abominable. Thus, Jews were required to avoid anything that could pollute them, either physically or spiritually. In his *Guide for the Perplexed*, Maimonides noted that "the dietary laws train us in the mastery over our appetites; they accustom us to restrain both the growth of desire and the disposition to consider the pleasure of eating and drinking as the end of man's existence." This concept is illustrated in the *Sifra* (11:22): "Let not a man say, 'I do not like the flesh of swine.' On the contrary, he should say, 'I like it but must abstain seeing that the Torah has forbidden it'." In his allegorical Torah commentary *Akedat Yitzhak*, the 15th century Isaac ben Moses Arama wrote: "The reason behind all the dietary prohibitions is not that any harm may be caused to the body, but that these foods defile and pollute the soul and blunt the intellectual powers, thus leading to confused opinions and a lust for perverse and brutish appetites that lead men to destruction, thus defeating the purpose of creation."

Nevertheless, commentators have suggested some health benefits for following the Jewish dietary laws. As a physician, Maimonides observed that, "all food which is forbidden by the Law is unwholesome." Sefer ha-Chinuch noted, "The injurious effect of some forbidden foods is not known to us, or even to physicians. The True Faithful Doctor who has commanded us in all these things is infinitely wiser than we. How petty and foolish is the man who thinks that only those things which his understanding grasps are true, and everything else, everything unknown to him, is not true."

As part of kosher slaughtering, a careful examination of the lungs and intestines was required to reject meat from animals with an underlying disease. Similarly, biblical commandments prohibited the consumption of animals that died a natural death (Lev. 22:8) or those that died following the attack of another animal (Exod. 22:31). The eating of blood was also strictly forbidden (Lev. 3:17; 7:26; 17:14; Deut. 12:23).

The biblical proscription against eating pork had substantial health value in protecting against trichinosis. Nevertheless, Maimonides observed that pork "contains more moisture than is necessary (for human food) and too much superfluous matter. The principal reason why the Law forbids swine's flesh is that the habits and food of the swine are very dirty and loathsome. . . . A saying of the Sages declares: 'The mouth of a swine is as dirty as dung itself'" (Ber. 25a).

A kosher fish must have both fins and scales, which excludes creatures whose scales are not clearly defined such as shellfish, shark, catfish, and amphibians. According to Nachmanides, fish with fins and scales can swim close to the surface and, on occasion, come up for air. This warms their blood so that they are able to remove excess fluids and other impurities from their bodies. In contrast, those lacking fins and scales swim close to the sea bottom, cannot purify their bodies, and thus can be harmful to humans if eaten.

# TALMUD

~: :~

Agreeing with the rabbinic view of study as the best medicine, Joshua ben Levi used various biblical verses to prove that this activity is the perfect cure for headache, sore throat, abdominal pain, bone pain, and even generalized pain throughout the body (Er. 54a). When a human being administers a medicine to his friend, it may be beneficial to one limb [organ] but harmful to another. Not so God, who gave the Torah to Israel as a life-giving remedy for the entire body" (Er. 54a).

The Talmud attacked faith healing or magical incantations, labeling those who relied on them as idolaters (Sanh. 11:1). Although it is forbidden to magically try to cure oneself by reciting Torah verses to drive away evil spirits, it is permitted to do so as prayers for continued health and to prevent illness (Shev. 15b).

## REMEDIES AND PREVENTATIVES

The Rabbis suggested a variety of home remedies. For example, "Six things heal a sick person of his disease with a permanent cure: cabbage, beetroot, water distilled from dry moss, the stomach and womb of an animal, and the large lobe of the liver. Some add small fish, which also make fruitful and invigorate a man's whole body" (Ber. 57b). "Bread with salt [the ordinary meal of the poor] and a jug of water will prevent all illness" (BK 92b). In contrast, "Ten things bring a man's sickness on again in a severe form: eating beef, fat meat, roast meat, poultry and roasted egg; shaving; eating cress, milk or cheese; and bathing. Some add nuts and cucumbers" (Ber. 57b). The Talmud (Git. 69b) offers recommended remedies for a host of conditions, including diarrhea and constipation, tapeworms, asthma, catarrh, and angina. For asthma, the Rabbis recommended fennel, mint, and wormwood. These substances in spirits were used as treatment for convulsions after childbirth (Av. Z. 29:1).

Ginger and cinnamon were used as remedies for toothache (Shab. 65a), and a clove of garlic soaked in olive oil and sprinkled with salt was considered an effective treatment for scurvy (Yoma 84a). "One who regularly takes black cumin will not suffer from heartburn" (Ber. 40a). A person who "takes mustard seed regularly once in 30 days keeps sickness away from his house" (Ber. 40a). However, the Rabbis cautioned against taking it every day, "because it weakens the heart" (Ber. 40a). A recommendation for avoiding stomach trouble was "dippings" of bread or other food in wine or vinegar, taken regularly both summer and winter (Git. 70a). Demonstrating an understanding of addiction, Rav warned his son Hiyya, "Do not take drugs [even as a medicine, as they are habit forming]" (Pes. 113a).

"Anxiety [fear], travel, and sin drain a man's strength; eating, drinking, or having marital intercourse standing weaken a man's body" (Git. 70a). Conversely, "Three things restore a person's good spirits: beautiful sounds, sights, and smells" (Ber. 57b). "Eight things diminish the power of procreation: [excessive consumption of] salt, hunger, leprosy, weeping, sleeping on the [bare] ground, lotus, cucumbers out of season, and bloodletting at the lower part of the body, which is as bad as any two" (Git. 70a).

The Rabbis taught that garlic "satiates [satisfies the appetite], keeps the body warm, brightens the face, increases semen [potency], and kills intestinal worms. Some say it fosters love and removes jealousy [by producing a feeling of well-being]" (BK 82a). Considering it an aphrodisiac, the Jerusalem Talmud recommends that garlic be eaten on Friday evenings since "it promotes love and arouses desire" (JT Meg. 4:1, 75a).

Salt was deemed essential to life and eaten with every meal. "Salt lends a sweet taste to meat" (Ber. 5a). "After every food eat salt, and after every beverage drink water, and you will come to no harm. [However,] if one eats any kind of food without taking salt after it, or drinks any beverage without taking water after it, during the day he will be troubled with bad breath and during the night with croup" (Ber. 40a). According to the Jerusalem Talmud, "Salt is cheap and pepper dear; the world can exist without pepper but not without salt" (JT Hor. 48c). However, salt (and leaven) were among three things for which "a little is good but a large amount is harmful" (Ber. 34a), and salt was one of eight things that "decrease seminal fluid" (Git. 70a).

Vegetables constituted a substantial part of the diet during the Talmudic period. The statement, "No scholar should dwell in a town where vegetables are not available" (Er. 55b), indicates that they were considered an important and wholesome food. However, the Rabbis cautioned, "Woe to the house [i.e., stomach] through which vegetables are always passing!" implying that excessive amounts of vegetables are potentially dangerous. Deemed harmful when uncooked, "All raw vegetables make the complexion pale" (Ber. 44b).

The Rabbis recommended certain vegetables more than others. "Eating lentils once every 30 days prevented croup, but eating them every day caused bad breath" (Ber. 40a). "Horse-beans are bad for the teeth, but good for the bowels" (Ber. 44b), and thus must be well cooked and swallowed rather than chewed. "Cabbage is nourishing and beets are good for healing" ( Ber. 44b). R. Hisda stated, "A dish of beets is beneficial for the heart and good for the eyes, and even more so for the bowels," though Abaye said this applied to those that had been thoroughly cooked (Er. 29a).

Radish was termed a "life-giving drug" (Er. 56a), but "R. Hanina ate half an onion and half of its poisonous fluid and became so ill that he was on the point of dying. His colleagues, however, begged for heavenly mercy, and he recovered because his contemporaries needed him" (Er. 29b).

The Rabbis offered tips on how to counteract the dangers related to eating certain vegetables. "[To overcome the harmful effects of] lettuce, eat radishes; for radishes, eat leeks; for leeks, drink hot water." Indeed, drinking hot water was considered a panacea for treating the harmful effects of all vegetables (Pes. 116a).

For the Rabbis, "a soft-boiled egg is better than six ounces of fine flour" (Ber. 44b). They warned that "one should not converse at meals lest the windpipe acts before the esophagus and his life will thereby be endangered" (Ta'an. 5b).

The Rabbis recommended drinking large quantities of water with meals to prevent sickness. How much should one drink? "A cup of water to a loaf of bread" (Ber. 40a). "Eating without drinking is harmful and a source of intestinal ailments [indigestion]. If one eats without [afterwards] walking [at least] four cubits, his food rots [inside him] and leads to bad breath. If one eats when needing to relieve himself, it is like an oven that is heated over its ashes [new fuel being added without the old ashes being cleaned out], and this is the beginning of a [disagreeable] perspiration odor" (Shab. 41a). Drinking a pitcher of water after a breakfast of bread dipped in salt would prevent the "83 different kinds of illnesses connected with abnormalities of the gallbladder" (BK 92b).

The Talmud offered six signs as indications that the health of a sick person was improving – "sneezing, perspiration, open bowels, seminal emission, sleep, and dreaming" (Ber. 57b). According to the Rabbis, "Three things benefit the body without being absorbed by it – washing, anointing with oil, and exercise" (Ber. 57b). Concerning washing, "If one bathes in hot water and does not have a cold shower, he is like iron put into fire but not into cold water [i.e., just as the iron would not be fully tempered, so the body will not derive its full benefit]" (Shab. 41a). Conversely, ten things cause a severe relapse when convalescing from an illness: "eating beef, fat meat, broiled meat and poultry and roasted egg, shaving, and eating cress, milk or cheese, and bathing. Some also add eating nuts; others say eating cucumbers" (Ber 57b).

Ben Sira stressed the relationship between the emotions and health: "Do not give yourself over to sorrow, or distress yourself deliberately. A merry heart keeps a man alive, and joy lengthens his span of days [30:21–22] . . . Envy and anger shorten a man's life, and anxiety brings premature old age. A man with a gay heart has a good appetite and relishes the food he eats [30:24–25]." Rav's statement, "A sigh breaks half a man's body" (Ber. 58b), emphasized the danger of sadness and melancholy to a person's physical health.

The Rabbis considered the prevention of illness to be an important element in keeping healthy: "Pay heed to the physician while you are still healthy" (JT Ta'an. 3:6), and "People die prematurely because of self-neglect" (ARN 9). As the Jerusalem Talmud emphasized, "For each person who dies a natural death, 99 die due to their own negligence" (JT Shab. 14:14).

As a public health measure, the Midrash warns, "One should never expectorate where people pass" (Derch Eretz R. 10). Appreciating the danger of contagion during an epidemic, the Rabbis stressed the need to avoid crowds and to isolate and quarantine those who had been afflicted (BK 60b): "When infectious diseases are rampant, remain at home and do not venture out onto the street" (Mid. Ruth 1). Sanitation was considered both a virtue and a way to prevent disease: "Gnats, flies, and fleas are the curse of the earth" (Gen. R. 20). One recommended way to prevent contagious diseases was to rinse one's cup before and after drinking from it (Tem. 27b). One Rabbi, said to be knowledgeable in medicine, drank only boiled water (JT Ter. 8:5).

As a general rule, the Rabbis advised: "Do not sit too much, for prolonged sitting aggravates hemorrhoids; do not stand for a long time, because it can be harmful to the heart; do not walk too much, because it can be harmful to the eyes." They recommended: "Spend one third of your time doing each. Standing is better than sitting when one has nothing to lean against [i.e., a seat without back support]" (Ket. 111a).

## ANATOMY, PREGNANCY, AND GENETICS

According to the Mishnah (Oh. 1:8), "There are 248 members in a human body: 30 in the foot [six to each toe], 10 in the ankle. Two in the shin, five in the knee, one in the thigh, three in the hip, eleven ribs, 30 in the hand [six in each finger, two in the forearm, two in the elbow, one in the upper arm, four in the shoulder]. This makes 101 on each side of the body. Then there are 18 vertebrae in the spine, nine [members] in the head, eight in the neck, six in the chest, and five in the genitals (Nid. 31a).

Regarding the fetus, the Talmud states that "during the first three months the embryo occupies the lowest chamber [part of the uterus], during the middle ones it occupies the middle chamber, and during the last months it occupies the uppermost chamber; when it is time to emerge, it turns over and comes out, and this is the cause of the woman's pains." R. Eleazar explained that the reason why the pains associated with the birth of a female are worse than those for a male relates to the positions they assume during intercourse. Since all embryos develop face down, a female fetus must turn upward prior to being born, and this turning intensifies the pain (Nid. 31a).

According to the Rabbis, "During the first three months [of pregnancy], marital intercourse is injurious to the woman and also to the child. During the middle ones, it is injurious to the woman but beneficial for the child. During the last months, it is beneficial for both the woman and the child, since on account of it the child becomes well-formed and of strong vitality" (Nid. 31a).

The Talmud states that "there are three partners in creating a human being – God, the father, and the mother. The father supplies the semen of the white substance out of which are formed the child's bones, sinews, nails, the brain in his head and the white in his eye; the mother supplies the semen of the red substance out of which is formed his skin, flesh, hair, blood, and the black of his eye; and God gives him the spirit and the breath [soul], beauty of features, eyesight, the power [of the ear] to hear, the ability [of the mouth] to speak and [of the feet] to walk, understanding, and discernment" (Nid. 31a).

The Talmud notes that some prayers are not appropriate and thus invalid. The Mishnah labels a supplication to God to change the past as a "vain prayer" (Ber. 9:3), citing as an example a husband praying that his pregnant wife will bear a male. At the same time, however, the Talmud states that from the third to the 40th day (after conception), a man may pray that the child should be a male. This suggests that a definite gender is not assigned until that time, presumably related to chemical or endocrine reactions controlled by the Y chromosome that must take place before a definite gender is expressed, and for which some scientific evidence has been reported. Interestingly, there is a similar concept in Islam, which describes that the sperm and ovum fall into the uterus and remain there for forty nights, after which the angel in charge of fashioning it descends upon it and says, "Lord! Male or female?" Then Allah makes it male or female.[1]

A biblical legend regarding Dinah, the youngest child of Leah and Jacob, supports this notion of delayed gender determination. According to the Talmud, Leah "passed judgment" (*dinah din*) on herself out of compassion for her sister, Rachel. She knew that twelve tribes (sons) were destined to issue from Jacob. Leah already had six, and the handmaids each had two. If the child Leah was carrying would also be a male, Rachel would be fated to have only one son and thus not even be equal to one of the handmaids. When Leah prayed that the child in her womb would be a girl, the embryos were switched. Thus Joseph was moved into the womb of Rachel, and Dinah into that of Leah. (Ber. 60a; Targum Yonatan Ber. 30:21)

The Talmud (Yev. 64b) recognized the role of genetics. For example, if a woman delivered two boys, both of whom died from bleeding after circumcision, it was forbidden for this procedure to be performed on a third son. This presumably relates to the hereditary condition of hemophilia. The Talmud explains that the sons of her sisters must not be circumcised, whereas boys born to her brothers may be circumcised, indicating an understanding that hemophilia is transmitted through females yet only affects males. There was also an understanding that certain diseases run in families. On the same page, the Talmud prohibits marrying a woman from a family of epileptics or lepers.

## ENVIRONMENT

The Rabbis were sensitive to environmental concerns. A *midrash* relates that God led Adam around the Garden of Eden and pointed out the beauty and excellence of all His works: "For your sake I created it. See to it that you do not spoil and destroy My world, for if you do, there will be no one to repair it after you" (Eccles. R. 7:13). The Jerusalem Talmud states, "It is forbidden to live in a town that does not have a green garden" (JT 4:12). The Rabbis also emphasized the importance of public measures to protect the health of the population. According to the Babylonian Talmud, "[Animal] carcasses, cemeteries, and tanneries must be kept at a distance

---

1. http://www.livingislam.org/n/hfhl_e.html

at least 50 cubits [about 75 feet] from a town [because of their bad smell]. A tannery may only be set up on the east side of a town [because the prevailing wind comes from the west, and the gentle east wind will not carry a bad odor to the town]" (BB 2:9). Streets and market areas were required to be kept clean. To preserve open space, trees must not be planted closer than 25 cubits from a town. Carob and sycamore trees, which are very leafy, must be at least 50 cubits away (BB 2:7).

Regarding the problem of proper disposal of waste material, "The pious men of former generations used to hide their thorns and broken glass in the midst of their fields at a depth of three handbreadths [about 11 inches] below the surface, so that even a plough could not be hindered by them. R Shesheth [who was blind] used to throw them into the fire. Rava threw them into the Tigris" (BK 30a).

The Rabbis understood the desirability of separating businesses from residential neighborhoods: "If a person wants to open a shop in a courtyard, his neighbor may stop him on the grounds that he will be kept awake by the noise of people going in and out" (BB 20b).

Among the "ten special regulations that were applied to Jerusalem," several were related to environmental issues:

> No garbage dumps were to be made there because of the creeping creatures [which breed in garbage dumps and, when they die, become a source of defilement of the sacred offerings brought to Jerusalem]; no kilns be kept there because of the smoke [which would blacken the city walls and buildings and mar the beauty of Jerusalem]; neither gardens nor orchards be cultivated there [excepting the Garden of Roses,7 which existed from the days of the first prophets] because of the bad odor [from manure and rotting flowers and fruit]; no chickens be raised there because of the consecrated [meat for sacrifices]; and no corpses be kept there overnight [this is known by the oral tradition]. (BK 82b).

### VISITING THE SICK (*BIKUR CHOLIM*)

Visiting the sick is one of the aspects of righteous living that constitute the fundamental Jewish concept of *gemilut chasadim* (lit, "giving of lovingkindness"). Based on God's visiting Abraham when the Patriarch was recovering from his circumcision (Gen. 18:1), visiting the sick is listed as one of the deeds for which "a man enjoys the fruits in this world while the principal remains for him in the World to Come" (Shab. 127a). The

Rabbis observed that one who visits the sick "takes away a sixtieth of his pain" and recommended that "sixty people visit him and restore him to health." Moreover, "even a great person should visit a humble one" (Ned. 39b). Conversely, R. Akiva maintained, "He who does not visit the sick is like a shedder of blood" (Ned. 40a).

One should not visit too early in the morning, when a sick person is often being attended by a physician, nor too late at night, when the patient is tired. During the first three hours of the day, the patient feels much better and the visitor may think that prayer is unnecessary. Conversely, during the last three hours of the day, the patient feels worse and the visitor may feel that praying is hopeless (Ned. 40a).

One who visits the sick must offer spiritual comfort and be attentive to the patient's material needs. Prayers for the sick are vital and may be said in any language. Multiple visits to a patient are permitted as long as they are not too tiring. The Talmud recommends not visiting those suffering with "bowel trouble," so that they do not become embarrassed, or patients for whom the effort of speaking is too tiring; instead, it is preferable to remain in an adjacent room and ask whether one can be of assistance (Ned. 41a). The sick should not be told of the death of a relative or any other bad news, lest this delay their recovery because of being "distracted in mind" (MK 26b).

Is it permitted to visit the sick on the Sabbath, the day of joy on which sadness should not intrude? Beit Shammai prohibited the practice, but the *halachah* agrees with Beit Hillel, which permitted such visits. One visiting a sick person on the Sabbath should say, "It is the Sabbath, when one must not cry out, but [I wish for you that] recovery will come soon." According to R. Meir, one should say, "May [the Sabbath] have compassion [i.e., proper observance of the Sabbath will bring recovery in its wake]" (Shab. 12a).

## PHYSICIANS

During Talmudic times, patients visited physicians in their homes, rather than the Greek practice of doctors treating patients in the marketplace. This led to the enactment of a special regulation requiring that anyone renting space to a physician must first obtain the agreement of his neighbor, since the cries of visiting patients might disturb them (BB 21a). Physicians also were involved in legal decisions. They were required to judge the physical condition of a person sentenced to corporal punishment to determine how many lashes he could withstand (Mak. 22b). When a person was injured, physicians were asked to evaluate the type and extent of physical disability to determine the amount of damages.

In a bizarre text, the Mishnah states that "the best of doctors go to hell" (Kid. 82a). Taking a cynical or playful view of medical care, the Hasidic Reb Nachman of Bratslav maintained that when God created the Angel of Death, the latter protested that he was being given too much work for one angel; immediately, God assured him: "Don't worry. I have given you helpers called physicians!" In *The Book of Delight*, Joseph ibn Zabara relates that a philosopher went to a physician, who said that the philosopher was so sick there was no reason to treat him; the philosopher recovered and later met the physician in the street. "Have you returned from the next world?" asked the physician. After an affirmative response, the physician continued, "What did you see there?" When the philosopher described the terrible punishments visited on physicians because "they kill their patients," the physician was horrified. "Do not feel alarmed," reassured the philosopher, "because I swore to them that you are no physician!"

In a less satiric vein, Rashi argued that the statement refers to the physician who arrogantly believes that the recovery of a patient was due to his own skill, with God playing no role in the process.[2] Some have suggested that "hell" is the fate of those physicians who are convinced they know everything and never seek the advice of their colleagues. The Maharal of Prague said it referred to those doctors who deal only with the physical dimension of medical care and deny the spiritual aspect.

Commentators have noted that the prayer for healing in the *Amidah*, which designates God as the Ultimate Healer, is repugnant to the haughty doctor and so he deletes it, or recites it without sincere intent. "For him, the original eighteen blessings are reduced to seventeen – the numerical

---

2. http://www.talmudology.com/jeremybrownmdgmailcom/2016/5/22/kiddushin-82a-the-best
-doctors-go-to-hell.

value of the Hebrew word *tov* (good) – which is why "the Talmud sarcastically refers to him as 'the best.' "

## Abba the Surgeon (3rd century)

As the Talmud relates (Ta'an. 21b), "When he performed his operations [blood-letting], he would separate men from women, and in addition he had a cloak which held a cup [for receiving the blood] and which was slit at the shoulder. Whenever a woman patient came to him, he would put the garment on her shoulder in order not to see her [exposed body]. He also had a box out of public gaze where the patients deposited their fees which he would charge; those that could afford it put their fees there, and thus those who could not pay were not put to shame. Whenever a young scholar happened to consult him, not only would he accept no fee from him, but on taking leave of him he also would give him some money at the same time adding, 'Go and use this to regain your strength. One day, Abaye sent two scholars to test him. Abba received them and gave them food and drink, and in the evening he prepared woolen mattresses for them [to sleep on]."

## Hanina ben Dosa (Land of Israel *tanna*, 1st century)

A student of R. Yochanan ben Zakkai and famed for his piety and as a miracle worker, Hanina ben Dosa's prayers were said to have healed the children of both his teacher and Rabban Gamaliel II (Ber. 34b). There are two versions of the miraculous encounter between Hanina ben Dosa and a poisonous lizard. In the Jerusalem Talmud (Ber. 5:1), the sage was so focused on his prayers that he did not realize that he had been bitten by a poisonous lizard. When the lizard was found dead, his students exclaimed: "Woe to the man who is bitten by a poisonous lizard, and woe to the lizard that bites Hanina ben Dosa!" The text goes on to explain that the result of a lizard's bite depends upon which reaches water first; if the man, the lizard dies (and vice versa), and in the case of Hanina ben Dosa a spring miraculously opened under his feet. In the Babylonian Talmud (Ber. 33a), Hanina ben Dosa learned of a poisonous lizard that used to injure people. He asked to see its hole and put his heel over it; when the lizard came out and bit him, it died.

According to legend, after Hanina ben Dosa prayed for the sick he could predict which would live and which would die. "Are you a prophet?" the

Rabbis inquired. "No," he replied, "I am neither a prophet nor the son of a prophet, but I learned this from experience. If my prayer comes fluently, I know that it is accepted; but if not, I know that it has been rejected" (Ber. 5:5). When the son of Rabban Gamaliel II become ill, the sage sent two disciples to request that Hanina ben Dosa pray for his recovery. After praying in the upper chamber of his home, Hanina ben Dosa came down to the messengers and told them that the boy's fever had passed and he would recover fully. The disciples carefully noted the exact moment of Hanina ben Dosa's pronouncement and reported it to Rabban Gamaliel, who informed them that "at that very time the fever left him and he asked for water to drink." On another occasion, when Hanina ben Dosa was studying Torah with Yochanan ben Zakkai, the sage's son became ill and Hanina ben Dosa was asked to pray for him. Hanina ben Dosa "put his head between his knees and prayed for him and he lived." Yochanan ben Zakkai observed that had he stuck his head between his knees for the whole day, it would have been to no avail. When his wife asked if that meant that Hanina ben Dosa was greater than he, Yochanan ben Zakkai replied: "No; but he is like a servant before the king [who has permission to go to him at any time] and I am like a nobleman before a king [who appears before him only at fixed times]" (Ber. 34b).

---

### Hanina bar Hama                                    (Land of Israel *amora*, 2nd/3rd century)

---

Most often referred to simply as Hanina, but also known as Hanina ha-Gadol (the Great), he was born in Babylonia and came to the Land of Israel, where he settled in Sepphoris and became a wealthy honey trader (JT Pe'ah 7:4). One of the prominent disciples of Judah ha-Nasi, Hanina bar Hama was said to have built the academy at Sepphoris, which he directed, from the money he earned from one especially profitable transaction (JT Pe'ah 7:3).

One of Hanina bar Hama's most famous sayings is, "Everything is in the hand of God [lit., 'Heaven'] except the fear of God" (Ber. 33b), meaning that although all a person's qualities were fixed by nature, his moral character depended on his own choice. Although convinced that all was predestined – "no man bruises his finger here on earth unless it was so decreed against him by Heaven" (Hul. 7b) – Hanina bar Hama nevertheless declared that fevers and chills were exceptions (BM 107b), and that 99 out of 100 people died through their own fault in not avoiding colds (JT Shab. 14:3). Hanina bar Hama himself lived a long and healthy life – it was reported that at age 80 he was able to balance himself on one foot while taking off and putting on his shoes – which he attributed to the warm baths and oil treatments that he received as a child (Hul. 24b).

---

## Hisda         (Babylonian *amora*, 3rd century)

---

Born into a priestly family, Hisda's early years were spent in poverty. However, he became so wealthy as a brewer (Pes. 113a) that he was able to pay for the rebuilding of the academy at Sura, which he later headed for the last ten years of his life.

Hisda adopted an extreme attitude to modesty, stating that a man should not converse even with his own wife in the street (Ber. 43b). Hisda advised his daughters: "Act modestly in the presence of your husbands: do not eat bread before your husbands [you may eat too much]; do not eat greens at night [because of their odor]; do not eat dates nor drink beer at night [because of their laxative properties]. Regarding nutritious and inexpensive meals, Hisda recommended to his poor students: "When a scholar has but little bread, let him not eat vegetables, because it whets [the craving for food]. I did not eat vegetables when poor or when rich. When poor, because vegetables excite the appetite [which I could not satisfy]; when rich, because I would rather eat fish and meat [which are more nutritious]." However, when purchasing vegetables Hisda urged that they "buy long ones, for one bunch is like another [in thickness], and so the length comes of itself [i.e., the additional length is extra value, since presumably the price was not increased]" (Shab. 140b). He noted that, "A dish of beets is beneficial for the heart and good for the eyes and even more so for the bowels" (Ber. 39a). Hisda recommended that a scholar who has only a little bread should not divide it into small portions, but instead should eat it all at one time so that he would be satisfied at least once during the day. He accused one who can eat barley bread but instead consumes bread made from more expensive wheat as being wastefully extravagant and violating the commandment, "You shall not destroy" (Deut. 20:19). He also suggested: "If a scholar buys raw meat he should buy the neck, because it contains three types of meat [fatty, lean, and tough sinews]" (Shab. 140b).

---

## Joshua ben Levi         (Land of Israel *amora*, 3rd century)

---

Joshua ben Levi was head of the academy at Lydda. Agreeing with the rabbinic view of Torah study as the best medicine, Joshua ben Levi used various biblical verses to prove that this activity is the perfect cure for headache, sore throat, abdominal pain, bone pain, and even generalized pain throughout the body (Er. 54a).

---

## Samuel                                          (Babylonian *amora*, 2nd/3rd century)

---

Born Samuel ben Abba ha-Kohen in Nehardea, his ability to independently determine the beginning of the months resulted in his being given the appellation *Yarchina'ah* (the Astronomer, from the Hebrew word *yare'ach* meaning "moon") (BM 85b). Considered an expert in astronomy, "who knew the paths of the heavens as well as the streets of Nehardea," Samuel also studied medicine and became the physician of Judah ha-Nasi, whom he cured of an eye disease. His medical training led Samuel to permit kindling a fire on the Sabbath for a woman in childbirth and anyone who had been bled and felt chilly, even during the hottest period of the year (Er. 79b; Shab. 129a).

Samuel, the director of the Nehardea academy, and Rav, the head of the academy at Sura, were close friends and intellectual adversaries in halachic discussions. Their disputes on civil and ritual issues constitute the core of the Babylonian Talmud. As teachers of the highest rank in the Jewish world, Samuel and Rav established the intellectual independence of Babylonia, enabling aspiring young scholars to remain at home to study rather than being required to go to the Land of Israel.

As a physician, many of Samuel's opinions on health and diet are found in the Talmud. He opposed the contemporary belief that most diseases were due to the evil eye, declaring instead that they were caused by something noxious in the air (BM 107b). He attributed many disorders to a lack of personal cleanliness and wearing unclean garments (Shab. 133b) and others to a change in diet [i.e., a poor man used to eating only dry bread during the week may suffer from indigestion after eating meat and other expensive foods on Sabbaths and festivals] (BB 146a). Although he developed a well-known salve for eye ailments that were widespread in his area, Samuel declared: "A drop of cold water in the morning, and washing the hands and feet in hot water in the evening, is better than all the eye-salves in the world" (Shab. 108b). He cautioned, "He who washes his face and does not dry it well, will have boils scabs break out [on his face]. What is his remedy? Let him wash well in water [in which beets have been cooked]" (Shab. 133b).

The Talmud relates that once when his colleague was suffering from stomach pains, Samuel brought Rav to his home "and fed him barley bread and small fried fish with beer." Rav became so sick that "he did not cease from visiting the bathroom [from intense diarrhea]. Rav then cursed Samuel saying, "One who causes so much pain should not sire children." And Samuel remained childless throughout his life! (Shab. 108a).

---

## Simlai

Simlai was best known as the first sage to observe that "613 commandments were communicated to Moses [on Mount Sinai]; 365 negative commandments, corresponding to the number of days in the solar year, and 248 positive commandments, corresponding to the number of parts of the human body" (Mak. 23b).

Known primarily as an aggadist, Simlai delivered the following discourse:

> What does an embryo resemble when it is in the bowels of its mother? Folded writing tablets. Its hands rest on its two temples, its two elbows on its two legs, and its two heels against its buttocks. Its head lies between its knees, its mouth is closed, and its navel is open; it eats what its mother eats and drinks what its mother drinks, but produces no excrement because otherwise it might kill its mother. However, as soon as it sees the light of day [lit., 'went out to the air space of the world'], the closed organ [its mouth] opens and the open one [its navel] closes, for otherwise the embryo could not live even one single hour. A light burns above its head and it looks and sees from one end of the world to the other. . . . It is also taught all the Torah from beginning to end. . . . As soon as it sees the light, an angel approaches, slaps it on its mouth, and causes it to forget all the Torah completely (Nid. 30b).

---

## Yochanan

As head of an academy in Tiberias, Yochanan attracted large numbers of gifted students from both the Land of Israel and Babylonia, many of whom became major scholars and related his teachings. Yochanan's authority was accepted throughout the Jewish world, and few contemporary scholars opposed him.

The Talmud related examples of Rabbis bringing about a cure by taking the hand of a sick person. When R. Hiyya bar Abba fell ill, Yochanan went in and asked the ailing sage, "Are your sufferings welcome to you?" From his sickbed, R. Hiyya bar Abba replied, "Neither they nor their reward [i.e., the implication that if one lovingly submits to his sufferings, he will receive a great reward in the World to Come]." Then Yochanan cured his colleague by the touch of his hand. When R. Yochanan later became ill, R. Hanina performed a similar service. The Talmud asked why, if he could cure R. Hiyya bar Abba, Yochanan could not heal himself. The answer: "The prisoner cannot free himself from jail [and similarly, the patient cannot cure himself]" (Ber. 5b).

# JEWISH PHYSICIANS
# IN ISLAMIC LANDS

∾: ∾

## THE GEONIC ERA

Following the initial editing of the Babylonian Talmud by Rav Ashi and Ravina around 500 CE, the *savoraim* completed the final editing a half century later. The *savoraim* were the disciples of the last *amoraim*, who interpreted the Mishnah and applied it to case law to form the Gemara, and were their immediate successors at the Talmudic academies of Sura and Pumbedita. The reopening in the year 589 of these pre-eminent educational institutions, which had been forced to close for a short period under government pressure, ushered in the Geonic Era.

*Gaon* (pl., *geonim*) was the formal title of the heads of the academies of Sura and Pumbedita. Known for their scholarship and wisdom, the *geonim* were considered the intellectual leaders of the entire Diaspora. They were responsible for interpreting Talmudic principles to arrive at practical halachic decisions of Jewish law and procedure, which had absolute legal authority in most Jewish communities. Similar weight was given to their *responsa*, replies to written questions sent to them from all parts of Babylonia and throughout the Jewish world. The *geonim* also exercised legislative power by issuing *takanot* (enactments), rabbinic regulations not derived from any biblical commandment but issued jointly by both academies to cope with new socioeconomic or historical situations or to improve compliance with existing *halachah*. The *geonim* were sent financial gifts from throughout the Diaspora to support their various activities.

## THE RISE OF ISLAM

During the first six centuries of the Christian era, Western Europe suffered through barbarian invasions, natural disasters, and epidemics. When combined with the rabidly anti-Hellenic outlook of the Catholic Church, this led to the loss of much of the classic Greek and Roman writings in philosophy and medicine that had constituted the basis of Western civilization. Fortunately, the rise of Islam in the 7th century resulted in the translation and preservation of much of the classic works of Greco-Roman knowledge.

Mohammed was born in the Arabian city of Mecca around 570. Influenced by exposure to Jewish thinking and the Hebrew Bible, Mohammad initially respected the Jews and borrowed some early teachings from Jewish tradition. However, the Jews refused to recognize Mohammed as a prophet, which resulted in his minimizing or even eliminating the Jewish influence on his beliefs. As examples, Mohammed shifted the direction of prayers from Jerusalem to Mecca, made Friday his special day of prayer, rejected Yom Kippur as a fast day and replaced it with the month of Ramadan, and renounced all the Jewish dietary laws except for the prohibition on eating pork. He retained the ancient Jewish practice of circumcision as a religious rite and adopted the Israelite stress of hygiene and cleanliness. By the time of his death in 632, Mohammed had succeeded in uniting all the Arabian tribes under the banner of Islam, a term meaning submission to the will of God (Allah).

Over the next century, Islamic forces assumed control of the Arabian Peninsula and Middle East, spreading into North Africa, Spain, and part of France. In 711, Arabs and Moors crossed the Straits of Gibraltar from Morocco. Within three years, they had conquered the entire Iberian Peninsula, which became known as the kingdom of Andalusia. Jews had inhabited this region since being brought there by Nebuchadnezzar of Babylonia after the destruction of the First Temple in 586 BCE, and by the Romans after the fall of Jerusalem in 70 CE. During the waning days of the Roman Empire in the early 5th century, Germanic tribes invaded the Iberian Peninsula from the north. After the Visigoth king adopted Catholicism in 589, restrictions were imposed on Jewish freedoms, a series of anti-Jewish laws were passed, and Jews were periodically given the choice between baptism and expulsion. Therefore, it is not surprising that the remaining Jews, many of whom had been forced to accept baptism publicly but still observed Judaism in secret, eagerly welcomed the Arab invaders and assisted them in conquering the land. In turn, the minority Arab rulers welcomed the services of their Jews subjects, who were valuable in administering the new government with its capital in Córdoba. With a tolerant new climate favorable to the development of a vigorous Jewish life, the Iberian Peninsula became the destination of numerous Jews from countries in North Africa and the Middle East, which eventually led to the so-called Golden Age of Spain.

A historical event that led to the spread of Jewish scholarship in the Diaspora, independent of the Babylonian academies, was the episode of the four captives, which probably occurred around 960. Four great Torah scholars from Babylonia, sent to collect contributions from the Diaspora, were captured by a Moorish-Spanish pirate, who decided to offer them for ransom to four different Jewish communities along the Mediterranean. To keep their price as low as possible, the rabbis kept their identities secret. The scholars who eventually gained their freedom were Moses ben Chanoch (and his young son Chanoch) in Córdoba (Spain); Chushiel ben Elchanan in Kairouan (North Africa); Shemariah ben Elchanan in Egypt; and a fourth captive whose identity and fate are unknown. These scholars established major Talmudic academies, so that by the close of the 10th century, important centers of Jewish learning had developed in Spain, North Africa, Egypt, and the Land of Israel that were independent of the scholars of Babylonia. In these communities, local teachings and decisions began to supersede those of the *geonim*. Of even greater importance, financial gifts from the Diaspora to the Talmudic academies of Babylonia steadily decreased and eventually stopped, as local communities preferred to support their own scholars and *yeshivot*.

The centuries of Jewish prominence in trade and commerce became of special value to the Arab conquerors. Because of the difficult and often contentious relations between Moslems and Christians, Jews served as convenient commercial and even diplomatic intermediaries. They permitted the transfer of textiles from Spain and Egypt and the spices and medicinal herbs of the Orient for the furs and timber of Christian Europe. Jews also played a vital role in the transmission of knowledge between the Arab- and Christian-dominated worlds.

The Arab conquerors were captivated by the advanced arts and sciences of the empires over which they assumed control – Greek, Roman, Persian, and Byzantine – and supported thriving centers of learning in Baghdad and Cairo, as well as in Córdoba, a major center in southern Spain. They supported translations of and commentaries on classic Greek and Roman works, amassing a large body of information in the fields of philosophy, mathematics, and science. This included books that no longer existed in their original languages, thus preserving these literary classics for subsequent generations.

Unlike the situation in Christian lands, where Jews were forbidden from treating Christian patients, in the early years of Islamic rule there was little prejudice against non-Muslims treating Muslims patients. Thus, some Jews became highly successful as practicing physicians. Many became renowned for their work as translators of classic Greek medical works into Arabic. They translated numerous major texts into Hebrew, making their wisdom readily available to Jewish physicians. Indeed, Christian scholars were forced to admit that their physicians were much less educated than their Jewish counterparts because they lacked a working knowledge of Hebrew and Arabic, in which most of the medical works of the time were written. Moreover, the close familial and commercial ties linking Jewish communities throughout Europe served as a pathway for swift communication of medical knowledge throughout the continent, enabling Jews to rapidly become aware of advances in medical knowledge and learn about drugs, plants, and remedies from various locales throughout the known world.

Jewish scholars often earned their livings as physicians. According to longstanding tradition, it was improper to accept payment for teaching Torah. Moreover, the philosophies and sciences of ancient and contemporary times often were incorporated into the curriculum of Talmudic academies. Consequently, many medieval Jewish physicians were simultaneously rabbis, scholars, scientists, translators, grammarians, or poets. Because of their wide range of general knowledge, Jews such as Hasdai ibn Shaprut often attained high official positions in the countries in which they lived.

Jews later were instrumental in bringing Arabic learning to the Latin-speaking Christian world. Having flourished during those periods in which an open and tolerant atmosphere existed in lands under Islamic control, Jews fully contributed to the expansion of secular and religious scholarship. Especially in Spain, where there were active contacts between Islamic and Christian cultures, Jews translated many Arabic and Hebrew medical writings into Latin, the language of Christian lands, thus returning classic Greek works to Western Europe. When the Jews of Islamic Spain fled persecution by the fanatical Almohades dynasty in Córdoba at the time of Maimonides in the 12th century, many fled north to various European centers of learning, especially in Salerno and Montpellier, bringing with them Arabic science and medicine.

## INFLUENTIAL ISLAMIC WRITERS ON MEDICINE

Two non-Jewish physicians from the Eastern portion of the caliphate and two from the west exerted a profound influence on the development of medicine in lands under Islamic rule during the Middle Ages.

Abū Bakr Muhammad ibn Zakariyyā al-Rāzī (c. 854–c. 925), was known in the West by his Latinized name, **Rhazes**. Through translation, his medical works and ideas became known among medieval European practitioners and profoundly influenced medical education in Western universities. Rhazes is best known for his *Al-Hawi* (*Continens Liber*, or Comprehensive Book) an encyclopedic compilation that summarized the medical and surgical knowledge of his time, adding commentary from his own extensive experience in medicine. He also wrote a pioneering work providing a clinical description of smallpox and measles, classifying them as two distinct infectious diseases.

Abū al-Qāsim Khalaf ibn al-'Abbās az-Zahrāwī (936–1013), known as **Abulcasis**, is considered the greatest medieval surgeon of the Islamic world. He was the author of major surgical textbooks, most prominently *Kitab al-Tasrif* (The Method), a 30-volume encyclopedia of medical practices. Albucasis developed new surgical instruments and procedures that influenced physicians for centuries.

Abū Alī al-Ḥusayn ibn 'Abd Allāh ibn Sīnā (980–1037), known as **Avicenna**, was a Persian prodigy who was reputed to have mastered the Koran by age 10 and became an expert in all the scientific knowledge of his time. By age 16, Avicenna quickly learned medicine and was called to cure the sultan of Bukhara, who had been suffering from an ailment that baffled the court physicians. Avicenna's medical masterpiece was *The Canon of Medicine*, a multivolume work structurally influenced by Aristotelian logic, which became the standard medical textbook used in universities in Christian Europe for 600 years. He also wrote influential works in science and philosophy.

Abū l-Walīd Muḥammad Ibn 'Aḥmad Ibn Rušd (1126–1196), known as **Averroes**, was born in Córdoba. A student of medicine, law, and philosophy, Averroes is best known for his extensive and clear exposition of the philosophy of Aristotle, which earned him the title of "The Commentator." His philosophic works had a major impact on Christian scholars, leading some to describe Averroes as the founding father of secular thought in Western Europe. Averroes' major medical work was the encyclopedic *Kulliyat*, which is known in its Latin translation as *Colliget* (Generalities, as in "general medicine"). Averroes also wrote a compilation of the works of Galen and a commentary on the *Canon of Medicine* by Avicenna.

---
### SPAIN
---

The Abbasid Caliphate remained in power in Córdoba from 750 until 1012, when it was defeated by an army of disgruntled Berber tribesmen who had been the major fighting force in the initial conquest of Spain but were relegated to an inferior status by the Arab aristocracy. With the Caliphate of Andalusia replaced by 23 small city-states, Grenada became the most important kingdom in the Iberian Peninsula. Samuel ha-Nagid ascended to the position of grand vizier, leading the army of Grenada to victory over surrounding communities. Within 50 years, however, Andalusia came under the control of the Almoravids, a Berber dynasty that had seized power in Morocco and spread its influence to the north. A large bribe enabled the Jewish community to flourish until a fanatical Arab sect, the Almohads, conquered the region and gave Jews the option of conversion to Islam or emigration. Maimonides and his family were among the many Jews who fled from Muslim Spain to Morocco and then to Egypt. Others went in the opposite direction to the neighboring Christian kingdoms of Spain and southern France.

With Arab Andalusia divided into multiple small states, Christian armies progressively moved southward and conquered these Muslim kingdoms, which contained substantial Jewish populations. By the mid-13th century, the Christian conquest of Spain was almost complete, with only Grenada remaining under Islamic control.

---

### Ibn Shaprut, Hasdai (Hisdai)                         (Spain, c. 915–975)

---

Hasdai ibn Shaprut studied Hebrew, Arabic, and Latin, at that time usually known only by the higher clergy of Spain. His medical skills led him to be appointed physician at the courts of Caliphs Abd al-Rahman III and his successor, al-Hakim II, where it is reported that he discovered a universal panacea called *al-faruk*. Hasdai ibn Shaprut eventually became a trusted confidant of the Muslim leader. Although not receiving the title of vizier, Ibn Shaprut was a skilled diplomat who essentially became the foreign minister responsible for arranging political and commercial alliances between the Muslim Caliphate and Christian kingdoms.

Hasdai ibn Shaprut used his diplomatic and financial resources in tireless efforts to secure religious liberty and improved living conditions for oppressed Jews in many countries. As head of the Jewish community in Spain, he used his own funds to establish schools and academies for Torah

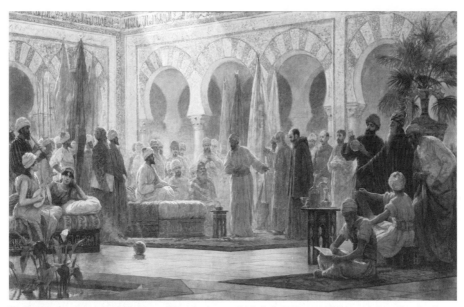

Painting by Dionisio Baixeras Verdaguer of Abd al-Rahman III receiving the Ambassador at the Caliphate in Córdoba, 1882. (*Wikimedia / University of Barcelona Virtual Museum*)

study and invited renowned Talmud scholars to teach there. Learning of the existence of the Khazars, a Central Asian kingdom that had converted to Judaism and is the subject of Judah Halevi's classic *Kuzari*, Ibn Shaprut corresponded with their king to learn more about the origin of their tribe and how they had designed their political and military structure.

Hasdai ibn Shaprut sent generous gifts to the Talmudic academies of Sura and Pumbedita, which awarded him the honorary title of *Rosh Kallah* (Chief of the Assembly). At the same time, he was instrumental in transferring the center of Jewish theological studies from Babylonia to Spain by appointing Moses ben Chanoch, one of the "four captives" stranded in Spain, as rabbi of Córdoba and founder of a Torah academy. Having in their midst such an illustrious scholar who had been given authority by Ibn Shaprut over all religious matters of the community, the Spanish Jews were able to decrease their dependence on the Babylonian academies, since they no longer had to consult them on issues of Jewish law and such matters as the calendar and dates of the festivals. Ibn Shaprut gathered other important Jewish scholars and poets around him, including Menachem ben Saruk and Dunash ben Labrat, both of whom composed poems for their patron. He also secured copies of important works for use by Spanish scholars, requesting Dosa (son of Saadia Gaon) to write a detailed biography of his famous father and Dunash ibn Tamim to send his treatise on astronomy and the process for adding an extra month in the calendar for leap years. Under the influence of Hasdai ibn Shaprit, Jewish scholarship, Hebrew poetry, and Andalusian culture flourished, marking the beginning of the Golden Age of Spanish Jewry.

Hasdai ibn Shaprut, together with a learned monk, translated Dioscorides' work on botany from Greek into Arabic, making this valuable book accessible to Arab-speaking physicians and naturalists.

## Moses ben Maimon                                              (Spain, 1135–1204)

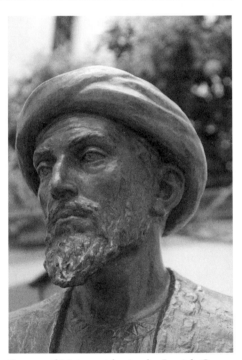

The most illustrious and influential figure in medieval Judaism and one of the greatest Jewish scholars of all time, Moses ben Maimon is generally known as Maimonides, or by the Hebrew acronym, *Rambam*. The pre-eminent philosopher, Talmudist, and codifier of the Middle Ages, Moses ben Maimon was born in Córdoba, where his father was a judge on the religious court. Following the Almohad conquest in 1148, the young Maimonides and his parents fled first to Fez, Morocco, and finally to Egypt, where he settled in Fostat near Cairo in about 1168. Supported for many years by his younger brother David, a wealthy dealer in precious stones, Maimonides devoted his time to in-

Statue of Maimonides in the Jewish Quarter of Córdoba. (*Wikimedia*)

tense study. However, after his brother was drowned at sea, Maimonides earned his living practicing medicine, eventually becoming court physician to the Grand Vizier, while also serving as the revered head of the Jewish community.

Maimonides' first major literary effort was the *Mishneh Torah* (Repetition of the Law), his only work written in Hebrew. This massive tome is divided into 14 books, each representing a distinct category of the Jewish legal system. It is a model of logical sequence and concise and clear expression, demonstrating the extraordinary learning of the author, who gathered together all the binding laws from the Talmud and incorporated the opinions of the *geonim*. Maimonides' other most famous work is *Moreh Nevuchim* (Guide of the Perplexed), which was designed for the Jew who was firm in his religious beliefs and practices but, having studied Aristotelian philosophy, was perplexed by the literal meaning of biblical anthropomorphisms and needed an explanation for how to harmonize philosophy with religion to provide a spiritual meaning that applies to God. In an introduction to the *Mishneh Torah*, Maimonides offers his own listing of the 248 positive and 365 negative commandments, along with extensive comments.

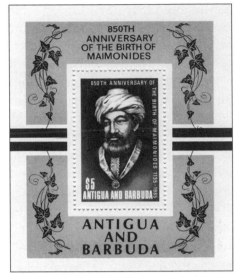

Stamp from Antigua and Barbuda honoring 850th anniversary of the birth of Maimonides. (*Author's private collection*)

As a brilliant physician, Maimonides stressed treating the patient rather than the illness, espousing moderation and disease prevention. He offered a six-point plan for preventing disease and preserving health in his "Treatise on Asthma." Stressing the Aristotelian ideal of moderation, Maimonides cited the importance of (a) clean air (anti-pollution), (b) diet (high-fiber, low-fat), (c) exercise (a sedentary existence leads to constipation, aches and pains, and decreased strength), (d) regular excretion, (e) ample sleep, and (f) regulation of emotions (direct link between body and soul).

Maimonides authored nine other medical treatises, including volumes on poisons and their antidotes, hemorrhoids and digestion, and cohabitation and health promotion, as well as a glossary of drug names in Arabic, Syriac, Greek, Spanish, Persian, and Berber.

Maimonides emphasized the critical role of developing good health habits so that they become "second nature." He wrote that whole grains were superior to white flour for digestion, and that "thick meat" should be avoided since its digestion is "hard on the stomach," while stressing that fruits and vegetables should be a regular part of the daily diet. Maimonides recommended eating poultry and small saltwater fish. However, he warned against consuming large amounts of fish, presumably because in the absence of refrigeration fish were preserved in salt, which he identified as posing a danger to health. Maimonides recommended dairy products because they are digested easily, but warned that they were "harmful for those suffering from headaches." He suggested drinking cool water some two hours after eating, when digestion had already begun. Maimonides also provided advice on how to exercise, bathe, sleep, and have sexual intercourse.

Although advocating regular and balanced meals, Maimonides did not always comply with this policy. He worked so hard as a physician in the sultan's palace that when he arrived home in the nearby town of Fostat, "I would find the antechambers filled with gentiles and Jews. . . . I would go to heal them and write prescriptions for their illnesses . . . until the evening . . . and I would be extremely weak."[3] Some have suggested that Maimonides' tireless devotion to his patients resulted in declining health and led to his death.

Maimonides translated the voluminous *Canon of Medicine* by Avicenna into Hebrew and compiled a collection of the aphorisms of Hippocrates and Galen in Arabic. Translations of his writings into Hebrew and Latin were widely read throughout Christian Europe. *The Oath of Maimonides* is a document stating medical values that is recited upon graduation by some Jewish physicians as a substitute for the Hippocratic Oath.

> The eternal providence has appointed me to watch over the life and health of Thy creatures. May the love for my art actuate me at all time; may neither avarice nor miserliness, nor thirst for glory or for a great reputation engage my mind; for the enemies of truth and philanthropy could easily deceive me and make me forgetful of my lofty aim of doing good to Thy children.
>
> May I never see in the patient anything but a fellow creature in pain.
>
> Grant me the strength, time and opportunity always to correct what I have acquired, always to extend its domain; for knowledge is immense and the spirit of man can extend indefinitely to enrich itself daily with new requirements.
>
> Today he can discover his errors of yesterday and tomorrow he can obtain a new light on what he thinks himself sure of today. Oh, God, Thou has appointed me to watch over the life and death of Thy creatures; here am I ready for my vocation and now I turn unto my calling.

---

3. From a famous letter sent to Samuel ibn Tibbon in 1199 (cited in The New York Jewish Week, 2014; http://jewishweek.timesofisrael.com/the-maimonides-effect/

## Zerachiah ben Shealtiel (Spain, 13th century)

A Jewish physician and philosopher, Zerachiah ben Shealtiel was a prolific translator of medical and philosophical works from Arabic to Hebrew. In addition to medical works of Galen, these included philosophical texts of Aristotle and commentaries on them by Averroes, and parts of *The Canon of Medicine* by Avicenna.

## NORTH AFRICA

During the Second Temple period, Alexandria in Egypt was one of the most populous Jewish communities in the world. However, Jewish settlement in Egypt was destroyed in the second century CE, when the Jews joined their co-religionists in the Land of Israel in the failed Bar Kochba rebellion. Jewish communities also existed in Second Temple times in Tunisia and Libya. In Morocco, many Jews crossed the straits of Gibraltar from Spain to escape the oppressive conditions under Visigoth rule.

The Arab conquest of North Africa in the 7th century was accompanied by a major influx of Jews into this region. Important Jewish communities with vibrant Talmudic academies were established in Fostat (Old Cairo), situated south of the modern Egyptian capital, Kairouan ("the camp") in Tunisia, and Fez in Morocco. Arab rule initially was lenient in all areas until the rise of the fanatical Almohads, who often gave the Jews the choice of accepting Islam or death. With the downfall of the Almohads in 1269, the fortunes of the Jewish communities in North Africa improved. Their ranks in the west were swelled by Spanish Jews escaping the persecutions of the late 14th century and then the mass exodus from Spain (1492) and Portugal (1497). However, Morocco was not sufficiently prepared to absorb the refugees or provide for their physical needs. Despite receiving government permission to enter the country, many Jews died of hunger or were killed.

## Dunash ibn Tamim (Tunisia, 10th century).

Like his teacher, Isaac Israeli, Dunash ibn Tamim was a physician at the court of the Fatimite caliphs in Kairouan (Tunisia). One of the earliest proponents of scientific study among Arabic-speaking Jews, he wrote a treatise on astronomy that discusses the nature of the spheres, astronomical calculations, and the paths of the stars, as well as another work (dedicated to the caliph) that demonstrates weak points in the principles of astrology.

Dunash ibn Tamim believed that Aramaic and Arabic were only corrupt derivatives of Hebrew and not separate languages with their own grammatical rules. As he wrote, "If God assists me and prolongs my life, I shall complete the work in which I have stated that Hebrew is the original tongue of mankind and older than Arabic; furthermore, the book will show the relationship of the two languages, and that every pure word in Arabic can be found in Hebrew; that Hebrew is a purified Arabic; and that the names of certain things are identical in both languages."[4]

Dunash ibn Tamim's only surviving work is a commentary on *Sefer Yetzirah* (Book of Creation). Unfortunately, the Arabic original has been lost and the manuscripts of the Hebrew translations vary greatly.

---

### Ephraim ibn al-Zafran                                      (Egypt, 11th century)

---

Ephraim ibn al-Zafran was a Jewish physician living in Cairo who served at the court of the caliph of Egypt. An author and bibliophile, Ephraim ibn al-Zafran was renowned for his extensive library of more than 20,000 books, many of which were medical and other scientific texts.

---

### Moses ben Maimon (Maimonides) – *see under* Spain

---

4. https://wikivisually.com/wiki/Dunash_ibn_Tamim.

## PERSIA

In 586 BCE, the Babylonians under Nebuchadnezzar destroyed the First Temple in Jerusalem and exiled the Jews to the region of present day Iran. A quarter century later, Cyrus the Great became king of the small state of Persia, which within 30 years had replaced the mighty Babylonia Empire. Unexpectedly, Cyrus told the Jews that they could return to their homeland in the Land of Israel and rebuild the Temple. Although some accepted the royal offer, a majority remained in what had been Babylonia. Unlike other exiled people, however, the Jews built a thriving culture in their new home and did not disappear through assimilation and intermarriage. With the destruction of the Second Temple by the Romans in 70 CE, the center of Jewish scholarship moved to Babylonia. There the extensive rabbinic discussions and interpretations of the Mishnah in the great academies of learning became the basis for the multi-volume Talmud, which has exerted a profound influence on Jewish life and thought ever since.

With the Islamic conquest of Persia in 634, the Jews (along with Christians and Zoroastrians) were given the status of *dhimmis*, non-Muslim subjects of the Islamic empire who were permitted to practice their religion but were required to pay special taxes to the state. Nevertheless, the Jews of Persia had significant economic and religious freedom when compared to their co-religionists in European nations. Many served as doctors, scholars, and craftsman, gaining positions of influence in society.

In 1258, the Mongols captured Baghdad and established their capital in Tabriz. They abolished the inequality of *dhimmis*, considering all religions as equal. One Mongol ruler even appointed Sa'd al-Dawla (a Jew) as his vizier, an act that provoked the anger of the Muslim clergy. Soon after the death of the ruler, al-Dawla was murdered, and the Persian Jews in Tabriz suffered a period of violent Muslim-incited persecutions. After the conversion of Ghazan Khan to Islam in 1295, Jews again were relegated to the status of *dhimmis*. His successor destroyed many synagogues and decreed that Jews had to wear a distinctive mark on their heads. These actions pressured many Jews to convert to Islam, including Rashid al-Din, a famed physician, historian, and statesman, who adopted Islam to advance his career but later was executed for allegedly poisoning the ruler.

## Asaph Judaeus                                      (7th century)

Pages from *Book of Remedies* by Asaph Judaeus Ha-Rophe, the oldest known medical work written in Hebrew. (*Courtesy of the National Library of Israel*)

The reputed author of the earliest known medical book written in Hebrew, also known as Asaph ben Berechiah and Asaph ha-Rofe (Asaph the Physician), he probably lived in Mesopotamia in the 7th century. *The Book of Asaph* is based on the Greek medicine of Hippocrates (5th–4th centuries BCE) and Galen (129–217 CE), but also contains the then-known wisdom of Babylonia, Egyptian, and Persian medicine. It makes no mention of Arabic medicine, suggesting that it was written before the Moslem conquest of the region. *The Book of Asaph* includes the oldest known Hebrew translation of the *Aphorisms* of Hippocrates and chapters of the work of Dioscorides (40–90 CE).

After a legendary account of the history of medicine, *The Book of Asaph* discusses such topics as the four humors; anatomy, embryology, and physiology; nutrition and the healing powers of herbs; fever and pulse lore; urinology and diseases of various organs and their treatment. The book concludes with an oath similar to that of Hippocrates, in which Asaph Judaeus stresses the ethics of medicine and the confidentiality of medical information. Unlike the Hippocratic Oath, which begins "I swear by Apollo, Physician and Asclepius and Hygieia and Panaceia and all the gods and goddesses," the Oath of Asaph opens with a statement of faith in the One God, the Lord of Israel and the entire world, the true Healer of the sick.[5]

Along with Johanan ben Zavda, Judah ha-Yarchoni, and other Jewish scholars, Asaph Judaeus founded a medical school. The Israeli hospital Assaf ha-Rofeh, east of Tel Aviv, is named in his honor.

## Masarjuwayh of Basra (c. 8th century)

Following the Arab conquest of the Middle East and Spain, Jews were instrumental in translating a large number of medical works from Greek and Syriac (a dialect of Aramaic) into Arabic. Masarjuwayh of Basra is mentioned as the first in this long list of Jewish physicians.

## Rabban al-Tabari, Sahl and Ali (Persia, 9th century)

A noted Jewish physician, mathematician, and astronomer, Sahl Rabban al-Tabari eventually converted to Islam. He was the first to translate Ptolemy's *Almagest* from Greek into Arabic. This 2nd century mathematical and astronomical treatise developed the geocentric model of the apparent motions of the stars and paths of the planets. One of the most influential scientific texts of all time, its conclusions were accepted for more than 1,200 years until the heliocentric model of Copernicus.

Sahl Rabann al-Tabari's son, Ali, who was also a convert to Islam, served as the court physician to the Abbassid caliphs for almost 30 years. Ali al-Tabari was an ophthalmologist who is best known as the teacher of Rhazes (Abū Bakr Muhammad ibn Zakariyyā al-Rāzī), the celebrated alchemist who is considered the greatest Arab physician of his era. Ali al-Tabari was the author of *Paradise of Wisdom*, one of the first original Arabic medical textbooks, which was based on Greek sources and dealt with medicine, embryology, astronomy, and zoology.

## Rashid al-Din (Persia, 1247–1318)

Rashid al-Din was born into a Jewish family in Hamadan, a vibrant Jewish cultural center and home to a prominent rabbinical college that he may have attended. The son of a Jewish court apothecary, Rashid al-Din

5. https://www.britannica.com/topic/Hippocratic-oath

was trained as a physician. Also known as Rashid Tabib (Rashid the physician), he joined the court of the Mongol ruler of Persia, Abagha Khan. Converting to Islam by age 30, Rashid al-Din became the powerful vizier (chief minister) of the Mongol Ilkhanate under Ghazan Khan, a kingdom encompassing modern Iran and Iraq. He enacted sweeping financial and administrative reforms, which protected the populace from the extravagances of the Mongol elite. Amassing tremendous power and wealth and owning property throughout the Mongol Empire, Rashid al-Din used his personal fortune to build schools, hospitals, and other public and educational institutions in many places, especially in the capital city of Tabriz.

Serving under several Mongol rulers, Rashid al-Din was the focus of palace intrigues and false accusations by enemies determined to drive him from power. Finally, he was accused of deliberately prescribing a purgative that worsened rather than improved the condition of Ojeiru Khan. When the ruler died, his son accepted the charge that Rashid al-Din had poisoned his father and ordered the grand vizier to be executed. Despite the fact that Rashid al-din had conveniently converted to Islam 40 years before, his decapitated head was carried around Tabriz for several days, with his enemies shouting, "This is the head of the Jew who abused the name of God; may God's curse be upon him!"[6]

For the Asiatic Mongols, Rashid al-Din represented an unusual combination of knowledge of rabbinic theology and Jewish-Arabic medicine and its Greco-Roman roots. Consequently, he was commissioned by Ghazan to write the *Jami al-Tawarikh* (Compendium of Chronicles), which initially was to be a history of Genghis Khan and the Mongol dynasty but gradually expanded into a comprehensive and universal history of the world since the time of Adam. This monumental work, several sections of which have been lost, was completed between 1307 and 1316. It was written down by a team of skilled calligraphers and lavishly illustrated.

### Sa'd al-Dawla ibn Hibbat Allah ibn Muhasib Ebheri (Persia, c. 1240–1291)

After their conquest of Eurasia in the 13th century, the Mongols generally allowed the local authorities of subject areas to continue in power (under Mongol governors) and recruit talented individuals to administrate their territories. These included Jews, among whom was the physician-scholar

---

6. David Littman, *Jews Under Muslim Rule: The Case of Persia* (Institute of Contemporary History, 1979), p. 3.

Sa'd al-Dawla (Arabic for "Felicity of the Empire," an honorific title he assumed when becoming grand vizier).

According to a historical account, Sa'd al-Dawla cured Arghun Khan and, having gained his confidence, demonstrated his knowledge of the Mongolian language and existing conditions in the province, informing the governor of the corruption of Baghdad officials. Sa'd al-Dawla soon was named general controller of the finances of Baghdad, and in 1289 he was appointed grand vizier (chief minister). Sa'd al-Dawla instituted a variety of financial regulations that increased revenues and regulated taxes. He also issued a decree forbidding the employment of Muslims in the official bureaucracy, employing only Jews and Christians. It was alleged that his own relatives filled a substantial share of the positions.

His rapid rise to power and the rules he instituted earned Sa'd al-Dawla many enemies. The Mongolian officials hated him because they could no longer divert large amounts of state money to their own use. The Muslims were humiliated by having a Jew placed over them, especially since Sa'd al-Dawla had a proud and haughty manner. When Arghun Khan became ill, opponents of Sa'd al-Dawla accused the grand vizier of poisoning him. After it became clear that Arghun Khan was dying, Sa'd al-Dawla's enemies took advantage of the opportunity and had him murdered at the royal camp, after serving only two years in office. His goods were confiscated, and Sa'd al-Dawla's family and the Jews in general were persecuted.

# JEWISH PHYSICIANS
# IN CHRISTIAN LANDS

∼: :∼

THE CATHOLIC CHURCH AND local rulers periodically issued regulations forbidding Jewish physicians from treating Christians, holding official positions, or studying at universities. Nevertheless, Jewish physicians continued practicing their professions. Some held high positions at the courts of the same clerical and royal authorities who strenuously preached against them, indicating the high level of respect for their medical skills. In Catholic Spain, virtually every Christian monarch in Castille had a Jewish doctor, even Queen Isabella who expelled the Jews from her country in 1492. Many prominent Jewish physicians focused on translating classic medical works from Arabic to Hebrew and Latin.

Jewish doctors often were accorded special privileges. When ecclesiastic authorities in the early 13th century required their Jews to wear special badges and pointed caps, physicians were often exempted and even permitted to assume the same professional attire as their Christian colleagues. Some prominent Jewish physicians were exempted from paying special taxes imposed on their co-religionists. When the Jews were expelled from Venice at the end of the 13th century, physicians were specially permitted to remain.

## SPAIN

In the 11th century, a series of civil wars in the Islamic-controlled area of Spain led to the breakup of Andalusia, which was divided into multiple small states. Christian armies progressively moved southward, conquering Toledo in 1085 and overrunning most of the small Muslim kingdoms. By the mid-13th century, the Christian conquest of Spain was almost complete, with only Grenada remaining under Islamic control. The territories captured by Christian forces contained substantial Jewish populations.

The Christian rulers tolerated their new Jewish subjects, elevating educated and cultured Jews to influential positions. Despite the longstanding Church tradition of persecuting Jews under their control, the Jews in Spain lived under much better conditions than their co-religionists in Central Europe and were spared the ravages of the Crusades. However, once the conquest of Spain was almost complete, with only Grenada remaining under Islamic control, the situation of the Jews in Spain dramatically changed for the worse. In 1263, Nachmanides was forced to represent the Jews in a public disputation, and Jews were compelled to listen to repeated synagogue sermons urging them to convert. In 1391, economic instability and religious fanaticism encouraged by the government led to anti-Jewish violence in the major cities in Castille and Aragon, leading thousands of Jews to convert to Christianity. Christian hostility recurred in the early 15th century after a prolonged public disputation in Tortossa (1412–1414), and thousands more Jews converted. By the middle of the century, about a third of Spanish Jewry had converted, creating a large New Christian (*converso*) community that generally lived alongside the Jewish one. In 1469, Isabella of Castile married Ferdinand of Aragon, and within 10 years the Catholic Monarchs ruled all of Spain except for Granada and Navarre. Tens of thousands of Jews were forcibly converted to Christianity, though many of them continued to practice Judaism in secret. The Inquisition was revived to eradicate any trace of Jewish allegiance and observance among the secret Jews, who had been baptized voluntarily or under duress. Those who were caught were ruthlessly tortured and then burned at the stake. With the conquest of Grenada in 1491, Ferdinand and Isabella no longer had need for Jewish finances to support their military exploits in the Iberian Peninsula. Even the political efforts and large bribes of Don Isaac Abrabanel were of no avail. Ferdinand and Isabella signed an edict expelling all Jews from Spain, ostensibly to prevent them from contaminating the Christian community through ongoing contacts with the *conversos*. The final decree took effect on Tisha b'Av, the fast day commemorating the destruction of the First and Second Temples. Up to 150,000 Jews left Spain, and the most powerful and influential medieval Jewish community in the world had ceased to exist. Ironically, on the same day in 1492, three small ships sailed from the Spanish port of Cadiz on an expedition largely supported by Jews and *conversos* – the voyage of Christopher

Columbus to the land that would one day be the home to the largest Jewish community in the world.

## Abraham of Aragon       (Spain, 13th century)

Abraham of Aragon was a Jewish physician specializing in diseases of the eye. Although a law forbade Christians from being attended by Jewish doctors, Alphonse Capet of Poitier, the virulently anti-Semitic brother of Louis IX, asked Abraham of Aragon to treat him for an eye infection. Abraham of Aragon refused, arguing that even the brother of a king was not exempt from this decree. Only after the persistent pleading of the Lord of Lunel did Abraham of Aragon relent and agree to cure the prince.

## Aldabi, Meir ben Isaac       (Spain, 14th century)

A native of Toledo who moved to Jerusalem, Meir Aldabi was the grandson of the renowned halachist Asher ben Yechiel (the Rosh). After receiving a comprehensive education in biblical and rabbinic literature, Aldabi turned to philosophical and scientific studies. Although not a physician, Aldabi had extensive knowledge of medicine and astronomy, in addition to theology.

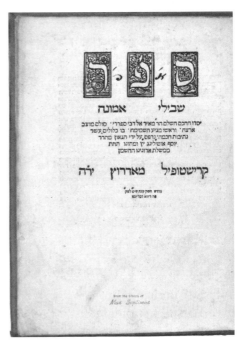

Frontispiece of *Shvilei Emunah* by Meir ben Issac Aldabi, published in 1887, Warsaw.

Aldabi is best known for his major work, *Shvilei Emunah* (Paths of Faith), which was written in 1360 and divided into ten chapters: the existence of God, His attributes, His immateriality, unity, and immutability that are unaffected by prayer or even by miracles (in which he includes a kabbalistic discussion of the names of the Deity); the creation of the world and astronomy; human embryology and the generative functions; human anatomy, physiology, and pathology; recommendation for health and long life;

the soul and its functions; exaltation of the soul through fulfilment of the commandments and their ethical value; truth of the Torah and the Oral Law; reward and punishment, paradise and hell, immortality of the soul and its transmigration in human beings; and the redemption of Israel, the resurrection, and the world to come.

## Alfakhar, Joseph and Judah (Spain, 12th and 13th centuries)

Physician members of one of the most distinguished Jewish families in Christian Spain, the Alfakhars fled from Granada in the wake of the Almohad invasion and settled in Toledo. Joseph ibn Alfakhar was the court physician to Alfonso VIII, who made him the *Nasi* (Prince) over the entire Jewish community. His son, Judah ibn Alfakhar, served as physician to Ferdinand III of Castile and succeeded his father as *Nasi*. The only Spanish doctor opposed to the attempts of Maimonides to reconcile Torah revelation with philosophy, Judah ibn Alfakhar was one of the major forces in the Maimonidean controversies and maintained a written dispute with David Kimchi, the primary defender of Maimonides.

## Benveniste, Isaac ben Joseph (Spain, d. 1224)

A physician living in Barcelona and serving the court of Aragon in the early part of the 13th century, the highly esteemed Isaac Benveniste was honored with the title *Nasi* (Prince). In 1215, he was a leading figure in the convention of representatives from multiple Jewish communities to select delegates to send to Rome in a vain attempt to rescind the decision of the Lateran Council that Jews be required to wear a special badge. However, Benveniste was successful in arranging that the provisions of this law were not strictly enforced in Aragon. On the recommendation of King Jaime I, Pope Honorius issued a papal order exempting Benveniste from such an indignity in recognition of his medical services and abstention from usury. It also further stipulated that the Jews of Aragon were not to be forced to wear special badges (though later rulers and popes restored this obligation).

## Benveniste, Sheshet ben Isaac ben Joseph (France, c.1131–1209)

Born in Narbonne, Sheshet Benveniste was a renowned physician in the Kingdom of Aragon, first in Barcelona and then in Saragossa. Granted the title *Nasi* (prince) like his esteemed father, he was the author of an important medical work on gynecology in Arabic. His reputation as a doctor was so great that patients came from long distances to seek his advice (with Solomon ben Hananel said to have journeyed from Mainz to consult with him).

In addition to his medical activities, Benveniste was a trusted political advisor to the king and served as a diplomatic envoy. Playing an active role in the fiscal administration of the kingdom, he received revenues from the state in return for loans to the royal treasury. Like other nobles, Benveniste was exempted from taxes and even enjoyed legal immunity from the jurisdiction of the state authorities and the local Jewish community.

## Caslari, Abraham ben David                    (Spain, 14th century)

A Jewish physician living in Catalonia, Abraham Caslari was considered among the most skillful doctors of his time. He is best known as the author of *Aleh Refuah* (Leaf of Healing), a five-part treatise on fevers (1326). Almost a quarter century later, Caslari authored a work on pestilential and other fevers, at a time when the Black Death was destroying much of the population of Provence, Catalonia, and Aragon.

## Crescas, Abiathar                    (Spain, 15th century)

A Jewish physician and astrologer serving King Juan II of Aragon, Abiathar Crescas was a prominent oculist. He is best known for having restored the eyesight of the king by performing two surgical procedures to remove cataracts. This procedure, known as "couching," is an ancient technique in which a sharp instrument is used to dislodge the cloudy lens (representing the cataract) and pushing it to the bottom of the eye.

## El'azar Benardut                    (Spain, 14th century)

Born in Huesca, El'azar succeeded his father as the major physician at the court of King Alfonso IV of Aragon, which had a long tradition of Jews in medicine attending to Christian rulers. In this position, El'azar effectively became the principal minister for all matters dealing with the Aragon Jewish community. After the death of Alfonso, El'azar continued as court physician under his son, Pedro III, joining the monarch on a military campaign against Majorca and representing the king in secret diplomatic missions throughout Spain.

## Falaquera, Nathan ben Joel (Spain, 13th century)

Nathan Falaquera was a Spanish physician who authored a medical book in Hebrew on the theory and practice of medicine, therapeutics, herbs and drugs, and hygiene. Entitled *Tzori ha-Guf* (Balm of the Body), it was a compilation of the opinions of Hippocrates, Galen, Averroes, Avicenna, and Maimonides, to which Falaquera added all the medical and botanical terms he could find in the Talmud. When these were not available, he employed technical Arabic expressions, which he then translated into the vernacular. Falaquera's book was a valuable contribution for those Jewish physicians who did not read Arabic,

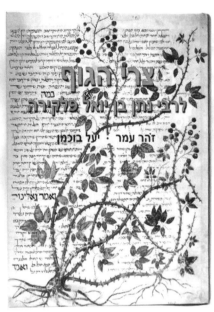

Cover of *Tzori Ha-Guf* by Nathan ben Joel Falaquera.

providing them with access to contemporary Islamic medical learning.

## Judah ben Moses ha-Kohen (Spain, 13th century)

Born in Toledo, Don Judah ben Moses was a physician-astrologer who led a team of Jewish scholars at the court of Alfonso the Learned of Castile in translating medical works from Arabic into the vernacular. In addition to Hebrew, Joseph ben Moses was literate in Arabic, Castilian, and Latin. He also was the rabbi of the synagogue in Toledo.

## Judah Halevi (Spain, 1075–1141)

A renowned philosopher and physician and generally acclaimed as one of the greatest Hebrew poets, Judah Halevi was born in either Toledo or Tudela. As a youth he moved to Grenada, the center of Jewish literary and intellectual life at the time, and received a comprehensive education in traditional Jewish scholarship, Arabic literature, Greek sciences and philosophy, and medicine. The dramatic decline in Jewish life in Grenada following the 1090 invasion by the Almoravides, a fanatical Islamic sect from North Africa, led Halevi to move to Toledo, where his reputation as both a poet and doctor preceded him, and he became a successful court physician.

Judah Halevi's masterwork is *Book of Refutation and Proof on Behalf of the Despised Religion*, popularly known as the *Kuzari*. Originally written in Arabic and translated into Hebrew by Judah ibn Tibbon, the *Kuzari* expresses Judah Halevi's concept of traditional Jewish teachings, which he defends against the attacks of non-Jewish philosophers, Christians and Muslims, and members of heretical sects (primarily the Karaites) who seceded from the

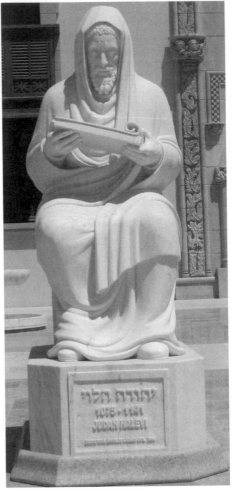

Sculpture of Judah Halevi in the *Ralli Museum of Modern Art* in Caesaria. (*Wikipedia*)

great majority of the Jewish people. Based on the well-known historical fact of the conversion of the Khazar kingdom to Judaism almost 400 years earlier, Halevi constructs multiple dialogues to examine all of the relevant issues that he believed could have led to the Khazar's decision to convert to Judaism.

Fearing the ultimate demise of Jewish life in Spain in the wake of holy wars between the increasingly fanatical Christian and Muslim worlds, Halevi wrote about the return of the Jewish people to the Promised Land, believing that a perfect Jewish life was possible only in the Land of Israel. In 1140, Halevi left for Egypt, where he received an enthusiastic welcome and was urged to remain. It is unclear whether Judah Halevi actually reached the Holy Land before his death. Tradition maintains that he did arrive in Jerusalem, where he fell to the ground in a state of ecstasy. However, as he kissed the soil of his beloved Land of Israel, the poet was trampled and killed by an Arab horseman.

## Nafuci, Isaac (Spain, 1336–1387)

Living in Majorca, Isaac Nafuci was a physician-astronomer and favorite of King Pedro IV of Aragon. He developed extremely accurate clocks and quadrants that could be used as celestial navigation devices by the Spanish and Portuguese explorers of the 14th and 15th centuries. In recognition of his service to the crown, in 1360 Nafuci was named as rabbi of the Jewish community of Majorca. However, after the anti-Jewish riot of 1391, Nafuci converted to Christianity, taking the name of Jaime Corretger. He later repented and returned to his Jewish faith before moving to the Land of Israel.

## Vizinho (Vecinho), José (Portugal, 15th–16th century)

Born in Covilhã, Jose Vizinho was a physician at the court of John II. A pupil of Abraham Zacuto, under whom he studied mathematics and cosmography, Vizinho was sent by the king to the coast of Guinea to measure the altitude of the sun using the improved astrolabe of Jacob ben Machir. When Christopher Columbus in 1484 proposed to the king his plan for a western route to the Indies, Vizinho was part of the commission that recommended against it, with the state agreeing on this decision based on Vizinho's criticisms. Nevertheless, Columbus obtained from Vizinho a translation of Zacuto's astronomical tables to take with him on his voyage in 1492. It was Vizinho's translation of Zacuto's tables that was published by the Jewish printer Samuel d'Ortas under the title *Almanach Perpetuum* in 1496.

## Yuceff Faquin (Spain, 14th century)

According to a document of King James IV of Majorca (1334), Yuceff Faquin of Barcelona (also known as Joseph the Physician) had circumnavigated the entire known world on the orders of the king. His experiences, combined with those of Marco Polo, intrepid Jewish traveler Benjamin of Tuleda, and Arab sources, were used by Jewish cartographer Abraham Crescas in producing the beautiful Catalan Atlas that displayed all the known world with unparalleled accuracy. This was critical to the age of exploration, when Portuguese and other European mariners began their adventures to India and the East.

## Zabara, Joseph ben Meir                              (Spain, 13th century)

Born in Barcelona, Joseph Zabara studied in Narbonne (France) under Joseph Ḳimchi, a famed grammarian and biblical commentator who had fled his native southern Spain after Moorish persecution. As a physician, Zabara served at the court of Jaime I of Aragon.

Zabara is most famous as the author of *Sefer Sha'ashu'im* (The Book of Delights), a collection of social satires, dialogues, and observations written in Hebrew. Many of these stories relate to the wickedness and guile of women, such as the woman who professes endless love for her late husband but eagerly marries another man, and the account of a death row criminal who is offered a royal pardon if he marries a wicked woman, but instead chooses to die rather than suffering "many deaths each day." Among Zabara's ironic observations are: "A doctor and the Angel of Death both kill, but the former charges a fee;" and "Never send for a doctor, for one cannot expect a miracle to happen."

## Zacuto, Abraham ben Samuel                           (Spain, 1452 –1515)

Born in Salamanca and receiving an excellent Jewish education, Abraham Zacuto (also known as Diego Roderigo) was a physician who studied mathematics and astronomy and was appointed as a university instructor. At the request of his patron, the bishop of Salamanca, Zacuto wrote his major astronomical work, *Ha-Hibbur ha-Gadol* (The Great Book), which is composed of extensive tables in almanac format that chart the positions of the sun, moon, and five known planets. This work revolutionized ocean navigation by making it possible for sailors to correct for "compass error" (the deviation of magnetic north from true north) using the declination of the sun, rather than the previous system assessing the quadrant and the North Star. It also permitted more accurate calculation of solar and lunar eclipses.

Once translated from Hebrew into Latin as the *Almanach Perpetuum* (*Perpetual Almanac*), Zacuto's astronomical findings were invaluable in

Spanish and Portuguese maritime discoveries. Christopher Columbus used his tables on his voyages, which proved lifesaving during his third expedition to America. Faced with starvation when the Indians of Hispaniola (modern Haiti and the Dominican Republic) refused to sell him food, Columbus knew from Zacuto's tables that there would soon be an eclipse of the moon (February 29, 1504). Threatening the natives that he would forever cover the moon and the sun unless they sold him provisions, Columbus and his crew were able to survive. Indeed, a copy of Zacuto's tables with Columbus' notes is preserved in Seville.

Astronomical Table from *Almanach Perpetuum* by Abraham ben Samuel Zacuto. (*National Library of Portugal*)

Zacuto also designed the first astrolabe made of copper, rather than wood, which enabled sailors to determine the position of the sun with greater precision at sea, unlike the earlier device that was only intended for use on land. Vasco da Gama, the famous Portuguese explorer, used Zacuto's astrolabe and maritime charts on his first trip to India in 1497.

When the Jews were expelled from Spain, Zacuto sought refuge in Portugal, where King John II appointed him as the Royal Astronomer. (The lunar crater *Zagut* was named in his honor.) However, Zacuto was forced to flee his home again when the Jews of Portugal were forced to convert to Christianity. After twice being taken prisoner on his journey, Zacuto finally arrived in Tunis. There he completed his most important Jewish work, *Sefer ha-Yuchasin* (Book of Genealogy), a chronicle of Jewish history from the creation of the world until his time. It contains a comprehensive, alphabetical listing of all the *tanna'im* and *amora'im* mentioned in the Talmud and Midrash, with citations of the places where material about them is found. Far more detailed than any prior work, *Sefer ha-Yuchasin* became an essential resource for future scholarly research on the subject.

## PROVENCE

The southern region of modern France, Provence was ruled by local counts or kings during medieval times. In 1113, the area was annexed by the count of Barcelona and became a haven for Jews fleeing Almohad persecution in Arab Andalusia. Spanish influence pervaded the area, and traditional Jewish scholarship was enhanced with the study of poetry, Hebrew grammar, philosophy, and science. Major centers of Jewish learning were established in various cities in southern France, such as Avignon, Lunel, and Montpellier. Although Jews were still subjected to periodic persecutions, restrictions, and even expulsions during the next several centuries, Jewish physicians generally were able to practice their profession. As with their co-religionists in Spain, a major role of Jewish physicians in southern France was the translation of Arabic works into Hebrew and Latin, the latter language making them available to doctors in Christian Europe. In addition to Arabic translations of the writings of Hippocrates and Galen, this also included the works of Averroes, Avicenna Avenzoar, and Rhazes, as well as those of Isaac Israeli and Maimonides. In some cases, the original Arabic works had been lost, so that they were preserved only through their Hebrew translations.

Founded in the 12th century, the prestigious medical school of the University of Montpellier was one of the oldest in the world, and many of its earliest teachers were Jewish scholars from Spain. Through their relations with their co-religionists all over the world, the Jews of Montpellier played a major role in the commercial growth of the city, as well as contributing substantially to the development of the school of medicine established there. To a large degree, the school owed its success to the policy of permitting any licensed physicians to lecture there, with no fixed limit to the number of teachers. Consequently, the number of lecturers increased rapidly, thus providing a wide choice of teachers who attracted large numbers of students from around the Mediterranean region. Many Jewish scholars apparently were able to study Hebrew law, science, and medicine at the university in exchange for a specified fee. The fame of its Jewish graduates was such that Jacob ben Machir ibn Tibbon (a Jew known as Profatius Judaeus, in Latin) was appointed regent of the faculty of medicine.

When some universities in Christian Europe were closed to Jews in the 15th and 16th centuries, Hebrew translations were made of classic Arabic and Greek medical texts specifically for the use of Jewish medical students.

## Anatoli, Jacob (France, c. 1194–1256)

Born in southern France and a rabbi, Jacob Anatoli was invited to Naples by the Holy Roman Emperor, Frederick II, to translate scientific Arabic literature to Hebrew, thus making Arabic learning accessible to Western readers. Not only was this of value for Jewish physicians and scholars, but since many monks knew Hebrew, they were subsequently able to translate the Hebrew texts into Latin.

Jacob Anatoli's most important medical translations were of seminal texts by the physician-philosopher Averroes. These included an encyclopedia on general medicine, a compilation of the works by Galen, and commentaries on the works of logic by Aristotle and *The Canon of Medicine* of Avicenna.

Anatoli was the son-in-law (and possibly also the brother-in-law) of Samuel ibn Tibbon, the famed translator of the works of Maimonides. As such he was heavily influenced by the philosophy of the Rambam, which he incorporated in *Malmad ha-Talmidim* (which can be translated as either "Teacher of the Disciples" or "Goad to the Students"). Divided into brief chapters according to the weekly Torah portions, it urges readers to learn classic languages and delve into "profane" (i.e., non-Jewish) branches of learning. As Anatoli wrote, "the Greeks had chosen wisdom as their pursuit; the Romans, power; and the Jews, religiousness."[7]

## Ibn Tibbon, Jacob ben Machir (France, 13th and 14th century)

Also known by the Latinized version of his name, Prophatius Judaeus, Jacob ibn Tibbon was born in Marseilles and studied medicine, mathematics, and astronomy at the University of Montpellier. A descendant of the famed translator, Judah ibn Tibbon, Jacob ibn Tibbon translated into Hebrew many Arabic versions of Greek mathematical and astronomical works, including volumes by Euclid and Ptolemy. In the preface to his translation of Euclid's *Elements*, Jacob ibn Tibbon noted that he translated this seminal book on geometry into Hebrew "in order to avoid the mockery of the Christians, who say that we [the Jews] lack all sciences."

Jacob ben Machir ibn Tibbon also wrote original works in mathematics and astronomy, including *Jacob's Quadrant*, which contains a table of 11 fixed stars to be used in the construction of the instrument that was later called the *quadrans novus* (new quadrant), to differentiate it from the tradi-

---

7. https://en.wikipedia.org/wiki/Jacob_Anatoli#cite_note-Jewish-1.

tional one. He also wrote *Almanach Perpetuum*, which included astronomical charts for the longitude of Montpellier for the year 1300.

## Ibn Tibbon, Judah ben Saul                    (Spain, c. 1120–1190)

Born in Granada, Judah ibn Tibbon was the progenitor of a family of several generations of rabbis, living mainly in Provence, who were renowned for their translations of important Jewish works from Arabic into Hebrew. Forced to leave Spain with his family in 1150 to escape the persecutions of Jews by the fanatical Almohad sect, Judah ibn Tibbon settled in Lunel in southern France.

While practicing as a physician, Judah ibn Tibbon was asked by his close friend, Meshullam ben Jacob, to translate Bachya's ibn Pakuda's classic *Duties of the Heart* from Arabic into Hebrew. Among the important philosophical works that Judah ibn Tibbon translated from Arabic to Hebrew over the next 25 years were *The Improvement of the Moral Qualities* and *Choice of Pearls* of Solomon ibn Gabirol, the *Kuzari* of Judah Halevi, *Book of Roots* of Jonah ibn Janach, and *Book of Beliefs and Opinions* of Saadia Gaon.

In the introduction to his translation of *Duties of the Heart*, Judah ibn Tibbon states that he prefers

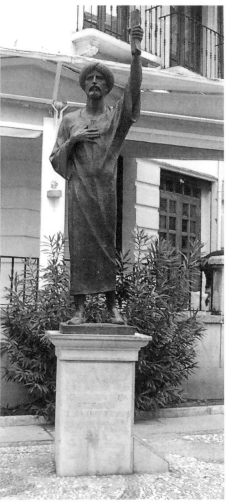

Statue of Judah ibn Tibbon in Grenada. (*Wikimedia / Svenholly*)

to give a literal rather than a free translation because he believes that this more accurately preserved the ideas of the author. His translations were regarded as far superior to others, leading Judah ibn Tibbon to be called the "father of translators."

The sole existing work of Judah ibn Tibbon is an ethical will addressed to his only son, Samuel, who also became a famed scholar and translator. He recommends that his son practice writing in Arabic, since Jews such as Samuel ha-Nagid attained rank and position only because they were able to write in that language. Moreover, Judah ibn Tibbon urges his son to study both Torah and secular disciplines (including medicine), pay attention to his diet lest he frequently become sick, and always act in a moral and ethical manner. He also notes that he had amassed a large library so that Samuel would never have to borrow a book from anyone, encouraging him to look them over every few months and to keep the library in order, so that he would never have to search for a book. Judah ben Tibbon also admonishes his son to "cover the bookshelves with beautiful curtains, protect them from water from the roof, from mice, and from all harm, because they are your best treasure."[8]

## Ibn Tibbon, Moses                                    (France, 13th century)

Born in Marseille and the son of the illustrious Samuel ibn Tibbon who translated the works of Maimonides, Moses ibn Tibbon was a member of the famed family of Jewish physicians and scholars known for translating works written in Arabic into Hebrew. With other Jewish physicians of Provence, Moses ibn Tibbon was restricted by the order of the Council of Béziers (May 1246), which prohibited Jewish doctors from treating Gentiles.

## Ibn Tibbon, Samuel ben Judah                        (France, c. 1150–1232)

Samuel was the second generation and most influential of the Ibn Tibbon family, which had a long and illustrious tradition of translating Jewish philosophical works from Arabic into Hebrew. Born in Lunel, an active rabbinic center in southern France, his father (Judah ben Saul) taught Samuel both classical Jewish subjects (Hebrew language, Bible, rabbinic literature) and secular disciplines such as philosophy, medicine, and Arabic language, poetry, and calligraphy.

At the request of Jonathan of Lunel, Samuel ibn Tibbon translated Maimonides' *Guide of the Perplexed* into Hebrew, including a glossary of philosophical terms in an appendix. During this process, he sent part of

---

8. J. Hillaby, *The Palgrave Dictionary of Medieval Anglo-Jewish History* (UK: Palgrave Macmillan, 2013), p. 201.

the translation to the Rambam for approval. Although Maimonides suggested that readers would prefer a free translation, Samuel ibn Tibbon followed the approach of his father (when translating the *Mishneh Torah*) that a literal approach is more accurate and faithful to the ideas of the original. Later scholars agreed, and Samuel ibn Tibbon's translation was highly favored over the free translation of Judah Alharizi. Other major works of Maimonides that Samuel ibn Tibbon translated into Arabic were the *Thirteen Articles of Faith* (originally part of the Mishnah commentary to the tenth chapter of tractate Sanhedrin) and his commentary on *Pirkei Avot*, including the philosophical introduction entitled *Shemonah Perakim* (Eight Chapters). Samuel ibn Tibbon also produced the first Hebrew versions of Arabic translations of Greek philosophers (Aristotle, Galen) and original short works of Avarroes and Avicenna.

In several works, Samuel ibn Tibbon explains his method of translation. The first step is to prepare a reliable original text, which requires collecting and comparing manuscripts to eliminate corruptions. When encountering difficult terms, he would consult a reliable Arabic dictionary as well as previous translations by his father and others; when a Hebrew term already existed, he followed established convention, even if he disagreed. The Arabic translation of the Bible by Saadia Gaon was also a valuable source. When feasible, as with works by Maimonides, Samuel ibn Tibbon would address questions to the author himself, though he generally ignored the Rambam's advice. At times, he would be forced to coin new Hebrew terms.

In addition to his translations, Samuel ibn Tibbon wrote the first full Aristotelian explication of the book of Ecclesiastes in Hebrew and a lengthy allegorical-philosophical interpretation of a single verse in Genesis (1:9). His son (Moses ibn Tibbon) and son-in-law (Jacob Anatoli) continued the family tradition of translating Arab-language works into Hebrew.

## Kalonymos ben Kalonymos                                    (France, 1286–after 1328)

Born into a prominent Jewish family in Provence and, like his father, bearing the honorific title *Nasi*, Kalonymos ben Kalonymos studied medicine (in addition to philosophy and rabbinic literature) but never practiced it. Instead, he devoted himself to the translation of Arabic scientific works into Hebrew. In addition to medicine, his translations included writings on philosophy, mathematics, natural sciences, and astronomy, including such authors as Galen and Averroes and the *Principles of Medicine* by Ibn Ridwan.

## Levi ben Gershom                    (France, 1288–1344)

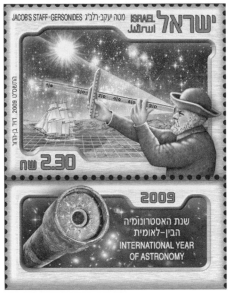

Generally known as Gersonides (his Latinized name) or by the Hebrew acronym, *Ralbag*, Levi ben Gershom was a court physician, philosopher, Talmudist, mathematician, astronomer, and astrologer. He was born in Provence, where the Jews were treated leniently by the popes of Avignon, and which had become the cultural center of Jewish intellectual activity with the decline of Spanish Jewry in the 13th century. Gersonides was greatly influenced by Aristotle, which the Jews of Provence learned through the commentaries of Averroes (12th century Muslim philosopher) and Maimonides. Indeed, his work has been described

Israel stamp with tab commemorating the International Year of Astronomy, 2009. (*Author's private collection*)

as an attempt to integrate the teachings of Aristotle, as mediated through Averroes and Maimonides, with Jewish thought in an attempt to demonstrate that philosophy and Torah, reason and revelation, are co-extensive. Nevertheless, Gersonides believed that reason and Torah cannot be in opposition, so that reason is the criterion for achieving truth: "The Law cannot prevent us from considering as true that which our reason urges us to believe."[9] As an example of his rationalist bent, Gersonides argued that the biblical account of Saul speaking to the dead prophet Samuel represented the king's mental illness, rather than reflecting the sorcery of the Witch of En Dor.

Gersonides' major work is *Sefer Milchamot ha-Shem* (The Wars of the Lord), which took 12 years to write and was completed in 1329. Modeled after the *Guide of the Perplexed* of Maimonides, it focuses on such topics as whether the rational soul is immortal, the nature of prophecy, God's knowledge of facts and providence, the nature of astronomical bodies and the theory of astrology, and whether the universe is eternal or created.

As one trained in mathematics and astronomy, Gersonides developed

---

9. Stanford Encyclopedia of Philosophy. https://plato.stanford.edu/entries/gersonides/.

a complex system of astrological principles to explain the connection between celestial and terrestrial events. He developed an instrument, the
so-called Jacob's staff, to measure the heights of stars above the horizons.
He also was the only pre-modern astronomer to have estimated the vast
distances between the earth and the stars, dismissing the classical view that
the stars were situated on a rotating sphere just beyond the outer planets.
The lunar crater "Rabbi Levi," is named after him. In his *Ma'aseh Hoshev*
(Work of Calculation), also known as *Sefer ha-Mispar* (Book of Numbers),
Gersonides deals with a variety of complex arithmetical operations. A later
book, *On Sines, Chords and Arcs*, is devoted to the analyses of trigonomet-
ric functions.

## Sarah of St. Giles                                    (France, 14th century)

Sarah of St. Giles was one of the very few medieval women physicians who
were teachers of medicine. A Marseilles manuscript written in 1326 records
an agreement between Sarah of St Giles, widow of Abraham, and Salvetus de Burgonovo, in which she would teach Salvetus "the art of medicine
and physic" and clothe, lodge, and feed him for seven months. In return,
he would pay Sarah fees for her services and turn over to his teacher all
the fees he earned during that period as a physician treating the sick. The
terms of the agreement appear to indicate that Salvetus already had some
medical training and was receiving advanced tutoring from Sarah.[10]

## ITALY

One of the oldest Jewish communities in the Diaspora, by the time of Julius Caesar in the first century BCE it is estimated that Jews comprised up
to 10 percent of the population of Rome. With the Roman conquest of
Jerusalem, large numbers of Jews were sold as slaves and brought to the
capital. Jews eventually spread to the south, establishing communities in
such port cities as Naples, Pompeii, and Brindisi. The conversion of Emperor Constantine to Christianity led to a variety of anti-Jewish restrictions, but Italian Jews of the time were spared the expulsions and massacres
suffered by their European brethren.

---

10. L. Whaley, *Women and the Practice of Medical Care in Early Modern Europe, 1400–1800.* (New York:
Palgrave MacMillan, 2011).

The 11th century conquest of Sicily by the Muslim rulers of Kairouan (Tunisia) exposed the Jews of Italy to the Arabic influences (Greek philosophy, poetry, astronomy, medicine) experienced by their co-religionists in Spain and the Middle East. During this period, Talmudic and kabbalistic scholarship flourished. With the Norman conquest, Jews assumed important positions at court, and Jewish scholars were asked by the ruling monarchs to translate major works from Arabic into Latin. Unfortunately, the Angevine conquerors from northern France brought with them intolerance for Jews and accusations of blood libel. Given the choice between baptism and death, a large percentage of the Jewish community of southern Italy converted to Catholicism.

In northern Italy, many Jews studied secular topics, with some becoming physicians to popes and kings. Menachem Recanati penned one of the most important early kabbalistic commentaries to the Torah, and Hillel of Verona was a major defender of the philosophy of Maimonides. The immigration of German Jews in the 15th century led to the development of a vibrant Ashkenazic community in Italy, with major *yeshivot* established in Padua and Naples. Many Jews expelled from Spain found safety in Italy, which became one of the pre-eminent centers of Torah scholarship in Europe.

## Salerno Medical School

The first modern medical school in Christian Europe, based on a revival of the ancient Greek and Latin tradition, was established in Salerno at least by the 10th century, and it became a model for subsequent medical schools throughout Europe. Despite the presence of the nearby Benedictine monastery of Monte Cassino, the wealthiest and intellectually most advanced abbey of Europe, there was little clerical control. According to a five-volume history published by Salvatore De Renzi in the 1850s, the medical school was founded by four physicians – Pontus, a Greek; Adale, a Saracen; an unnamed native of Salerno; and Elinus, a Jewish rabbi. The presence of a Jewish physician as one the founders of the medical school should not be that surprising, since a community of Jewish physicians had flourished in Salerno since ancient Roman times. Moreover, although the Dark Ages stifled scientific progress in Christian Europe, Arabs and Jews were translating the classic works of Hippocrates, Aristotle, and Galen, with commentaries by such scholars as Avicenna and Maimonides. In the 11th century, the medical school at Salerno reached a high point with the arrival of Constantine the African. Born in Carthage and the most prolific

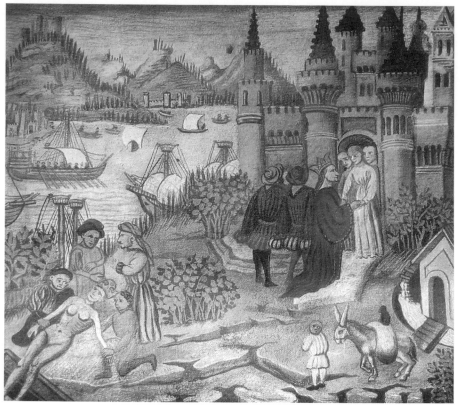

Miniature depicting the Salerno Medical School, from a copy of *Avicenna's Canons*. (*Wikimedia / Library of the University of Bologna*)

translator of his time, Constantine was a convert to Christianity, possibly from Judaism.

The curriculum required for becoming a physician at the Salerno medical school included three years of humanities followed by five years of medical school itself. In addition to learning the works of classical writers, students at the Salerno medical school received practical instruction in history taking and physical examination, as well as lectures in anatomy, fevers, blood-letting, material medica, and surgery. Upon successful completion of their final examinations, they were awarded the title of Magister (at that time, the title of Doctor was used exclusively to indicate professorship).

In addition to Salerno, there were only three other major Italian universities founded during the Middle Ages – Bologna (11th century), Padua (13th century), and Pisa (14th century) – with only Padua regularly admitting Jews. Because of very small class sizes, only a small percentage of physicians, both Jewish and Christian, were university-trained. Consequently, even those who obtained their medical education outside of university study were eligible to take the equivalent of a medical board examination. Although some Jews mastered the required medical theory from courses offered at *yeshivot*, most medieval Jewish physicians learned their trade by serving as apprentices to accredited Jewish physicians. This also was much less expensive than the cost of university training. For some families, medical knowledge was transmitted from father to son for generations; some sons-in-law even received medical training as part of the dowry agreements provided by the physician fathers of their brides.

## Bonet de Lattes (Provence, d. 1515)

Also known as Jacob ben Immanuel, Bonet de Lattes was forced to leave his homeland when the Jews were expelled and settled in Carpentras. From there he went to Rome, where he became physician to Popes Alexander VI and Leo X. On one occasion, Johannes Reuchlin, the Christian Talmudist, wrote a Hebrew letter to Bonet de Lattes, begging him to use his influence at the papal court to protect Reuchlin's book from proscription by the Dominicans of Cologne; Bonet de Lattes' intercession seems to have been successful.

Bonet de Lattes served as the rabbi of the Jewish community of Rome. A contemporary account describes the top part of Bonet de Lattes' house as being a synagogue containing the ark, hidden by a curtain, and books, lamps, and prayer shawls. He also was a judge of the highest Italian court of appeal. Bonet de Lattes is best known as the inventor of an astronomical instrument, by means of which solar and stellar altitudes can be measured and the time determined with great precision at night as well as during the day.

## Donnolo, Shabbetai (Sabbato) (Italy, 913–982)

Born in Oria, at age 12 Donnolo and his family were captured by Saracen raiders, but he was ransomed by his relatives and spent the remainder of his life in southern Italy. As he writes, Donnolo devoted himself to the study of medicine and astrology, seeking knowledge of the sciences of the Greeks, the Ishmaelites, the Babylonians, and the Indians. Well versed in multiple languages, including Hebrew, Greek, and Latin, Donnolo was first person in Christian Europe to write about medicine. His *Sefer ha-Yakar* (The Precious Book), written in Hebrew, summarizes his 40 years in medicine and includes specific instructions for making 120 medical remedies. The book is based on Greek and Latin sources and shows no indication of Arabic influences.

Donnolo also wrote a commentary to the mystical *Sefer Yetzirah* (Book of Creation), filled with astrologic and cosmologic observations and including a table of the position of the heavenly bodies in the month of Elul, 946.

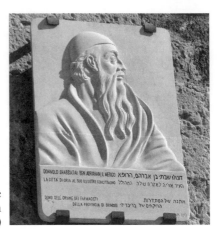

Bas relief of Shabbetai Donnolo on the right side of the Door of the Jews in Oria, Italy. (*Wikimedia / Laura Buccolieri*)

## Elia di Sabbata da Fermo                                      (Italy, 15th century)

Elia di Sabbata da Fermo, the most illustrious of Jewish physicians of the time, practiced medicine for more than 50 years and gained international fame. Known as Master Elia, he attended Popes Innocent VII, Martin V, and Eugenius IV. Master Elia was invited to Milan, a city that did not permit Jews within its borders, to become the personal physician of the duke, who later awarded him the distinction of being one of the first European Jewish knights. Recognized with the status of Roman citizen, Master Elia also was summoned to England to treat King Henry IV. A teacher of medicine at the University of Pavia, he was the first Jew recorded on the faculty of a European university. In 1436, Master Elia and some of his relatives received permission to travel to the Holy Land, when such pilgrimages were officially forbidden to any Jew.

## Faraj ben Salim (Moses ben Solomon) of Girgenti          (Italy, 13th century)

After studying medicine at the University of Salerno and becoming the personal physician of Charles I of Anjou, king of Naples and Sicily, Faraj ben Salim was asked by the monarch to translate several medical treatises from Arabic into Latin. The most important of these was the vast medical encyclopedia of Rhazes (al-Razi), written in Persia in the 9th–10th century, which in the Latin version is known as *Liber Continens* (Comprehensive Book). Consisting of 20 parts, the translation was completed in 1279 and first printed in 1486.

Faraj ben Salim also translated into Latin *De medicinis expertis*, attributed to Galen.

---

## Grapheus, Benvenutus (Jerusalem, 12th or 13th century)

Little is known about the life of Benvenutus Graphaeus other than his *Practica Ocularum*, a treatise on the theory and practice of ophthalmology that provides an indication of the medical knowledge of the eye during the Middle Ages. Translated into many European languages, it was the most popular textbook on ophthalmology during this era.

According to some sources, Grapheus was probably a Jew who was born in Jerusalem and converted to Catholicism. The name "Grapheus" may have derived from "*ha-rophe*," a Hebrew term meaning "the physician." As a medical specialist in diseases of the eye, Grapheus practiced in Southern Europe and may have taught at the medical school in Salerno.

---

## Hillel ben Samuel (Italy, 13th century)

Born into a rabbinic family, Hillel ben Samuel studied medicine at Montpellier. He established a successful medical practice in Rome, where he was a friend of Maestro Gajo, the court physician of the pope. Hillel ben Samuel then lived in Naples and in Capua, where he continued to practice medicine and studied philosophy with the famed kabbalist, Abraham Abulafia. He became an enthusiastic admirer of Maimonides and ardently defended him against all challenges during the Maimonidean controversies.

Hillel ben Samuel translated many philosophical texts from Latin into Hebrew. His major philosophical work is *Tagmulei ha-Nefesh* (The Rewards of the Soul), which was completed in 1291. Rebutting the theory of Averroës, Hillel ben Samuel argued that the soul is composed of "formal substance" that derives from the universal soul. As he wrote, the chief purpose of this work was "to explain the existence of the soul, its essence and its rational faculty, which continues to exist externally after death."[11]

---

11. Routledge Encyclopedia of Philosophy, https://www.rep.routledge.com/articles/biographical/hillel-ben-samuel-of-verona-c-1220-95/v-1.

## Isaac ben Mordecai (Italy, 13th century)

Known as Maestro Gajo, Isaac ben Mordecai was a distinguished rabbi and medical scholar, who served as the personal physician of Pope Nicholas IV.

## Leo (Italy, 15th century)

Probably the first physician from Western Europe to enter Russia, Leo was court physician to Grand Duke Ivan III Vassilivich. Prior to the 1473 arrival in Moscow of Sophia Paleologus (the niece of Constantine, the last Byzantine emperor) to become the second wife of the grand duke, there was little contact between Western Europe and Russia. In 1490, when the brother of the grand duchess, Prince Andreas of Morea, and the Russian ambassador to Rome visited the court of Moscow, among those they brought with them was Leo, a physician from Venice. Soon after his arrival, Leo was summoned to treat Ivan III's son for gout. Unfortunately, Leo was so confident in his ability to produce a cure that he pledged to forfeit his life in case of failure. Although he treated the patient with herbs and dry cuppings, the prince became worse and died. Convinced of the infallibility of medical science, Ivan III and his court accused the unsuccessful physician of wrongdoing. After the 40-day mourning period for the prince, Leo was publicly beheaded at Bolvanov Place.

## Leon, Judah ben Yechiel (Italy, 15th century)

The honorary title by which he is generally known, Messer (Sir) Judah Leon, was bestowed on him by Emperor Frederick III during his first visit to Italy, in acknowledgment of his eminence as both a philosopher and physician. The term *Messer* (Maestro), was similar to knighthood, while "Leon" was the equivalent of Judah, based on the phrase "lion of Judah." Excelling in both rabbinic and secular studies, Messer Judah Leon introduced this combined educational approach in the *yeshiva* he established as rabbi in Ancona.

According to one tradition, Messer Judah Leon initially had a close relationship with Joseph Colon, Italy's foremost Judaic scholar and Talmudist at the time, which for some unexplained reason degenerated into a bitter conflict. This became so inflammatory that the duke of Mantua was forced to intervene and ban both scholars from the city. Leon then moved to Naples, where he established a Talmudic academy and remained for the rest of his life.

As a halachist, Messer Judah Leon urged Italian Jews to adopt the stricter Ashkenazic tradition, based on Judah ben Asher's *Ba'al ha-Turim* that was espoused by French and German scholars migrating into northern Italy, instead of the more lenient practices based on the *Mishneh Torah* of Maimonides that were predominant at the time. This resulted in his unpopular call for stricter rules regarding family law and a controversial ban of the Torah commentary of Gersonides, which he deemed a subversive influence that deviated from traditional halachic thought.

Messer Judah Leon wrote commentaries on the Logic, Ethics, and Physics of Aristotle, as well as the analyses of Averroes on these works. He also developed three textbooks on grammar, logic, and rhetoric, which were considered essential areas of study during the Renaissance for advanced courses in humanities, philosophy, and medicine. For Jews, he addressed these areas in Hebrew textbooks on grammar (*The Pavement of Sapphire*), logic (*The Perfection of Beauty*), and rhetoric (*The Honeycomb's Flow*). These were designed to convince his co-religionists that Jews, rather than being hostile to secular studies, should use them to better appreciate their own literature.

---

### Maestro Manuele and his son Angelo                    (Italy, 14th century)

---

In the early 13th century, laws were enacted requiring Jews to wear special badges and pointed caps. Although church law had forbidden Christians to receive medical treatment from Jewish doctors, many ecclesiastic leaders quietly ignored this policy and entrusted their health to Jewish physicians. On some occasions, authorities would officially eliminate these restrictions for especially prominent Jewish physicians. A prime example occurred in 1376, when the Roman Senate relieved the Jewish physician Maestro Manuele and his son Angelo and their families from all taxes and the requirement to wear the Jewish badge, "because of their great experience in their profession and of the valuable services they had rendered and were rendering daily through their art to the citizens of Rome."[12] In 1392, the new Pope Boniface IX issued a papal decree in which he appointed "his beloved son" Angelo as his court physician and confirmed the rights and privileges previously granted to Angelo and his late father.

---

12. Harry Friedenwald, "Jewish Physicians in Italy: Their Relation to the Papal and Italian States." *Publications of the American Jewish Historical Society*, no. 28, 1922, p 149.

## Moses of Palermo                                         (Sicily, 13th century)

Moses of Palermo was one of a group of Jewish translators from southern Italy, employed by Charles of Anjou, who continued the tradition of Jewish translation that flourished during the reigns of Frederick II and his son Manfred. According to a contemporary document from 1277, the king ordered Maestro Matteo Siciliaco to teach Moses of Palermo the Latin language, so that he could translate Arabic medical works preserved in the royal residence. Among these was a presumed lost work on diseases of horses by Hippocrates (whose name means "chief of horses"), which for centuries was a major text in veterinary medicine.

## Nathan ben Eliezer ha-Me'ati                              (Italy, 13th century)

Fluent in multiple languages, Nathan ha-Me'ati used this skill to translate scientific and especially medical works from Arabic into Hebrew, becoming known as the "Prince of Translators." This allowed Jewish physicians and scholars to have access in Hebrew to the medical works of Hippocrates, Galen, and other Greek authors, which had been preserved only in Arabic translations. In this way, Jewish physicians could be well versed in the medical science of the era and practice at a high level.

Among the major translations of Nathan ha-Me'ati are *The Canon of Medicine* by Avicenna (1279), to which he added a glossary, Galen's commentary on Hippocrates' *On Airs, Waters, and Places*, and the aphorisms of Maimonides.

## PORTUGAL

Jews made important contributions to Portugal's Golden Age of Discovery in the 13th and 14th centuries, comprising almost 20% of the population. They were engaged in all phases of exploration, from financing the Portuguese sailing fleets to making valuable scientific discoveries in mathematics, cartography, and medicine. Unlike in Spain, the Portuguese Catholic rulers protected their Jews both from waves of anti-Jewish violence and the fanaticism of the Inquisition, which devastated the community of their co-religionists in the rest of the Iberian Peninsula. Members of the Ibn Yachya family held important positions at court, and Don Isaac Abarbanel was the powerful minister of finance under Alfonso V (1438–1481). However, soon after John II assumed the throne, Abarbanel was falsely accused of conspiracy against the king and forced to flee, entering the royal service of Ferdinand and Isabella in Spain. Several years after the expulsion of the Jews from Spain, Manuel became the new Portuguese king and determined to unite the entire Iberian Peninsula into a single realm. In return for the hand in marriage of the daughter of Ferdinand and Isabella and heiress to the throne of Aragon and Castille, Manuel promised to expel all the Jews from Portugal, which by 1497 was fully accomplished. In 1531, the Inquisition was introduced into Portugal to seek out crypto-Jews (*conversos*), leading many to flee the country and seek haven in the Netherlands, where they established flourishing Jewish communities in Amsterdam and The Hague.

---

### Abrabanel, Judah Leon ben Isaac                     (Portugal, c. 1460–1523)

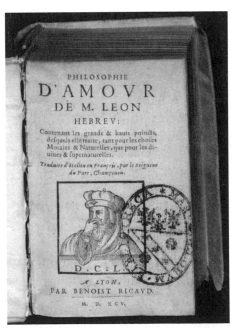

Eldest son of the illustrious Don Isaac Abrabanel, a renowned statesman, financier, and defender of the Jewish faith, Judah Abrabanel was born in Lisbon. Alternatively known as Leone Ebreo or Leo Hebraeus, he eventually moved to Spain. Well connected at court, Abrabanel was one of the physicians who attended the royal family. After the edict of expulsion was issued, Ferdinand and Isabella requested that Abrabanel remain in Spain, though this would require that he convert to Christianity. Judah and his immediate family, including his father, were forced to escape to Naples, where he practiced medicine at the university. When the city was captured by the French, Abrabanel

Frontispiece of Judah ben Isaac Abrabanel's *Dialoghi d'amore*. (*Wikimedia / BEIC Foundation*)

and his family again were forced to flee, first to Genoa, then to Barletta, and eventually back to Genoa.

A poet and philosopher, Judah Abrabanel's masterwork is *Dialoghi di Amore* (Dialogue of Love), a popular book that was one of the first original philosophical compositions published in the vernacular (Italian) rather than Latin. One of the most important philosophical works of its time, *Dialoghi di Amore* employs three dialogues between Philo, representing love or appetite, and Sophia, reflecting science or wisdom (combined as philo-sophia), to examine the philosophical nature of spiritual and intellectual love. Abrabanel demonstrates that love permeates the entire universe and is the dominant principle of all life, illustrating how it operates among human beings. He spiritualizes human love by connecting it to Divine love, arguing that it is necessary to go beyond physical union to a merger of minds and souls. From these underlying premises, Judah Abrabanel derives insights into such topics as ethics, metaphysics, mysticism, psychology, cosmology, and astrology.

## Gedaliah ibn Yaḥya ben Solomon          (Portugal, 15th century)

Born in Lisbon around 1400, Gedaliah ibn Yaḥya ben Solomon served as doctor and astrologer at the court of Joao I and his son Duarte, earning the title Mestre Guedelha Fysico e Astrologo (Master Guedelha, Physics and Astrology).

## ASHKENAZ (NORTHERN FRANCE AND WESTERN GERMANY)

Medieval Jews applied the name Ashkenaz (from Gen. 10:3) to Northern France and Western Germany, which formed a substantial portion of the Holy Roman Empire under Charlemagne. Within a half century of his death, however, the area was divided into three kingdoms that soon became fragmented into smaller territories. Living in a feudal society, the Jews of each town developed independent, self-governing units known as the *kehilla*. Jewish studies flourished in northern France, featuring such luminaries as Rabbeinu Gershom, whose method of learning was followed by Ashkenazic Torah academies for centuries; Rashi, who studied in German academies and compiled the classic commentaries on the Pentateuch and Talmud; and the tosafists, primarily Rashi's sons-in-law and grandsons. Major centers of Jewish studies developed in the Rhineland cities of Mainz and Worms in Germany, and in Troyes and Sens in Northern France.

Unlike the bicultural environment of Spanish Jews, which produced renowned philosophers, kabbalists, scientists, and statesmen, the unicultural society of Ashkenaz focused completely on Jewish values and scholarship. In Christian Europe, Jews were not allowed to dwell, trade, or work to-

gether with non-Jews, instead living in an encapsulated Jewish environment. In the *kehilla*, life was based on tradition, the belief that Torah was
the all-inclusive truth. The entire school curriculum was based on the
Talmud, which was considered as containing everything worth knowing.
Unlike in the Sephardic world, the study of secular subjects (mathematics,
physics, and literature) and philosophy was strictly forbidden. Ashkenazic
society was tightly stratified socially and economically, with each person
having a pre-defined role. The only path to upward mobility was rabbinic
scholarship, which could allow a poor but intelligent boy to be ordained
a rabbi and marry into the leadership of the community.

As in Spain, the Jews of Ashkenaz suffered periodic persecutions, massacres, and blood libels abetted by the Catholic Church and secular leaders.
In northern France, there were episodic expulsions, with the Jews permitted to return in exchange for a large bribe when the Crown ran short of
money. However, the expulsion of 1394 proved more long lasting, with
the Jews only allowed to return in the 17th century. With the absence of
a central authority in western Germany, Jews lived in small areas at the
pleasure of the local rulers. Consequently, when the Jews were banished
from one place, they were able to move to a neighboring town. In this
way, the Jews of Germany were spared the calamity of a general expulsion
that devastated their co-religionists in France and Spain.

The individual Jews and entire communities martyred in western Germany during the Crusades inspired the composition of *Av ha-Rachamim*
(Father of Mercy), a memorial prayer inserted into the Sabbath service
calling for God to exact punishment on those who forced Jews to die *al
Kiddush ha-Shem* (for the sanctification of the Name [of God]). In northern France, an accusation by an apostate that the Talmud contained blas-
phemies against Jesus and Christianity eventually led to the 1242 public
burning in Paris of 24 cartloads of manuscripts of the Talmud. Persecution
of the Jews of Ashkenaz was exacerbated during the Black Death (bubonic
plague), which devastated Europe from 1348–1351 and killed up to half the
population. A perception that Jews were suffering less from this scourge
than their Christian neighbors, presumably because of higher levels of
hygiene and ritual hand washing, led to the vicious accusation that the
Jews, even though they drank the same water, were poisoning the wells –
resulting in mob violence against them.

In the late 14th and 15th centuries, large numbers of Jews emigrated
east from Ashkenaz and settled in Poland, where they were welcomed by
the kings of the land.

Unlike the high level of science and medicine in Spain and southern
Europe, superstition and folk medicine ran rampant in the Jewish com-

munities of Germany and Eastern Europe. Among the German population of the Middle Ages, demons were widely accepted as the cause of disease. Bizarre "dirt pharmacy" cures – in which the ill were treated with such unpleasant substances as urine, spit, semen, and sweat – were based on the reasoning that the pathogenic evil spirits could be made to suffer so much by exposure to these noxious materials that they would willingly allow themselves to be expelled from the body. A strange custom among Jews in Germany (and Eastern Europe) was for the community to change the name of a person who was gravely ill as a last desperate measure. They reasoned that if, for example, God had ordained that a person by the name of David was to die, the Divine judgment might not extend to an individual by the name of Moshe. A copy of the Hebrew Scripture would be opened at random, and the sick person would be given the name of the first meritorious Jew that appeared. Charity would be donated on behalf of the invalid, along with a blessing for his/her recovery. If the patient recovered, the individual would carry the new name from then on.

---

### Balovignus                                               (Germany, 14th century)

---

Balovignus was a Jewish physician living in Neustadt, Germany, as the Black Death was raging throughout Europe. In 1348, after being tortured on the rack, Balovignus confessed that the Chief Rabbi of Toledo had sent him a poisoned powder, ordering him under threat of excommunication to contaminate the wells, but only after warning his fellow Jews. This led to vicious pogroms against the Jews in Europe. The kings of Castille and Aragon and the pope in Avignon took steps to protect the Jews, who were blamed for the outbreak of the plague. However, by the time the slaughter and pestilence subsided two years later, the population of Jews in the Iberian Peninsula had been decreased to about one quarter of its former size.

---

### Sarah of Würzburg                                        (Germany, 15th century)

---

Sarah of Würzburg was one of the few women permitted to practice medicine in Bavaria. In 1419, she received a license from Archbishop Johann II von Nassau, which enabled her to build a profitable medical practice. Other Jewish women physicians during this era included the oculist, Rebekah Zerlin of Frankfurt, and the Parisian practitioner Sarah La Migresse (late 13th century). In most instances, women physicians were limited to treating other women.

# AFTER THE EXPULSION
# FROM SPAIN

~: :~

THE EXPULSIONS FROM SPAIN (1492) and Portugal (1497) were momentous events marking the beginning of a new era in the history of Jews in medicine. Spanish Jews primarily settled in countries along the Mediterranean Sea. The largest number moved to Turkey, but significant numbers immigrated to Italy, Egypt, and Morocco. Many Jews from Portugal moved to Amsterdam and The Hague in the Netherlands.

A major council of the Church held in Basel in the mid-15th century developed a series of restrictions against the Jews, among which was a decree prohibiting Jews from receiving a university degree. Those Jews admitted to universities were forced to pay special fees and even forced to listen to lectures urging them to convert. After graduation, they were generally forbidden to treat Christian patients.

A key technologic development around 1450 was the invention of the printing press using movable type by Johannes Gutenberg. This soon eliminated the previous painstaking and time-consuming process of copying manuscripts by hand, leading to the availability of thousands of copies of printed books and the widespread dissemination of medical scholarship. Improved transportation made travel between countries much easier and more common. The expulsions of Jews from several countries led to major migrations of populations, with Jews coming in contact with co-religionists having different traditions.

The 16th century was a period of extensive exploration, discovery, and progress. In 1543, Andreas Vesalius published *The Fabric of the Human Body*. In this seminal work, filled with exact desriptions and ilustrations, the young Flemish professor of anatomy in Padua demonstrated how nerves penetrated muscles, the structure of the brain, and the relationsip among the various organs in the abdomen. For all the anatomic structures he described, Vesalius provided Hebrew names in addition to their Greek and Latin equivalents, using terms from the Hebrew translation of Avicenna's classic *Canon of Medicine* and even from the Talmud.

Successful Jewish physicians were often subjected to verbal attacks by their jealous Christian counterparts. This led some Jewish physicians, especially David de Pomia, Benedict de Castro, and Isaac Cardoso, to publish reasoned treatises in which they defended their co-religionists and issued scathing attacks against their detractors.

By the late 17th century, Jews in Western Europe became exposed to the era of great social and cultural changes known as the Enlightenment (*Haskalah*). This age of rationalism and unparalleled scientific achievement led philosophers in England and France to question the existing order dominated by the Church, the State, and the privileged aristocracy. It introduced new concepts of freedom, natural human rights, religious tolerance, equality, and reliance on reason rather than tradition. Jewish proponents of this movement (*maskilim*) eagerly welcomed this opportunity to adopt the language, manners, and culture of their Gentile neighbors and immerse themselves in secular knowledge. Others challenged this belief, attacking it as a threat to Jewish traditions and institutions. Indeed, acceptance of Enlightenment thinking did result in widespread assimilation in Western and Central Europe, as large numbers of Jews decided that the opening of new opportunities required them to renounce their Judaism. Some even became baptized as Christians, considering this their ticket to societal advancement in the arts and the professions.

## SPAIN AND PORTUGAL

Those Jews remaining in Spain and Portugal had been forced to convert to Christianity. Tens of thousands became *conversos*, crypto-Jews who practiced their Judaism in secret. Those whose hidden allegiance to Judaism was discovered by the Inquisition – the Church body charged with uprooting heresy – were ruthlessly tortured and then burned at the stake in a ceremony known as the *auto-da-fé*. Some *conversos* fled far from the Iberian peninsula – to India, Japan, and even what would become the United States – while others remained living in Spain and Portugal for centuries.

## Acosta, Cristóbal          (Portuguese Cape Verde, 1515–1580)

Born into a *converso* family living in the Portuguese colonial empire in Africa (and thus known as "the African"), Cristóbal Acosta studied medicine at a Spanish university, probably Salamanca. Traveling to India as a soldier, Acosta met Garcia de Orta, the great scholar of Indian medicinal plants. After returning to Portugal for a while, Acosta came back to India to rejoin his former captain, physician Luis de Ataide, the newly appointed viceroy of Portuguese India. Named physician to the royal hospital in Cochin, Acosta collected botanical specimens throughout India. Returning to the Iberian Peninsula,

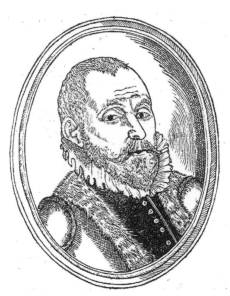

Christopher Acosta "Africanus," 1578. (*Wikimedia*)

Acosta settled in Burgos (Spain), working first as a surgeon and finally as a doctor hired by the municipality.

A pioneer in plant pharmacology, Acosta is best known for his *Treatise of the Drugs and Medicines of the East Indies*, published in 1578 and written in Spanish. Acknowledging his debt to the earlier work of Garcia de Orta, Acosta offers detailed descriptions and illustrations of numerous East Asian plants and drugs, including some mentioned by his predecessor. It concludes with a treatise on the Asian elephant, probably the first to appear in Europe.

Acosta also wrote a study of the herbs, plants, fruits, birds, and animals of the East, but this work has been lost.

## Cardoso, Isaac (Fernando)          (Portugal, 1604–1683)

*Converso* physician and Jewish apologist, Isaac Cardoso was raised and educated in Spain, where he lived for several decades as a nominal Christian. After studying medicine, philosophy, and natural sciences at Salamanca, Cardoso taught at the University of Valladolid before moving to Madrid, where he became a physician at the royal court of King Philip IV. In

1648, at the height of his fame, Cardoso abruptly left Spain to escape the Inquisition. Arriving in Venice, Cardoso openly embraced Judaism and changed his name to "Isaac." He soon moved to Verona, practicing as a physician in the ghetto.

*Philosophia Libera in Septem Libros Distributa* (1673) is Cardoso's comprehensive work on cosmogony, physics, medicine, philosophy, theology, and natural sciences. It includes a critical discussion of various philosophical systems, opposing kabbalah and the false messiah, Shabbetai Zvi. Cardoso then wrote *Las Excelencias y Calcuminias* (distinguishing characteristics and calamaties) *de los Hebreos*, a passionate defense of the Jew and Judaism. He discusses their selection by God, the divinely mandated commandments that separate them from other peoples, and some of their special attributes (faith, chastity, philanthropy, compassion for the sufferings of others), while attacking the unjustified charges made against them. Among these were such malicious charges that the Jews smelled bad, were hard and unfeeling toward other people, caused the Black Plague in France by poisoning the wells, and killed Christian children to use their blood for such ritual purposes as baking matzah for Passover.

---

### Garcia de Orta                                    (Portugal, c. 1501–1568)

A *converso* physician of Spanish descent, Garcia de Orta studied medicine, arts, and philosophy at the Universities of Alcala de Henares and Salamanca in Spain. Returning to Portugal, Garcia de Orta practiced medicine and became a lecturer at the University of Lisbon and royal physician to King John III. Fearing the increasing power of the Portuguese Inquisition, Garcia de Orta evaded the ban on emigration of New Christians by sailing to India in 1534 as Chief Physician with the Por-

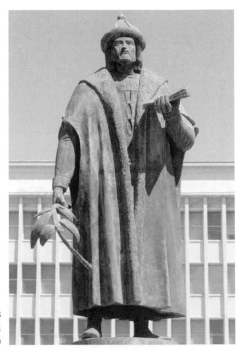

Statue of Garcia de Orta by Martins Correia at the Institute of Hygiene and Tropical Medicine, Lisbon. (*Wikimedia*)

tuguese fleet. He settled in the Portuguese island colony of Goa, off the western coast of India, where he established a substantial medical practice that treated Portuguese and Indian patients, including prominent leaders in both communities.

Garcia de Orta was a pioneer of tropical medicine, pharmacology, and ethnobotany. His extensive collection and classification of Indian medicinal plants was the basis for his major work, *Conversations on the Simples* (herbs used singly), *Drugs, and Medical Substances in India*. Published in 1563, this multivolume treatise was the first scientific work in the Portuguese language. Written in the format of a dialogue between Portuguese and Indian physicians, it detailed the names and medicinal properties of individual plants, offered case studies of various diseases, and introduced Indian medical knowledge to Europe. Later translated into Latin by Flemish physician and botanist Carolus Clusius, Garcia de Orta's work was widely used in Europe as a standard reference text on medicinal plants.

Soon after publication of his magnum opus, the Inquisition was introduced into India, with active persecution of *conversos* and Hindus. Although his sister was executed for continuing to practice Judaism secretly, Garcia de Orta died before becoming the victim of serious persecution. Nevertheless, he was condemned posthumously and his bones exhumed and burned (along with an effigy) at an *auto-da-fé* in 1580.

---

### Henrique Jorge Henríques                      (Portugal, c. 1555–1622)

A *converso* graduate of the medical school in Salamanca, Henríques practiced medicine in the Castilian court under the powerful protection of the house of Alba and remained outwardly Catholic until his death. Nevertheless, his relatives and servants were then denounced to the Inquisition, prosecuted, and imprisoned for two years, under the charge that they had buried his body according to Jewish rituals.

Henríques is best known as the author of *Retrato del Perfecto Medico* (Portrait of the Perfect Physician), published in 1595. It is an example of the 16th century literary genre, often written by *converso* physicians, that analyzes the link between medical and political authority. Despite being anchored in the prevailing values of the Counter-Reformation Spain, Henriques criticized the lack of training physicians received in the classical arts, the low educational standards in Castilian medical faculties, the dearth of travel experience among medical practitioners, the lack of control of health practices and practitioners by the political authority, and the social promotion of inefficient practitioners at the expense of competent ones.

This last issue attacked the serious discrimination inherent in applying "purity of blood" statutes, rather than merit, to the selection of medical practitioners in charge of municipal and public jobs.

---

## Huarte, Juan                                    (Spain, 1529–1588)

---

A *converso* born in Lower Navarre, Juan Huarte de San Juan studied medicine at the University of Alcala. Huarte is most famous as the author of *Examen de Ingenios Para las Sciencias* (Inquiry into the Nature and Kinds of Intelligence), which was published in 1575. Translated into multiple languages, the book earned him a reputation throughout Europe. Considered the first attempt to show the connection between psychology and physiology, it nevertheless was based on the ancient medicine of Galen.

According to Huarte, a person may only have a single talent in which he excels and must find a profession that is appropriate to that talent. Moreover, each talent is associated with a temperament that corresponds to the physique of the person. Children should be studied while they are young to evaluate their abilities and determine the area in which they excel, so that at a young age they can begin to acquire knowledge related to their special talents. Huarte believed that this approach also would enable children to learn language earlier, and logic when they were older.

Employing the concept of humoral temperaments, Huarte posited that levels of heat, cold, moistness, and dryness had an effect on differences in memory and understanding. According to his theory, memory depended on moistness, and understanding on dryness. Consequently, he believed older people had brains that were dry (understanding), but also indicated a poor memory. Conversely, children had moist brains well suited for memory tasks, but poor for understanding. Huarte was convinced that, for everyone, memory is better in the morning and worsens throughout the day, because brains accumulate moisture while sleeping and dry out during waking hours.

---

## Lopez, Roderigo                              (Portugal, 1517–1594)

---

The son of a Portuguese royal physician of Jewish descent, Roderigo Lopez was baptized and raised in the Catholic faith as a *converso*. After becoming a physician, Lopez was accused by the Inquisition of secretly practicing Judaism. According to legend, he was captured on the high seas by Sir Francis Drake and forcibly brought to England. Lopez settled in London,

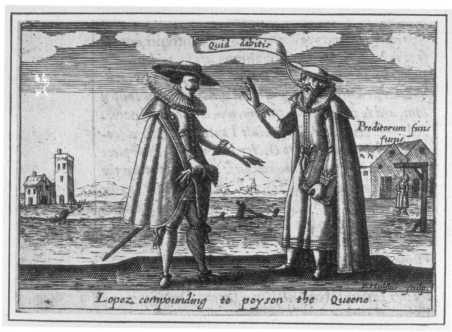

*Quid dabitis*

*Proditorum finis funis*

*Lopez compounding to poyson the Queene.*

Engraving of Roderigo Lopez by Esaias van Hulsen. (*Wikimedia / Wellcome Trust*)

anglicizing his first name as "Roger," joined the Church of England, and became the first house physician at St. Bartholomew's Hospital and a distinguished Fellow of the College of Physicians. Lopez developed an excellent reputation as a careful and skilled physician. In 1581, he served as physician-in-chief to Queen Elizabeth I of England. In return, he was granted a monopoly on the import of anise seed and sumac.

Early in 1594, the Earl of Essex falsely accused Lopcz of conspiring to poison the Queen. Despite vigorously protesting his innocence, Lopez was convicted of high treason in February and hanged, drawn, and quartered in June. The only royal doctor in English history to have been executed, it is generally believed that Lopez was the prototype for the character of Shylock in Shakespeare's *The Merchant of Venice*, which was written within four years of his death.

## Ludovicus Mercatus               (Portugal, 16th century)

Also known as Luis de Mercado, Ludovicus Mercatus was a renowned Jewish physician, personal doctor of Kings Felipe II and Felipe III, and the first professor of medicine at Valladolid. A disciple of the teachings of Galen, Ludovicus Mercatus's *Opera Omnia* (Complete Works) covered all the medical knowledge of his time. He also authored *On the Conditions of Women*, which is considered the most important gynecological treatise published in early modern Europe. In addition to general gynecology, this four-volume work dealt with sterility and pregnancy-related problems, diseases that affect newborn children, and the proper way to breast feed, as well as a detailed description of monstrous births. Ludovicus Mercatus also provided pioneering descriptions of angina, diphtheria, and syphilis.

---

## Luis d'Almeida                                    (Portugal, c. 1525–1583)

---

Born in Lisbon, Luis d'Alameida was a *converso* physician, the son of forcibly converted Jewish parents. Seventeen years after his birth, Portuguese traders were the first Europeans to discover Japan. In 1557, d'Almeida set sail for the east, and one year later he joined the Jesuit order in Japan. In his letters, d'Almeida observed that the upper classes had "exquisite cleanliness" that afforded hygienic benefits, but the lower classes lacked medical care. He was appalled by the Japanese practice known as *mabiki* (thinning our seedlings), which meant getting rid of unwanted children by abortion, infanticide, or exposure. Consequently, d'Almeida used much of his substantial fortune to establish a hospital for orphans in Funai. While teaching medicine at this facility, d'Almeida raised money to expand this unique Western hospital in Japan to also care for lepers and syphilitics, as well as arranging for herbs and other medications to be imported from the Portuguese colony of Macao.

---

## Lumbrozo, Jacob                                    (Portugal, 17th century)

---

Born in Lisbon, Jacob (originally João) Lumbrozo was a *converso* who arrived in Maryland on January 24, 1656, becoming probably the first physician and first openly practicing Jew in the British colony for which there is documented evidence. Lumbrozo became very wealthy, both on the basis of a thriving medical practice and the grant of a commission to trade with the native Indians. Although at one time arrested by some religious zealots for "blasphemy" (denial of the Trinity), Lumbrozo was quickly released as part of a general amnesty issued by a new governor.

## Nunez, Alvares (Portugal, 16th century)

A member of a *converso* family expelled from the Iberian Peninsula, Alvares Nunez served as Professor of Medicine at the Louvain University and set up a private medical practice in Antwerp for 30 years. He and fellow Portuguese *converso* physicians residing in Antwerp were instrumental in raising the level of medicine, because they brought with them Arabic-Islamic sources that provided exposure to the classic Greek medical tradition. This also was enhanced by the thriving printing activities in the city.

## Nunez (Nonnius), Luis (Ludovicus) (Portugal, 1553–1645)

Born in Antwerp into a *converso* family and the son of the Professor of Medicine at Louvain University, Luis Nunez was a highly successful physician and cofounder of the first medical society in the southern Netherlands. He was a friend of artist Peter Paul Rubens, who painted Nunez's portrait and several times sought his medical advice, especially his dietary prescriptions. Nunez is often considered the founder of medical dietetics, and he was the first to systematically study foods from a medical and hygienic point of view and develop the basic principles of a healthy diet. In his major book on dietetics, Nunez argued the health benefits of eating fish, described four kinds of bread, listed varieties of vegetables and fruit (indicating their action on the body humors), and praised the universal preserving quality of salt. Nunez described several types of wine, but advised against mixing them, and he also advocated the importance of the curative properties of mineral water to prevent kidney stones.

## Viega, Thomas Rodrigo da (Portugal, 1513–1579)

A *converso* physician, Thomas Rodrigo da Viega was the son of the personal doctor of King Joao III, who had permitted the pope to bring the Inquisition to Portugal. A philosopher and the first professor at the University of Columbra, his writings address problematic passages in the classic works of Galen.

## Villalobos, Francisco Lopez de (Spain, 1473–1549)

Born in Zamora, Francisco Lopez de Villalobos was a *converso* who descended from a family of physicians. Trained at the University of Salamanca, Villalobos served as court physician to the Duke of Alba and King Ferdinand. In 1519, Villalobos was named chief physician of Emperor Charles I, in whose service he remained until his retirement in 1542.

Villalobos' first work was *The Summary of the Medicine* (1498), which included the first detailed description of syphilis as well as Avicenna's *The Canon of Medicine* in verse. Villalobos defined the primary, intermediate, and secondary symptoms of syphilis, declaring it a "new and contagious" disease that had first attracted attention only a few years earlier.

## Zacutus Lusitanius, Abraham (Portugal, 1575–1642)

Born Manuel Alvares de Tavara and the grandson of the physician-royal astronomer Abraham Zacuto, Zacuto Lusitanius was a *converso* physician who studied medicine at the universities of Coimbra and Salamanca and developed a successful practice in Lisbon. Forced at age 50 to leave Portugal to escape the Inquisition, Zacutus Lusitanius and his family immigrated to Amsterdam, where he openly returned to Judaism, was circumcised, and took the name Abraham. In this new environment, Zacutus Lusitanius began writing his six-volume history of medical history (*De Medicorum Principum Historia*; a History of the Great Physicians), comparing and contrasting his observations on various diseases with both earlier and contemporary physicians. In an era when autopsies were rare, Zacutus Lusitanius relied on post-mortem examinations for his anatomic observations on a broad spectrum of diseases, ranging from heart disease and urinary stones to malignant tumors and the plague. He also published a book of

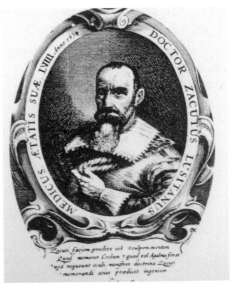

Zacutus Lusitanius, 1634. (*Photo of exhibit at the Diaspora Museum, 2011*)

rare and extraordinary medical cases, a code of ethics, and a manual for practicing physicians.

## TURKEY

Jews were living in Turkey and the Balkans as early as the Second Temple, but persecutions under Christian Emperors of the eastern part of the Roman Empire had resulted in a small Jewish community with no scholarly significance. This situation changed dramatically in 1453, when Constantinople, the capital of the Byzantine Empire, was captured by Mehmet II and renamed Istanbul. The Turkish ruler welcomed all Jews to what became known as the Ottoman Empire. This provided a safe haven for many of the Jews expelled from Spain and Portugal, and large and thriving Jewish communities with newly established *yeshivot* soon developed in Constantinople, Salonika, and Smyrna. In 1516, Selim I conquered Syria and the Land of Israel, leading to an influx of Jews from Turkey into their ancient homeland. There were close relations between these two areas, with the Jews of Constantinople aiding their co-religionists in the Land of Israel in times of need, while scholars from the Land of Israel served as rabbis in the Turkish capital. The extremely wealthy Dona Gracia Mendes, a *converso* living in Venice, founded and financed a *yeshiva* in Constantinople and established a Hebrew printing press that published many scholarly works.

During the 16th and 17th centuries, the Jews of Turkey were the most prosperous of any of their co-religionists in Europe and the Middle East. Many served as private physicians to the ruling sultans. In return for supporting Selim II, the winning candidate to succeed Suleiman the Magnificent, the new sultan dedicated the depressed area of Tiberias and its environs for redevelopment as a Jewish region, even planting mulberry trees for raising silkworms to provide an economic base. Many Jews expelled from the Papal States soon settled in this area.

## Ashkenazi, Solomon ben Nathan                    (Italy, c. 1520–1602)

Born in Udine, Solomon Ashkenazi studied medicine at the University of Padua. He moved to Cracow, where he served for 16 years as physician at the court of Sigismund II. In 1564, Ashkenazi settled in Constantinople, where he soon became the personal physician of Marcantonio Barbaro, the Venetian *bailo* (diplomatic representative of the Venetian "nation"), and then physician to Mehmet Sokollu, the grand vizier. Sokullo also used Ashkenazi as an advisor on international affairs, entrusting him with many delicate commissions. Ashkenazi displayed great diplomatic skill and effectively managed the foreign affairs of Turkey.

## Brudo, Manuel (Portugal, 16th century)

The son of Dionysus Brudus, a Portuguese court physician and author of books of Galenism and phlebotomy, Manuel Brudo was a *converso* physician who practiced medicine in Venice, London, and Flanders. He eventually settled in Turkey, where he served as a physician in the royal court of the sultan and openly returned to Judaism. His popular study on diets, *De Ratione Victus* (Essential Food; 1544), discusses the proper foods for those suffering from febrile disease and offers insights into living conditions of the *conversos* who escaped to England. He describes how they fried fish, first sprinkling it with flour and then dipping it in eggs and bread crumbs – probably the origin of the first part of the famed British combination of fish and chips. For the sultan, Brudo translated his book into Turkish (*The Walking Stick of the Old*) dealing with the maladies of old age and their cures.

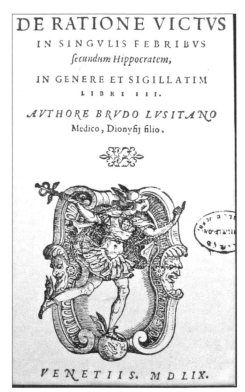

Frontispiece of *De Ratione Victus* by Manuel Brudo, 1559. (*Photo of exhibit at the Diaspora Museum, Tel Aviv, 2011*)

## Cohn, Tobias

(Poland, 1652–1729)

Born in Metz, Tobias Cohn was the son and grandson of Eastern European physicians and received a *yeshiva* education in Cracow. He was one of the first Jews to be allowed to study at the medical faculty in Frankfurt. However, for more than two centuries there had been a law in that region forbidding a Jew from receiving an academic diploma. Consequently, to get his medical degree, Cohn was forced to move to Padua, an Italian university with a long history of welcoming Jews (and Protestants) into its nominally Catholic medical school. After practicing several years in Poland, Cohn moved to

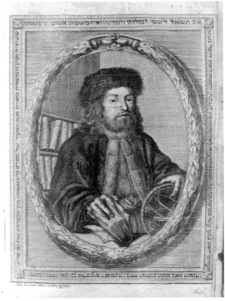

Tobias Cohn. (*Wikimedia / Wellcome Trust*)

Adrianople, where he served as the personal physician to five successive Ottoman sultans. In 1715, Cohn made *aliyah* to the Land of Israel, dying in Jerusalem.

Familiar with ten languages, this broad linguistic knowledge enabled Cohn to write his encyclopedic *Ma'aseh Tuviyah* (Work of Tobias), which was published in Venice in 1707. Written in Hebrew, it is divided into eight parts – theology, astronomy, medicine, hygiene, syphilitic conditions, botany, cosmography, and an essay on the four elements. The large medical section contains a full-scale engraving comparing the human body to a house. The head is a superstructure on the roof; the eyes are windows; the mouth, an open lattice; the shoulders, a lower roof; the lungs, a ventilated balcony; the heart, a pump; and the stomach a boiling cauldron.

*Ma'aseh Tuviyah* is strikingly different from *Otzar ha-Hayim* (The Treasury of Life), an influential medical text written a quarter century earlier by Jacob Zahalon of Rome. Zahalon's goal was to produce a medical book somewhat analogous to the *Shulchan Aruch* (Set Table) of Joseph Caro, the authoritative code of Jewish law published more than a century previously. He aimed to present the "accepted and correct view" in a handbook addressed to doctors and patients alike, so that any person could "easily" master the art of healing. Zahalon presented his medical prescriptions with absolute certainty and no hint of controversies or alternative courses of action reflecting contemporary challenges to classical medical therapy.

Conversely, according to David B. Ruderman, Cohn writes from "a deep-seated feeling of cultural inferiority," related to the anti-Jewish hostility he experienced while a student in Frankfurt. His goal was to include the "latest and most serious scholarship in the medical sciences" that demonstrated the high level of Jewish learning, and as such comprehensible only to Jews literate in Hebrew and impossible for the general public to understand.[13] Cohn had no qualms about including disagreements about medical theories and therapies, resulting in a book that "reads more like a Talmudic discussion than a *Shulchan Aruch*, a simplified code of prescribed procedure" (ibid.). Cohn attacked those who claimed the ability to treat patients but had never studied academic medicine, arguing that becoming a successful physician "involved years of painful devotion to study, intense exposure to rabbinics as well as to the secular sciences" (ibid.). Rather than needing to read a single medical manual such as Zahalon's, a person using Cohn's textbook would realize the difficulty of becoming an effective physician, given the complexity and uncertainty inherent in the profession. Yet Cohn always stressed that this could be accomplished just as well by Jewish students as by Gentiles, as long as they had the intense commitment to succeed and were given the proper training.

## Hamon, Moses (Spain, c. 1490–c. 1567)

Born in Granada, Moses Hamon became the personal physician of Sultan Suleiman the Magnificent and the most influential Ottoman court physician of his time. Hamon accompanied the famous monarch on all his travels and military campaigns. A fine linguist who was versed in Arabic, Turkish, and Persian, Hamon was a patron of Jewish learning and a leader of the community. In Constantinople, the seat of the Ottoman Empire, Hamon arranged for the printing of several Hebrew works and built a Jewish school at his own expense.

In the mid-16th century, the Jews of Amasya were falsely accused of having murdered a Christian for ritual purposes. After several Jews had been executed for the crime, their innocence became clear when the missing man reappeared. A fearless advocate of his coreligionists, Hamon persuaded the sultan to issue a special decree prohibiting provincial judges

---

13. David B. Ruderman, *Jewish Thought and Scientific Discovery in Early Modern Europe* (New Haven: Yale University Press, 1995), pp. 235–236.

from trying cases of blood libel, instead referring them to the royal court for trial. Hamon also is believed to have interceded with Suleiman to exert pressure on Venice to facilitate the departure of the Mendes-Nasi family and to ensure their safe travel to Constantinople.

Hamon wrote a short treatise on dentistry, which was the initial Turkish work on this topic and one of the first published anywhere.

## ITALY

Expulsions starting in the last decades of the 15th century swelled the Jewish population of Italy. German Jews moved southward into the northern provinces of Italy, joining large numbers of Jews fleeing Spain and the Spanish island possessions of Sicily and Sardinia. The later acquisition by Spain of the duchy of Naples in southern Italy forced Jews to escape toward the north. Consequently, the focus of the Italian Jewish community became the central and northern parts of the country.

With the introduction of the printing press just north of the Alps, Venice and Florence became major centers of Hebrew publishing for several centuries. The first printed editions of such classics as the Mishnah, Talmud, *Mikra'ot Gedolot* (Rabbinic Bible), *Arba'ah Turim*, and *Shulchan Aruch* appeared in Italy.

The liberal spirit of the Renaissance was most evident in Italy, where especially the University of Padua permitted Jews to receive an excellent medical education at a time when most other European university medical schools were closed to them. Consequently, Jewish students throughout Europe flocked to attend the renowned medical school in Padua. Like other non-Catholics, Jews received their diplomas from a secularly appointed professor, rather than a local bishop, who served as chancellor of the university. Rather than the standard Padua diplomas that began with "In Christi Nomine Amen" and had dates listed as "Anno a Christi Navitate," the diplomas for Jews incorporated the terms "In Dei Nomine Aeterni" and "currente anno."[14]

However, the fortunes of Italian Jewry declined in the mid-16th century, with the Catholic response to the Reformation. In addition to a wave of persecutions, a series of popes issued anti-Jewish legislation in the Papal States of central Italy, which was also adopted by other provinces in the

---

14. Vivian B Mann, *Gardens and Ghettos: The Art of Jewish Life in Italy* (University of California Press, 1989).

region. The first ghetto was established in Venice in 1516, leading to Jews living in congested and squalid conditions. Copies of the Talmud were burned, and in 1655 the Jews of Rome were confined to a ghetto with limited opportunities for earning a living. In 1659, Jews were banished from the Papal States, except for Rome and Ancona.

---

## Cohen, Abraham ben Shabbetai                    (Crete, 1670–1729)

---

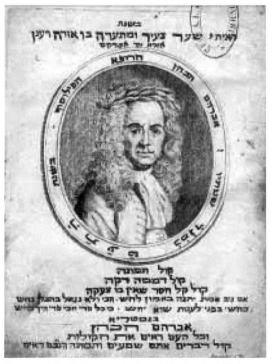

Engraved self-portrait from fly-leaf of *Kehunat Abraham*, by Shabbetai ha-Kohen, when he was 49 years old, 1719. (*Wikimedia*)

Abraham Cohen attended medical school at the University of Padua. He practiced medicine and lived most of his adult life in Zante, an Ionian island that was an overseas colony of the Venetian Republic. Also a rabbi and poet, in 1700 Abraham Cohen published *Derashot al ha-Torah*, a collection of sermons and commentary on the Pentateuch that is also known as *Kevod Hachamim* (The Glory of Wise Men). Two decades later, Cohen wrote *Kehunat Avraham* (The Priesthood of Abraham), a book of religious poems in metrical Hebrew verse, inspired by and written in the style of the Psalms.

## Cantarini, Isaac Hayim (Italy, 1644–1723)

Israel Cantarini was born in Padua, where he received both an excellent Jewish education and a medical degree from the University. In addition to an extensive medical practice, Cantarini often preached in synagogues (drawing many Christian listeners), taught in the yeshiva, and served as cantor on Yom Kippur. Well-versed in Talmud, Cantarini was often asked for his opinion on difficult halachic issues. The teacher of Isaac Lampronti, Cantarini trained his students in both rabbinic and scientific subjects.

Cantarini's best known Hebrew work is *Pachad Yitzchak* (The Fear of Isaac), which describes the internal conditions of the Jewish

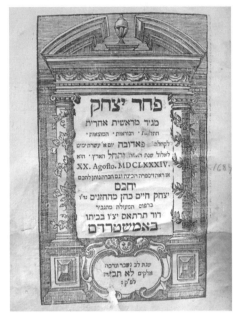

Frontispiece of *Pachad Yitzhak* by Isaac Hayim Cantarini, published 1684.

community of Padua in 1684, followed by a firsthand account of the attack on the Padua ghetto by the Christian populace. Cantarini was well regarded as a poet, basing his language on biblical style and allusions to biblical expressions, and he wrote paraphrases of many of the Psalms and a poem dealing with the coming of the Messiah (*Eit Ketz*; Time of the End).

## Conegliano, Solomon (Italy, 1642–1719)

An ordained rabbi and graduate of the medical school at the University of Padua, Solomon Conegliano was an esteemed teacher of medicine. He organized preparatory courses for young students, primarily Jews, who studied medicine at his alma mater. Among these was Tobias Cohn from Poland, whom Conegliano provided with both private tutoring to supplement his formal coursework in medicine and rabbinic studies to deepen his spiritual life. Conegliano later wrote the preface to Cohn's encyclopedic *Ma'aseh Tuviyah*.

Along with his younger physician brother, Israel, Solomon Conegliano

provided important diplomatic services to the Venetian court in its dealing with Turkish authorities. He and his brother were honored by being
granted Venetian citizenship and exempted from wearing the Jewish badge.

## David de Pomis                                          (Italy, 1525–1593)

The preface of his most famous work, *Tzemach David* (Branch of David),
states that David de Pomis was a descendant of four distinguished Roman
families which, according to an ancient tradition, were brought by Titus
from the Land of Israel after the destruction of Jerusalem in 70 CE. Born
in Spoleto, David de Pomis studied medicine and philosophy in Peru-
gia. Also a rabbi, he was forced to wander from place to place practicing
medicine in several noble courts to escape the 1555 edict of Pope Paul IV
prohibiting Jewish doctors to attend to Christian patients. David de Pomis
finally settled in Venice, where he published most of his works, including
*Tzemach David* (1587), a trilingual Hebrew, Latin, and Italian dictionary
that also contains numerous scientific and historical discourses.

An important work of David de Pomis is *De Medico Hebraeo Enarra-
tio Apologica* (Venice, 1588), in which he refutes the unjustified charges
brought against Jews in general and Jewish physicians in particular by a
1581 papal bull issued by Gregory XIII. After showing the common origins
of Judaism and Christianity and their belief in the same God, David de
Pomis cites biblical and Talmudic passages requiring the Jewish physician
to help every sufferer, regardless of religion. It relates numerous instances
in which Jewish doctors distinguished themselves by their work and their
loyalty. Rejecting centuries of false accusations of poisoning against Jewish
doctors, David de Pomis argues that they were merely based on common
prejudice. As he concludes, "When Christians accept falsehood for truth,
they harm themselves more than us, for this is completely contrary to the
teachings of Christ."

## Lampronti, Isaac Hezekiah                              (Italy, 1679–1756)

Born in Ferrara and a pupil of the preeminent Italian rabbis of his time,
Isaac Lampronti studied philosophy and medicine at the University of
Padua. Returning to Ferrara, he taught in the *talmud torah* of the Italian
and Sephardi communities, changing the curriculum to include study of
the humanities in addition to Torah. After further studies, Lampronti was
ordained as a rabbi and appointed head of the local yeshiva, giving him the

status of the senior rabbi in Ferrara. Throughout his career, Lampronti continued to practice medicine and was considered a superb physician, who provided free services for those unable to pay.

Living at a time of exciting scientific discoveries, Lampronti believed that educators, especially in the religious sphere, must be aware of developments in the intellectual ferment of modern European culture. In Judaism, for example, a debate raged over the effect that new scientific understanding should have on *halachah*. For example, traditional *halachah* maintained that lice were not living creatures, unlike fleas, and thus could be killed on the Sabbath. This was based on the assumption of spontaneous generation of creatures like lice from moisture or dung. However, as Lampronti wrote, contemporary science had indicated "that all living things originate from an egg," so that "any careful person who fears for his life would avoid such creatures and would not kill either a flea or a louse and not place himself in a situation of possibly being obligated to make a sin offering."[15] Nevertheless, many rabbinic authorities disagreed with Lampronti. His teacher, Judah Briel, argued that gentile scholars "knew and understood nature only in its superficialities regarding observable things and not in its internal nature as made known" to the enlightened rabbis – knowledge of the essence and not merely the appearance of things.[16]

Lampronti is most famous as the author of *Pachad Yitzhak* (Fear of Isaac), a phrase taken from Genesis (31:42). Constituting his life's work, *Pachad Yitzhak* is the most comprehensive and best known halachic encyclopedia. The entries are arranged alphabetically and include material from the entire spectrum of rabbinic literature (Mishnah, Talmud, commentaries of the *rishonim*, and decisions of the *posekim*), with special attention paid to the *responsa* of Italian rabbis. Originally planned to fill six volumes, only one and a half appeared during Lampronti's lifetime. The publication of the final volume was completed 127 years after the first one was printed.

Lampronti also edited three issues of a periodical focused on *halachah* and rabbinic literature, which included contributions from his students. Many of his *responsa* appear in collections of his contemporaries, but his popular sermons were not preserved.

---

15. David B. Ruderman, *Jewish Thought and Scientific Discovery in Early Modern Europe* (New Haven: Yale University Press, 1995), pp. 235–236.
16. Ibid.

## Lusitano, Amatus (Portugal, 1511–1568)

Born to *converso* parents in Castelo Branco, Amatus Lusitano studied medicine in Spain at the University of Salamanca. Returning to Portugal to pursue his practice, increasing hostility to *converso* physicians and fear of the Inquisition forced Lusitano to move to Antwerp in 1533. Three years later, Lusitano published *Index Dioscorides*, a translation and commentary on the classic text on herbal medicine and related medicinal substances written about 1,500 years previously, and the only book he published under his baptismal name, Joannus Rodericus. In 1540, Lusitano's great fame as a skilled physician and scientist prompted the Duke of Ferrara to appoint him Lecturer in Medicine at the University of Ferrara, a city where he had freedom to practice Judaism and to pursue scientific research.

Lusitano discovered the presence of venous valves and their function in the circulation of blood. However, he is best known for his seven-volume *Centuria*, a collection of the case histories of his most interesting 700 patients, which provides a unique insight into clinical medical practice in the 16th century.

With the accession of Paul IV as pope and his persecution of *conversos*, Lusitano fled to several places before finally taking refuge in Thessaloniki, a city in the Ottoman Empire with a large Jewish community where he could live openly as a Jew.

## Mantino, Jacob ben Samuel (Spain, c. 1490–1549)

A native of Tortosa, Jacob Mantino (also known as Mantinus) and his family moved to Italy after the expulsion of the Jews from Spain. He studied medicine and philosophy at the universities of Padua and Bologna. Mantino remained in Bologna as a professor of medicine, devoting much of his free time to translating scientific works from Hebrew and Arabic into Latin. This earned him an excellent reputation, which led to his being befriended by the highest dignitaries at the court of Pope Clement VII. When Paul III became pope in 1534, he appointed Mantino as his personal physician. Returning to Venice, Mantino accompanied (as physician) the Venetian ambassador to Damascus, but died soon after his arrival.

Mantino translated into Latin many of the commentaries of Averroes on works by Aristotle and Plato. He also translated several important medical works, including a general medical encyclopedia of Averroes, the first book of Avicenna's *The Canon of Medicine*, and the *Shemonah Perakim* (Eight Chapters) of Maimonides.

## Morpurgo, Samson ben Joshua Moses                    (Bosnia, 1681–1740)

After an intensive Jewish education at the *yeshiva* of Samuel Aboab in Venice, Samson Morpurgo studied medicine and philosophy at the University of Padua. Following graduation, Morpurgo devoted himself to the study of Talmud, traveling to Mantua to work with the outstanding scholar Judah Briel, who ordained him as a rabbi in 1709.

Morpurgo was a skillful physician who showed compassion to all, especially the suffering poor. During a devastating influenza epidemic in Ancona in 1730, Morpurgo distinguished himself in his care of the inhabitants of the town despite a Church ban against Jewish doctors treating the Christian sick. Consequently, Cardinal Lambertini publicly presented him with a document expressing gratitude and esteem for Morpurgo's devotion to the care of all members of the community.

Morpurgo was the author of a prayer beginning "*Ana ha-El ha-Gadol ha-Gibor v'ha-Nora*" (Please God, Who is great, mighty, and awesome) to be recited by persons visiting the cemetery.

## Provençal, David and Abraham                         (Italy, 16th century)

Rabbi of Mantua and linguist, David Provençal feared a decline in the study of Torah in Italy after the burning of the Talmud. In an appeal addressed to the Italian Jewish communities, he and his son Abraham called for the establishment of a college that would teach both Jewish studies (Torah, Oral Law, and Hebrew grammar, poetry, and philosophy) and secular subjects (Latin and Italian, grammar, astronomy, and medicine). This plan may have anticipated a papal bull by Pope Pius IV, prohibiting the admission of Jews to examinations for doctoral degrees. As written in their proposal, this program of study would make it possible "that anyone who wishes to become a physician need not waste his days and years in a university among Christians in sinful neglect of Jewish studies."[17] However, they were never permitted to open such a *yeshivah* university and had to settle instead for a Talmudic institute.

Abraham Provençal received doctorates in medicine and philosophy

17. http://www.jewishvirtuallibrary.org/universities.

from the University of Mantua, before serving as rabbi in various Italian towns (including Mantua and Ferrara) and earning the reputation as a superb physician.

## Rosales, Jacob Hebraeus                              (Portugal, c. 1588–c. 1668)

The son of a *converso* physician (Ferdinand Bocarro), Jacob Rosales studied medicine, mathematics, and classical languages at the University of Montpellier before returning to Lisbon, where he attained a considerable reputation as a physician and attended the Archbishop of Braga. Rosales later settled in Rome and came under the influence of Galileo, who encouraged the "learned astrologer" to write various books on the subject. Moving to Hamburg, where Emperor Ferdinand III bestowed upon him the title "Count Palatine," Rosales eventually resided in Livorno, where he lived as a Jew and assumed the name Jacob Hebraeus.

## Saladino Ferro d'Ascoli                              (Italy, 15th–16th century)

A physician who lived at the court of the Prince of Taranto, Saladino d'Ascoli was considered the leading pharmacist of his era. His classic *Aromatariorum Compendium* (1488) was regarded as the basic textbook of pharmacology until the 18th century.

## Yagel, Abraham ben Chananiah dei Calicchi        (Italy, 16th–17th century)

A member of a wealthy Italian Jewish banking family, Abraham Yagel was a physician, kabbalist, and naturalist who integrated an empirical study of nature with kabbalistic and rabbinic learning. He championed a modern approach to Jewish culture that underscored the religious value of the study of nature, reformulated kabbalist traditions in the language of scientific discourse so as to promote them as the highest form of human knowledge, and advocated the legitimate role of the magical arts as the ultimate expression of human creativity in Judaism.[18]

Many details of Abraham Yagel's life are recorded in his *Gei Chizayon* (Valley of Vision), written in prison where the author was confined after

---

18. David B. Ruderman, *Kabbalah, Magic and Science: The Cultural Universe of a Sixteenth-Century Jewish Physician* (Cambridge: Harvard University Press, 1988).

a bitter inheritance dispute. In this strange work, the author recounts a dream in which he narrates the events of his life and his innermost thoughts to his dead father. His father then tours him around *gehinnom* and shows him the denizens of the underworld, prominent among whom are bankers.

Abraham Yagel is best known for his *Lekach Tov* (Good Portion), written in the form of a conversation between a teacher and his student. Designed as a religious guide to the young, this book is an important work of *musar* literature that explains many fundamental tenets in Judaism. Influenced by contemporary Christian catechism, *Lekach Tov* describes faith, hope, and charity (love) as essential elements of a religious life. It discusses the seven "principal classes of sin" and then contrasts them with the seven major virtues.

Another work of Abraham Yagel is *Eishet Chayil* (Woman of Valor), a commentary on Proverbs 31, which was written as a guide to married life and discusses the virtues of a wife and her duties to her husband.

## Zahalon, Jacob ben Isaac (Italy, 1630–1693)

Jacob ben Isaac Zahalon was born in Rome to a family of Jews expelled from Spain and Portugal. An ordained rabbi and member of the rabbinical council of the community of Rome, Zahalon studied medicine at the University of Rome. He played an active role in caring for patients of the plague that spread throughout the city, including the Jewish ghetto. Later he served as rabbi in Ferrara until his death.

Zahalon is best known as the author of *Otzar ha-Hayim* (The Treasure of Life), an encyclopedic treatise published in 1683 that was designed to reflect contemporary medical practice. It was divided into 13 discrete sections: bodily hygiene and diet; fevers and their cures; the pulse, color of urine, and condition of the tongue; poison in plants and metals, and appropriate remedies; reasons for and diagnoses of diseases; simple and complex solutions; illnesses of the various parts of the head and remedies; the chest and limbs; internal illnesses; external illnesses; women's illnesses; children's illnesses; and mental illnesses.

*Otzar ha-Hayim* begins with a theological and legal justification for Jews to practice medicine, concluding that "the science of medicine is a commandment and a value."[19] As David B. Ruderman notes, Zahalon's handbook was designed to provide all readers with methods of healing the sick

19. David B. Ruderman, *Jewish Thought and Scientific Discovery in Early Modern Europe* (New Haven: Yale University Press, 1995), pp. 235–236.

in "the most correct, accepted, and tried manner."[20] Zahalon asserted that physicians could use his book like a *Shulchan Aruch* (Set Table), the authoritative code of Jewish law of Joseph Caro published more than a century previously, which provided the "accepted and correct view." As Zahalon added, the book could be used by anyone, even indigent sick Jews who did not have the funds to pay for the services of a "Gentile doctor." Unlike *Ma'aseh Tuviyah* (Work of Tobias), the encyclopedic tome written by Tobias Cohn a quarter century later, Zahalon did not include unresolved issues of conflicting views and alternative therapies. Instead, he asserted with conviction the correctness of his medical prescriptions and the belief that his book contained everything the doctor and patient needed to know.

Zahalon expressed confidence in classical medical therapy, constantly quoting the views of Galen, Hippocrates, Aristotle, and Avicenna. He occasionally referred to contemporary sources, especially those of Jewish ancestry, but only when they supported his position. Zahalon did not discuss the current challenges to classical medical thinking that were rife in the late 17th century.

*Otzar ha-Hayim* was the first general orientation to medicine published in Hebrew and had wide appeal. Zahalon also composed a prayer to be recited by the physician that stressed the religious aspects of his professional role: "You [God] are the physician, not me. I am but clay in the Potter's hand, in the hand of the Creator of all things, and as the instrument through which You cure Your creatures."[21]

## NETHERLANDS

In the 16th century, many *conversos* desiring to return to Judaism fled the Iberian Peninsula and were welcomed in Amsterdam, which had become independent from Spain. Some of the new Jewish immigrants were able to employ their skills as bankers, manufacturers, and printers to achieve economic success during the golden age of the Dutch republic. Well educated and often with university degrees, the *conversos* belonged to synagogues but often tended to have secular lifestyles. A small percentage, exemplified by Spinoza, became religious skeptics who rejected the norms of the Jewish community and its rabbis, convinced of the validity of forming their own religious identities based on rational thought.

---

20. Ibid, pp. 233–235.
21. Harry Friedenwald, *The Jews and Medicine* (Baltimore: Johns Hopkins Press, 1944), 1:273–277.

## Bueno, Ephraim Hezekiah (Portugal, 1599–1665)

Born into a medical family of *conversos* expelled from both Spain and Portugal, Ephraim Bueno studied medicine in Bordeaux. Not permitted to practice as a physician in France, Bueno settled in Amsterdam and became a court physician and a highly respected member of the Portuguese-Jewish community. In addition to his medical practice, Bueno was a biblical scholar who published poetry and translated the Psalms of David into Spanish. Bueno founded the Or Torah Academy in Amsterdam and in 1627 co-published the first Hebrew book in the city, on the press of his friend, Menashe ben Israel.

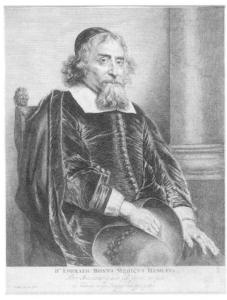

Portrait by Jan Lievens, 1656 etching. (*Joods Historisch Museum, Amsterdam*)

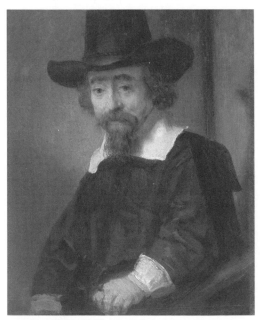

Portrait of a man, presumably Ephraim Bueno, by Rembrandt. (*Rijksmuseum, Amsterdam*)

Ephraim Bueno was the physician of Rembrandt and the subject of two of his etchings, the most famous of which is *The Doctor Descending the Stairs*, in which he is shown in expensive attire with an obvious ring on his index finger representing the insignia of the medical community. As an old man, Bueno also was etched by another famous artist, Jan Lievens, seated and wearing a *kippah*. Written at the bottom of the print is: "Dr. Ephraim Bonus, Medicus Hebraeus."

## De Castro, Balthazar (Isaac) Orobio                    (Portugal, 1617–1687)

Born into a *converso* family, Orobio de Castro studied philosophy before switching to the study of medicine and then opening a popular medical practice in Seville. Denounced by a vengeful servant he had punished for theft, de Castro was condemned by the Inquisition as a secret Jew. Despite denying the charge, he spent three terrible years in a dungeon, subjected to torture. When finally released, de Castro fled to Toulouse, where he became professor of medicine at the university. He eventually moved to Amsterdam, where he could practice Judaism openly, and adopted the name "Isaac." Well respected in his adopted country, de Castro was elected as a director of the Spanish-Portuguese congregation.

Although maintaining a friendly correspondence with Benedict Spinoza, de Castro wrote a work attacking the *Ethics* written by the latter. In addition to other books on philosophy and theology, de Castro was known for his *Friendly Discussions with a Learned Jew on Christianity* with the Dutch preacher Phillipp van Limborch, which Voltaire described as possibly "the first dispute between two theologians in which no insults are traded; on the contrary, the two adversaries treat each other with respect."[22]

## Menashe (Menasseh) ben Israel                    (Portugal, 1604–1657)

Born a *converso* in Lisbon or La Rochelle, Menashe ben Israel was baptized as Manoel Dias Soeiro. After his parents fled Portugal in 1610 to escape the Inquisition, the family settled in the welcoming haven of Amsterdam. Openly returning to his faith, his father took the name Joseph ben Israel, appropriately renaming his two sons Ephraim and Menashe.

Menashe ben Israel rapidly mastered a solid Jewish education, including Hebrew language and grammar and an understanding of Jewish thought ranging from the philosophical rationalism of Maimonides to the views of the late kabbalists. He also had a comprehensive exposure to secular studies, becoming fluent in ten languages and knowledgeable in classical literature, the sciences, and even the writings of early Christian theologians. A skilled physician, Menashe ben Israel was termed "Divine and Doctor of Physick" and, in Latin, *Medicus Hebraeus*. Among his many non-Jewish friends was the famous artist Rembrandt van Rijn, who made an etching of him.

In 1626, Menashe ben Israel founded the first Hebrew printing press in

---

22. Stanford Encyclopedia of Philosophy, https://plato.stanford.edu/entries/voltaire/.

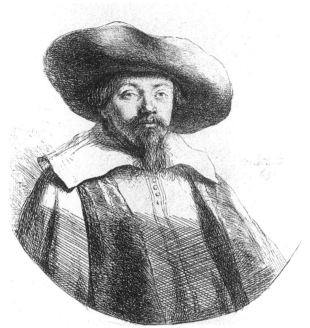

Portrait (etching) of Menashe ben Israel by Rembrandt, 1636. (*Rijksmuseum, Wikimedia*)

Holland, also publishing books in multiple other languages. Due to difficulty earning sufficient funds to support his family, he decided to move to Brazil, where many Jews had settled and business prospects were much better. However, when the Jewish community in Recife engaged their new spiritual leader Isaac Aboab de Fonseca as the rabbi of Amsterdam, the Amsterdam Jewish community promptly named Menashe ben Israel as his successor, solving his financial problems. Later, the Pereira brothers, two Jewish entrepreneurs, arrived in Amsterdam and established a *yeshiva* with Menashe ben Israel as its head.

In 1644, Menashe ben Israel met Antonio de Montesinos, who convinced him that the Andes Indians of South America were descendants of the Ten Lost Tribes of Israel. Already having a Messianic inclination, Menashe ben Israel believed that this discovery solved one requirement for the coming of the Messiah – the settlement of Jews in all parts of the known world. Now all that remained was to persuade the leaders of those countries barring Jews from living within their territory to repeal these discriminatory regulations and permit Jews to return. Menashe ben Israel focused his efforts on England, where the Jews had been expelled since 1290. He found much support among Christian Protestant theologians, especially after the publication of an English translation of his *Hope of Israel*, which described the discovery of the Ten Lost Tribes in the New World. Oliver Cromwell was sympathetic, both because of his beliefs in religious liberty and that the presence of Jewish merchants would improve English commercial ventures, but public opinion did not favor readmission of the Jews. To avoid a defeat in Parliament, the best Cromwell could do politically was to allow Jews to stay in England on an informal basis and practice their religion. It took another century until Jews were formally allowed to live in England and be granted English citizenship.

A Talmudic scholar and prolific author, many of Menashe ben Israel's works were directed at non-Jews in an attempt to present Judaism in a sympathetic manner acceptable to the Christian world. Among his writings are *El Conciliador* (The Mediator), which attempts to explain difficult passages in the Bible and reconcile apparent discrepancies, and *Nishmat Chaim* (Breath of Life), dealing with the nature of the soul, the concept of transmigration, and related issues. In view of his printing and literary activities, as well as his synagogue sermons to which non-Jewish scholars were invited, Menashe ben Israel was considered the leading representative of Jewish learning in Amsterdam.

Menashe ben Israel's most famous student was Baruch Spinoza, who was excommunicated by the rabbis of Amsterdam while his teacher was in London.

---

## Spinoza, Baruch                                    (Netherlands, 1632–1677)

---

One of the most influential rationalist philosophers in Western civilization, who laid the groundwork for such diverse areas as the Enlightenment, modern biblical criticism, and conceptions of the self and the universe, Baruch Spinoza was born in Amsterdam to Portuguese Jews living in exile in Holland. In addition to a traditional Jewish education, Spinoza received instruction in Latin and the physical sciences from a Christian phy-

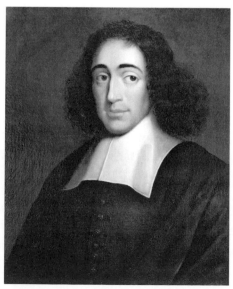

Oil portrait of Baruch Spinoza, circa 1665. (*Wikimedia*)

sician, Franz van den Ende. This gave him access to the medical books of Dr. Nichalaes Tulp, a renowned Dutch surgeon and mayor of Amsterdam (and the subject of Rembrandt's famous painting *The Anatomy Lesson of Dr. Nicolaes Tulp*). Others who had major roles in stimulating his free-thinking views were Jewish physician friends, especially the *converso* Spanish exile Juan de Prado.

Spinoza earned a living as a grinder of optical lenses and died of tuberculosis, which was apparently aggravated by constant occupational inhalation of fine glass dust. Although not a physician, he was employed in optometry, an allied medical

TRACTATUS
THEOLOGICO-
POLITICUS
*Continens*
Diſſertationes aliquot,
Quibus oſtenditur Libertatem Philoſophandi non tantum ſalva Pietate, & Reipublicæ Pace poſſe concedi: ſed eandem niſi cum Pace Reipublicæ, ipſaque Pietate tolli non poſſe.

Johann: Epiſt: I. Cap: IV. verſ: XIII.
*Per hoc cognoſcimus quod in Deo manemus, & Deus manet in nobis, quod de Spiritu ſuo dedit nobis.*

HAMBURGI,
Apud *Henricum Künraht.* cIↃ IↃ cLXX

Frontispiece of *Tractatus Theologico-Politicus* by Baruch Spinoza, published circa 1670. (*Wikimedia / Vanderbilt University Library*)

field. He also made an important contribution to anatomy, resulting from his dispute with Descartes over the importance of the pineal gland, a small structure deep within the brain. Rather than the French philosopher's concept of the pineal being the seat of the soul, from which it communicated to the physical body, Spinoza questioned whether this gland, or any other specific site within the brain, could be given this distinction.

Spinoza's controversial views of the nature of God caused him to be reviled as an atheist, because the Jewish community feared persecution by the Gentile authorities. After rejecting a substantial bribe in exchange for his silence, Spinoza was summoned before a rabbinic court and solemnly excommunicated from the community. Changing his name from the Hebrew Baruch to the Latin Benedict, Spinoza declined an offer of professorship at Heidelberg, preferring to maintain his intellectual independence and continue his studies alone.

In his *Tractatus Theologico-Politicus* (A Theological-Political Treatise),

Spinoza critiqued superficial popular religion and attacked the militant Protestantism of the House of Orange, which ruled Holland. He rejected a conception of God using anthropomorphisms on both logical and theological grounds. Spinoza proposed the use of modern historical-critical methods of biblical interpretation and supported political tolerance of alternative religious practices, convinced that Jews and Christians could coexist amicably if they could overcome the theological and cultural differences that divide them.

## NORTHERN EUROPE

The following were prominent physicians practicing and writing in various areas of Europe. Most were *conversos*, and many either graduated from the medical school in Padua or studied with illustrious graduates from that university.

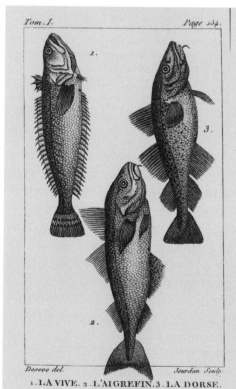

French edition of *Histoire naturelle des poisons*, by Marcus Bloch, 1801. (*Wikimedia*)

## Bloch, Marcus Elieser                                  (Germany, 1723–1799)

Born in Ansbach, Marcus Bloch's parents were so poor that they could barely provide him any education. Virtually illiterate in German until his late teens, Bloch had just enough knowledge of Hebrew and rabbinic literature to enable him to obtain a teacher's position in the house of a Jewish surgeon in Hamburg, learning German fluently and some Latin. With his enthusiasm for science aroused, Bloch completely devoted himself to the study of all branches of natural science and medicine, finally succeeding in earning a medical degree at Frankfort-on-the-Oder in 1747. Settling in Berlin, Bloch established a successful general medical practice.

Taking an intense interest in fish, Bloch is best known for his comprehensive and beautifully illustrated 12-volume work on ichthyology. His extensive collection of about 1,500 specimens is now preserved at a museum of the Humboldt University in Berlin.

## Castro Sarmento, Jacob Henriques de                  (Portugal, 1692–1762)

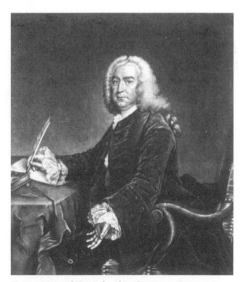

Born Henriques de Castro Sarmento into a *converso* family in Bragança, he studied medicine at Coimbra. To escape the persecutions of the Portuguese Inquisition, he left for London, where he changed his name to Jacob de Castro Sarmento and continued his studies in medicine, physics, and chemistry, becoming the first Jew to obtain a PhD in the United Kingdom. Well-versed in rabbinic studies, Castro Sarmento became the rabbi of the Bevis Marks Portuguese Jewish congregation in London. Castro Sarmento built an active medical practice and joined

Portrait of Jacob de Castro Sarmento. (*Wikimedia*)

the faculty of the University of Aberdeen. One of the first Jews to be admitted to the Royal College of Physicians, Castro Sarmento's development of a new medication for curing fevers led to his election as a Fellow of this medical organization.

A strong proponent of the philosophy of Isaac Newton, Castro Sarmento attempted to integrate it with Jewish theology. Unlike his mentor, David Nieto, Castro Sarmento was unable to rectify the natural science and religious world views, leading him to write a formal letter to the elders of the congregation announcing his intention to withdraw from the Jewish community.

---

## De Castro, Benedict                                    (Germany, 1597–1684)

The son of Rodrigo de Castro, Benedict de Castro was a member of an illustrious Sephardic Jewish family of Portuguese origin, whose members escaped the Inquisition by emigrating to Bordeaux, Bayonne, Hamburg, and various cities in the Netherlands. Known in Hebrew sources as Baruch Nachmias, de Castro studied medicine at the University of Padua. He practiced in Hamburg, acquiring such an excellent reputation that he was appointed physician to Queen Christina of Sweden in 1645.

De Castro's most famous medical work, under the pseudonym Philotheus Castellus, was a polemical defense of physicians of Portuguese origin against malicious attacks. The full title in translation is: "The Scourge of Calumnators, or Apology. In which the malicious charges of an anonymous author are refuted, the lust for lying of this person is disclosed, and the legitimate method of the most famous Portuguese physicians is commended, while the ignorance and temerity of empiric quacks are condemned as injurious to the commonwealth."[23] The preface was dedicated to the author by the famous Portuguese physician, Zacutus Lusitanus of Amsterdam. In the text, de Castro stresses the diagnostic abilities of Jewish physicians, arguing that "there is virtually no single part of medicine which cannot be traced to those old forefathers of the Hebrews."

---

## De Castro, Rodrigo                                     (Portugal, 1550–1627)

After studies in medicine and philosophy at Évora and Salamanca, Rodrigo de Castro practiced in Lisbon. As a *converso* physician escaping the persecutions of the Inquisition, de Castro and his family moved to Antwerp, northern Holland, and finally Hamburg in 1592. When the plague broke out in that city four years later, de Castro worked tirelessly to counteract it, writing a treatise on the disease that he dedicated to the Senate of Hamburg. A popular and well-known physician, de Castro was often summoned

---

23. Frank Heynick, *Jews in Medicine: An Epic Saga* (NJ: KTAV Publishing House, 2002).

by the magnates of neighboring countries, serving King Frederick II of Denmark and at the courts of the archbishop of Bremen and the dukes of Mecklenburg and Holstein. The full title of his most famous work, *Medicus politicus* is (in translation): "The Political Physician, or Treatise of Medical Political Skills . . . in which not only are the mores and virtues of good doctors explained and the frauds and impostures of bad ones unveiled but also very many useful and joyful things about this new topic are proposed. A work very useful for doctors, patients, and nurses and for everyone interested in letters and politics."[24]

An eminent gynecologist, de Castro wrote a lengthy two-volume treatise dealing with women's "nature" and diseases. The first volume deals with the anatomy of the uterus and breasts; semen and menses; coitus, conception, and pregnancy; and labor and breast feeding. The second volume focuses on women's diseases, including those that were then considered peculiar to widows and virgins; pregnancy and pregnant women; women in childbirth; and wet nurses.

For his first years in Hamburg, de Castro did not declare himself a Jew. However, a few years later his name appeared in the first list of Portuguese Jews published in the city council. Regarding chapter 38 of the apocryphal *Wisdom of Ben Sira* – "Show the physician the honor in view of your need of him, for the Lord has created him" – de Castro stressed the moral and religious role of the physician in the community. In another work, de Castro also discussed the use of music in healing, providing biblical citations to attribute this to the Psalms of King David.

---

**Delmedigo, Joseph Solomon**                      (Crete, 1591–1655)

---

Also known as *Yashar*, the Hebrew acronym for **Y**osef **Sh**lomo **R**ofe (physician), Joseph Delmedigo was the son of the rabbi of Crete and received both a traditional Jewish and secular education. Possessed of a photographic memory, Delmedigo entered the University of Padua at age 15, studying astronomy and mathematics under Galileo, as well as languages, philosophy, and medicine, while continuing his Jewish studies. Returning to Crete to practice medicine, Delmedigo began the ambitious task of writing *Ya'ar Levanon* (Forest of Lebanon), an encyclopedia of all the branches of knowledge studied at his time, which was never finished or published. Always restless, Delmedigo soon left for Cairo, where he easily bested a prom-

---

24. L. Whaley, *Women and the Practice of Medical Care in Early Modern Europe, 1400–1800* (New York: Palgrave MacMillan, 2011).

inent Muslim scholar who had challenged him to a public disputation on spherical trigonometry. His next stop was Constantinople, where Delmedigo became immersed in kabbalah under the tutelage of Jacob ibn Nehemias. Continuing his wandering, Delmedigo eventually settled in Vilna, where he became the personal physician of Prince Radziwill of Lithuania.

In response to a series of 12 general and 70 specific religious and scientific questions posed by a local Karaite scholar, Delmedigo wrote *Elim* (Trees). The precise number of questions inspired Delmedigo to select this name from two biblical verses (Exod. 15:27 and Num. 23:9), which describe the 12 foun-

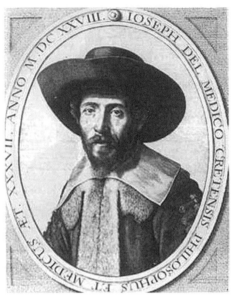

Engraving of Joseph Solomon Delmedigo by W. Delff after a painting by C. Duyster, 1628, from the frontispiece of *Sefer Elim*. (*Wikimedia / The Jewish Encyclopedia*)

tains and 70 palm trees that the Israelites encountered in Elim during their wanderings. The book spans the gamut of scientific and religious thought, including such diverse topics as astronomy, physics, mathematics, medicine, and music theory (string resonance, intervals and their proportions, and theoretical concepts of consonance and dissonance). Delmedigo maintains that the lack of Jewish participation in the Scientific Revolution reflected the domination of Ashkenazim, who focused their intellectual efforts solely on the Talmud, whereas Sephardim and the Karaites (for whom he had great affection) had greater interest in natural philosophy.

Joseph Delmedigo continued his travels, taking a rabbinic position in Hamburg and then becoming the rabbi of the Sephardic community in Amsterdam. There, *Elim* was published at the press of his rabbinic colleague, Menashe ben Israel.

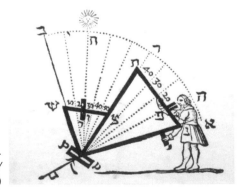

Image from *Sefer Elim* of Joseph Delmedigo, Amsterdam, 1629. (*Wikimedia / Diaspora Museum, Tel Aviv*)

## Falk, Hayim Samuel                    (Germany, 1708–1782)

Hayim Samuel Falk was a rabbi well-versed in practical kabbalah and alchemy. Almost burnt at the stake in Westphalia for sorcery, Falk was provided a haven by a German prince in Hozminden, where he gained renown for extraordinary powers by magically curing the daughter of a court Jew who had suffered from almost daily attacks of falling sickness. Moving to England, where he became known as Dr. Falkon, Falk perfected the art of master conjurer. His allegedly miraculous feats, including saving the Great Synagogue from fire by writing something in Hebrew on its doorpost, led some to refer to Falk as the "Baal Shem of London."

Falk kept a diary, written in cryptic Hebrew, which contained records of dreams and the kabbalistic names of angels. Rabbi Jacob Emden accused him of being a supporter of the false messiah, Shabbetai Zvi.

## Gumpertz, Aaron Solomon                (Germany, 1723–1769)

A graduate of the medical school at the University of Frankfurt and the first Prussian Jew to obtain a doctoral degree, Aaron Gumperz was especially known for being the philosophy teacher of Moses Mendelssohn and having inspired him with a love for literature. He also served as the role model for the Jewish hero of Gotthold Lessing's *Die Juden* (1749). In 1765, Gumpertz published an essay entitled *Ma'amar ha-Maddah* (Treatise on Science), which was designed to arouse the curiosity of contemporary Jews and encourage them to follow the dramatic developments in the field. Nevertheless, Gumpertz stressed that natural philosophy, especially the experimental type, had nothing in common with divine wisdom, which is not amenable to analysis and experiment because its elements are not subject to the senses. Consequently, science poses no threat to the Jewish faith.

## Herz, Marcus                          (Germany, 1747–1803)

Born in Berlin, where his father was a poor Torah scribe, at age 15 Marcus Herz left for Koenigsberg, where he worked as a clerk. Herz attended lectures at the University of Koenigsberg, becoming a pupil of Immanuel Kant, but was forced to discontinue his studies due to financial constraints. After a brief period traveling as a secretary for a wealthy Russian, Herz

returned to Germany and studied medicine at the University of
Halle. Following graduation, Herz
was appointed as a physician at the
Jewish Hospital in Berlin.

At age 30, Herz began delivering public lectures on medicine
and philosophy, which were well
attended by students, important
Prussian officials, and at times even
members of the royal family. For a
long time, his home was a meeting
place for the political, artistic, and
literary elite of Berlin society. Herz
wrote extensively on science and
philosophy and was a favorite pupil
and friend of philosopher Moses
Mendelssohn. His correspondence
with Immanuel Kant, collected
over many years, is considered to
be of importance to students of the history of philosophy.

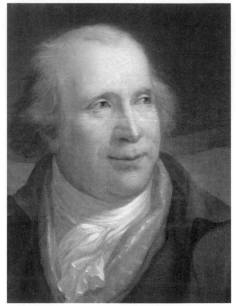

Coned image of portrait of Marcus Herz
by Friedrich Georg Weitsch, 1803. (*Wikimedia*)

According to scholars, the "Daily Prayer of a Physician Before He Visits His Patients," attributed to Maimonides and first appearing in print
around 1783, was probably written by Herz.

---

**Levison, George**                                (Germany, 1741–1797)

Born Mordecai Gumpel ben Judah Leib in Berlin, George Levison earned
a rabbinic diploma at an early age. Moving to England, Levison studied
medicine with two surgeon-brothers. After completing his course, Levison
received a medical degree from Marischal College in Aberdeen, the first
college in the British Isles to award medical degrees to professing Jews.
In London, he published *An Essay on the Blood* (1776) under the pseudonym, George Levison. Two years later, Levison wrote *An Account of the
Epidemical Sore Throat*.

Levison also wrote *Dissertation on Torah and Wisdom* (1771), a controversial philosophic treatise with radical tendencies, which so enraged the
authorities of the Great Synagogue that they expelled him from membership. He responded with a polemical attack that led to a vitriolic response
and the accusations of scandals in his past. Levison then left for Sweden,

where he became court physician and Professor of Medicine at the University of Ursula.

## Montalto, Philotheus (Elianus)                         (Portugal, 1567–1616)

Raised in the Jewish religion by his *converso* parents, Philotheus Montalto served as court physician to Grand Duke Ferdinand in Florence. Impressed by a cure he accomplished there, Queen Marie de Medici invited Montalto to become a physician in the French royal court, despite her husband, King Henry IV, having forbidden the practice of Judaism in his realm. Although the queen had previously engaged several *converso* physicians, they had hidden their Judaism. Previously, Montalo had refused several prestigious positions in Italy, including at the University of Padua, lest he not be able to fulfill his religious obligations. Therefore, Montalto stubbornly refused to come to France unless

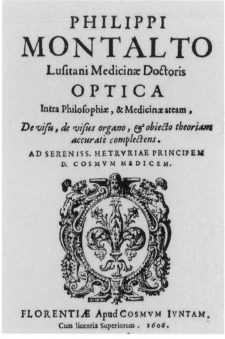

Frontispiece of *Optica* by Philotheus Montalto, 1606. (*Wikipedia*)

he was allowed to freely and openly practice his religion (including being exempted from any service on Saturday). Although King Henry strenuously objected to this condition, Queen Marie de Medici prevailed and even obtained a papal dispensation.

Montalto was the author of a major book on optics. His *Archipathologia*, describing various nervous system diseases and mental disturbances, was popular in his time and cited often by later medical writers. Steeped in the Jewish rationalist tradition, Montalto opposed claims of sorcery and superstition with regard to mental illness.

At his death, Queen Marie arranged for Montalto to be buried in Amsterdam, which had become a welcoming site for Jewish refugees and known as the "Jerusalem of the West."[25]

25. https://en.wikipedia.org/wiki/Jerusalem_of_the_West.

## Musaphia (Mussafia), Benjamin ben Immanuel          (Spain, c. 1606–1675)

A graduate of the medical school in Padua, Benjamin Musaphia practiced medicine in Hamburg and later was appointed royal physician to the Danish court by Christian IV. Also a biblical scholar and kabbalist, Musaphia's first literary work was *Zecher Rav*, an adaptation of the creation story in which all Hebrew word roots are used once, which he dedicated to his late wife. He also published a long medical treatise, which contained a controversial section on alchemy and the healing properties of gold, as well as possibly the first book by a Jewish author on medicine in the Hebrew Bible. After the death of his royal patron, Musaphia went to Amsterdam, joined the college of rabbis, and became involved in the movement that proclaimed Shabbetai Zvi as the messiah.

## Nieto, David          (Italy, 1654–1728)

Born in Venice, David Nieto was a rabbinic scholar and a graduate of the University of Padua, who practiced as a physician and served as a preacher and religious judge in Leghorn. In 1701, Nieto arrived in London to become the first rabbi of the Bevis Marks synagogue and the *hacham* of the Spanish and Portuguese synagogue, composed primarily of former *conversos*. One clause of his contract mandated that he could not practice medicine, since his role was to be exclusively as a religious leader and the primary spokesman of the Jews in England.

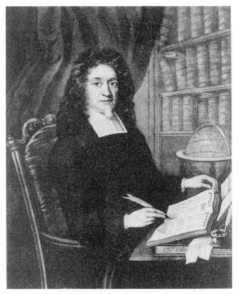

Portrait of David Nieto. From the *Jewish Encyclopedia*. (*Wikimedia*)

Influenced by the attempts of Christian theologians to relate the new advances in science to their understanding of the social and moral order of their faith, Nieto argued for the compatibility of scientific investigations and Judaism. He strove to identify areas in which science was not sufficient to provide ultimate answers and to show how the Jewish faith could enhance the moral and spiritual life of its adherents. Nieto's major work is *Mateh Dan* (1714), a comprehensive defense of the Oral Law and traditional Jewish faith and practice against the attacks of former *conversos* to whom the rabbinic tradition was both novel and unacceptable. Written in Hebrew and Spanish on the model of the *Kuzari* of Judah Halevi against the Karaites (though few members of this dissident group remained in Western Europe at the time), Nieto argued that science without religion cannot understand the totality of reality, thus providing only a partial truth. In *Esh ha-Dat* (Fire of a Law), Nieto wrote a scathing critique of Nehemiah Hiyya Hayon and his support of the heresies and false messianism of Shabbetai Zvi, which Nieto regarded as dangerous to Judaism.

*Pascalogia* (1702), Nieto's earliest work, describes the differences of calculation in the calendars of the Greek, Roman, and Jewish churches, especially in the relationship of Passover and Easter, demonstrating the errors that had crept into the calendar from the First Council of Nicaea in 325 CE. He later developed a calendar that fixed the time for the beginning of Sabbath eve for the latitude of England, which was used by the London Jewish community until the 19th century. In *De La Divina Providencia*, written in the form of a dialogue, Nieto expanded on a prior sermon to combat the deistic notion of "Nature" apart from God.

---

### Samuda, Isaac de Sequeira          (Portugal, 1681–1729)

Born in Portugal, Isaac de Sequeira Samuda was a physician best known for his contributions to astronomy. Forced to flee his native land to escape the Inquisition, Samuda arrived in London and became a conduit between the emerging world of Portuguese astronomy and the scientific community in England. In 1729, Samuda was the first Jew to be elected as a Fellow of the Royal Society.

---

### Sanchez, Antonio Riberio          (Portugal, 1699–1782)

A *converso* physician, Antonio Riberio Sanchez escaped the persecutions of the Inquisition and went to Holland, where he studied medicine at the University of Leiden under the eminent Herman Boerhaave. When asked by Empress Anna Ivanovna of Russia to send her a learned physician who would be competent to act as her medical adviser, Boerhaave recommended

Sanchez, who became Anna's personal physician. Known as a scholar as well as a skilled practitioner, Sanchez published several medical treatises, including an introduction to European physicians on the medical value of Russian steam baths. He also saved the life of a gravely ill young girl, whom other doctors had been given up for lost. This was the German Princess Sofia Frederika, bride of the heir to the Russian throne (Peter III) and later known as Catherine the Great.

When his Jewish origin became known at the Russian court, Sanchez was dismissed and retired to Paris, where he worked as a doctor among the poor. His financial situation deteriorated until Catherine the Great ascended the throne and granted a sizable life pension to the doctor who had saved her life.

---

**Sanchez, Francisco**                                    (Spain, 1551–1623)

Born in northwestern Spain of Sephardi Jewish origin, Francisco Sanchez was baptized in Portugal. As *conversos*, Sanchez and his family escaped the Inquisition by moving to Bordeaux, where he began his medical studies at the College de Guyenne. After several years of study in Rome, Sanchez returned to France to complete his medical degree at the University of Montpellier. After graduation, Sanchez joined several other Portuguese *conversos* at the University of Toulouse, becoming a professor of medicine and philosophy.

The major work of Francisco Sanchez is *Quod nihil scitur* (That nothing is known), published in 1581. In this critique of Aristotle and the scholastic system of knowledge and the syllogisms, Sanchez uses classical skeptical arguments in arguing that true scientific knowledge based on the Aristotelian concept of giving necessary reasons or causes for the behavior of nature is beyond human capability, because of the unreliability of the sense faculties and the nature of both objects and human beings. Rather than seek ultimate knowledge, the goal should be to gain limited knowledge that can be derived from observation, experience, and judgment. Consequently, Sanchez argued for a new rationality ("constructive skepticism") related to probabilistic conclusions based on empirical data as a realistic basis for human knowledge.

## Silva, Jean-Baptiste (France, 1682–1742)

Born in Bordeaux into a *converso* family of Spanish origin, Jean-Baptiste Silva studied medicine at the University of Montpellier. Moving to Paris, Silva's successful use of bleeding to cure the foot disease of Louis XV earned him a great reputation. Although his theories were refuted by other doctors, Silva became a fashionable physician in French society, especially among women.

Silva became the personal doctor of Voltaire, the French philosopher who usually had few good things to say about Jews. Referring to Molière's satirical play, *The Doctor Despite Himself*, Voltaire described Silva as "one of those outstanding physicians whom Molière neither could nor have dared to make ridiculous."[26]

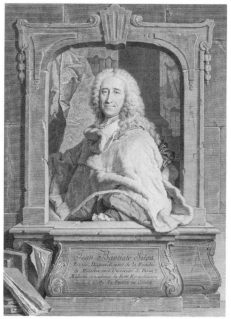

Engraving of Jean Baptiste Silva by Georg Friedrich Schmidt, 1742, after Hyacinthe Rigaud, 1740. (*Wikimedia / Wellcome Trust*)

## Teller, Issachar (17th century)

Although a barber-surgeon in Prague, rather than a physician, Issachar Teller had received medical instruction from Joseph Solomon Delmedigo, a prominent Jewish graduate of the medical school in Padua. He was the author of *Be'er Mayim Hayim* (The Wellspring of Living Waters), a popular medical self-help book written in Yiddish and published in 1655. It discusses the four elements, their influences, and the differences between men and women (such as women by nature being colder than men, except when having fever). This practical book also describes changes in a person related to age, seasons, and diet, and offers special medications for women and treatments for colic, warts, and other medical conditions.

26. Stanford Encyclopedia of Philosophy, https://plato.stanford.edu/entries/voltaire/.

## Wallich, Abraham ben Isaac                    (Germany, 17th century)

Born in Metz, Abraham Wallich studied medicine in Padua and was a fellow student of Tobias Cohn. Practicing as a physician in Frankfurt from 1657, Wallich is best known as the author of *Sefer Refu'ot* (Book of Cures), a Hebrew treatise on medicine. Known in Latin as *Harmonia Wallichis Medica* and published posthumously in 1700, the book describes many diseases (e.g., apoplexy, tuberculosis, dysentery, elephantiasis, pestilence) with recommendations for their treatment and prevention. He also includes advice on proper diet and a section on the treatment of small children with fever. Wallich attempted to prove that because ailments of the soul correspond to those of the body, they must be treated in the same way. Throughout the book, Wallich writes alternately as a physician and as a preacher of morals. He also includes recommendations for a doctor's proper bedside manner and that the doctor's prayer of Jacob Zahalon be recited before visiting a patient.

# MODERN ERA

~: :~

THE MODERN ERA OF medicine coincided with the removal of political and civic restrictions from Jews (Emancipation). This resulted from the ideas of the Enlightenment and the French Revolution (1789) which stressed equality and social reform and the integration of subgroups into the nation state. Natural results of the Enlightenment and Emancipation were acculturation and, in some cases, total assimilation. Many Jews abandoned their faith once permitted to adopt the secular culture and professions of their Gentile neighbors. Emancipation was achieved in Western and Central Europe during the 19th century, but in Eastern Europe it did not occur until the fall of the Russian Empire in 1917. The Emancipation resulted in a breakdown of Jewish communal and religious authority, which led to the development of the Reform, Conservative, and neo-Orthodox movements.

In 1782, Emperor Joseph II of the Habsburg Monarchy enacted a series of reforms to remodel Austria in the form of an ideal Enlightenment state. Reversing the often harsh dictates of his mother, Maria Theresa, the Edict of Tolerance extended religious freedom to Jews in the kingdom, permitting Jewish children to attend schools and universities, allowing Jewish adults to work as merchants and to open factories, and eliminated previous restrictions that had forced Jews to wear gold stars and to pay a tax that was only levied on Jews and cattle.

Throughout the 19th century, and continuing for the first three decades of the 20th century, Western Europe was universally acknowledged as the most advanced site for scientific medicine. French medical science developed in the hospital, while Germany pioneered medical science in the laboratory. Graduates of American medical schools flocked to Vienna, Berlin, Heidelberg, Paris, London, and Edinburgh for additional clinical or research training.

Although restrictions on Jews were officially lifted in Germany and Austria, some limitations persisted. Not permitted as university professors, a Jewish medical graduate could only aspire to become a *privatdozent*. This title has its origins in German-speaking countries in Europe before 1800 and referred to a lecturer who received fees from his students rather than a university salary. In effect, this academic title indicated that one had certain formal qualifications denoting an ability to teach a designated subject at a university level, but without holding a professorial chair.

In the United States, the Jewish population was the product of waves of immigration, primarily from communities in Europe. The first doctors in America were of Sephardi origin. In the century after it became an independent country, immigration to the United States was inspired by the business and religious opportunities offered by the New World. After the Civil War, the financial boom in the North led many German Jews to establish thriving commercial enterprises, including major department stores founded by former peddlers. Assimilation and intermarriage were special threats to the continuity of American Jewry, with few retaining a Jewish identity beyond the third generation. As in their native land, the vast majority of German Jews belonged to the Reform movement, which tended to be more radical than in Europe.

Persecution of Jews in Eastern Europe led to a dramatic change in the Jewish population of the United States in the late 19th century. The partitions of Poland in 1772 and 1793 effectively eliminated the country from the map. Some Polish territory went to Prussia and Austria, but the largest share was acquired by Russia, which became the country with the largest concentration of Jews in the world. Unfortunately, successive Russian rulers considered the Jewish presence in annexed Polish territory a problem that required a solution. More liberal ones emphasized assimilation, developing secular curricula for traditional Jewish schools and allowing graduates to attend universities, as well as permitting movement of Jews from areas to which they had been restricted. Most tsars, however, limited Jews to the Pale of Settlement, which had been established by Catherine the Great in 1791 in response to pressure to rid Moscow of Jewish business competition and the "evil influence" of Jews on the susceptible Russian masses. More than 90% of Russian Jews were forced to live in the poor conditions of the Pale, which included the territory of modern Latvia, Lithuania, Ukraine, Bessarabia, Belarus, and Poland. Representing only 4% of Imperial Russia, the Pale was effectively a large-scale ghetto, containing almost 5 million Jews by the turn of the century. The Jews were heavily taxed and forbidden to lease land, operate taverns, or receive higher education. The May Laws of 1882 restricted Jews in the Pale to urban areas, which were often overcrowded and offered limited economic opportunities. These deplorable conditions, combined with a series of vicious pogroms beginning in 1881, led to the mass emigration of more than two million Jews from Eastern Europe to the United States between that year and the start of World War I in 1914.

Emigration of Jews from Europe to the United States again increased sharply in the 1930s as the Nazis gained control in Germany. The passage of the Nuremberg Laws in 1935 deprived German Jews of their civil rights, and Jewish physicians and other academicians were discharged from their university positions. Jewish emigration was further increased by the German annexation of Austria in early 1938, as well as the escalation in personal assaults on Jews that culminated in the nationwide Kristallnacht (Night of Broken Glass) pogrom in November of that year and the subsequent seizure of Jewish-owned property. As an indication of the elevated academic levels of many Jewish physicians who fled Europe to escape from Nazi tyranny, of the 36 listed in the book, 14 subsequently received either the Nobel Prize or the Lasker Award.

With the decline of clinical and basic science research in the traditional centers of excellence in Europe, the United States became the world leader in science and medicine. Jewish physicians were welcomed to Jewish hospitals and later to major non-Jewish American medical centers, while basic scientists found research opportunities in prestigious foundations and universities. By the 1980s, there were far more Jewish physicians in the United States than in all other countries combined.

## AGE OF SPECIALIZATION

The modern era in medicine saw a dramatic increase in specialization. Initially, this development was opposed by many physicians and lay people, who feared that it would be harmful to patients by encouraging itinerant charlatans who specialized in treating only one type of illness. However, the rapid advance in medical information and the development of complex new instruments and techniques made it impossible for a single practitioner to master them all. Increasingly, patients were referred to physicians who devoted all their time to treating one type of illness or had developed expertise in one area of manipulation. For the individual physician, major incentives for becoming a specialist were the opportunity to charge higher fees and work fewer hours, as well as to gain the respect of being a recognized expert in a certain area.

To a large degree, Jewish physicians were excluded from the mainstream areas of internal medicine and general surgery. Consequently, they flocked to less popular clinical specialties that did not attract their non-Jewish colleagues, such as ophthalmology, dermatology, neurology, and psychiatry. In addition to clinical activities, many Jewish physicians became major figures in "microscopy," a term that at the time referred collectively to the more basic sciences such as biochemistry, anatomy, histology, immunology, hematology, and microscopic pathology. More recently, this list has expanded to DNA/RNA research. A Jewish preeminence in these fields has continued to the present day, as evidenced by Jews (plus a few of half-Jewish descent) having been the recipients of almost one-half of the prestigious Lasker Awards in Basic Medical Research.

# JEWISH HOSPITALS IN
# THE UNITED STATES

∻ ∼

ACCORDING TO EDWARD HALPERIN,[27] the word "hospital" comes from the same Latin root as the words "hospitality," "hostel," and "hotel." Consequently, the earliest hospitals developed as religious establishments maintained by Christian, Muslim, and Jewish organizations to serve as places of refuge for travelers, pilgrims, and the needy. By the early 11th century, European synagogues contained a room for the lodging of travelers, some of whom were both indigent and sick. Although many of those housed in these facilities could not be cured by the medical techniques available at the time, at least they could die in dignity in the care of their co-religionists. In medieval Spain and Germany, inns to care for sick strangers were funded by the community, benevolent societies, and charity boxes. In the 18th and 19th centuries, at the dawn of the era of modern medicine, major Jewish communities in Europe had established specific houses for the sick. In Poland, for example, there were 48 Jewish hospitals by the early 20th century, with one in Warsaw having 1,000 beds.

The story of Jewish hospitals in America begins with the 1654 arrival of a small French ship sailing into New Amsterdam (now New York City) carrying 23 Jewish refugees from Brazil. Peter Stuyvesant, the director–general, requested permission from his superiors at the Dutch West India Company in Amsterdam to refuse entry to what he termed "deceitful," "very repugnant," and "hateful enemies and blasphemers of the name of Christ."[28] However, company directors rejected Stuyvesant's request, because some of their major shareholders were Dutch Jews. Instead, he was

---

27. *The Rise and Fall of the American Jewish Hospital*; in T. Levitan, *A History of Jewish Hospitals* (New York, 1961).
28. http://jewishweek.timesofisrael.com/jewish-hospitals-are-becoming-extinct/.

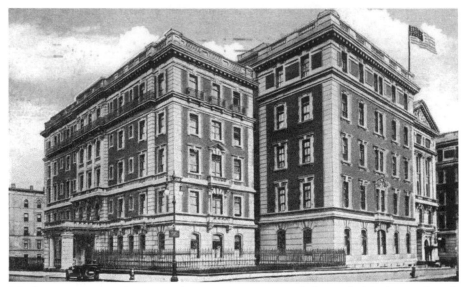

Manhattan – Postcard picture of Mount Sinai Hospital (formerly Manhattan Jewish Hospital) in New York City, sent in 1920. (*Wikimedia*)

ordered to admit the Jewish refugees, as long as they would pledge that "the poor among them shall not become a burden to the company or to the community, but be supported by their own nation."[29]

One of the most important of these American communal institutions was the Jewish hospital. The earliest arose in Cincinnati in 1854, founded by relatively secular German Jewish immigrants. Over the next 15 years, hospitals under Jewish auspices were established in Manhattan (later Mount Sinai Hospital), Baltimore, Chicago, and Philadelphia. The second wave of Jewish hospitals, beginning in the early 1880s, coincided with the immigration of millions of Jewish immigrants from Eastern Europe, who generally were more religiously observant.

Jewish hospitals developed for two major reasons, relating to both patients and physicians. They provided a unique environment compatible with the religious beliefs and customs of American Jews. As Halperin noted, Jewish hospitals "provided kosher food, an on-site synagogue, the comfort of a rabbi on the staff, and the placement of a *mezuzah* on the doorpost,"[30] as well as sparing Jewish patients from being forced to listen to Christians attempting convert them as they lay dying. Another major reason for the development of Jewish hospitals was rampant anti-Semitism in the medical profession. Medicine was a popular career choice for first- and sec-

29. Ibid.
30. Ibid.

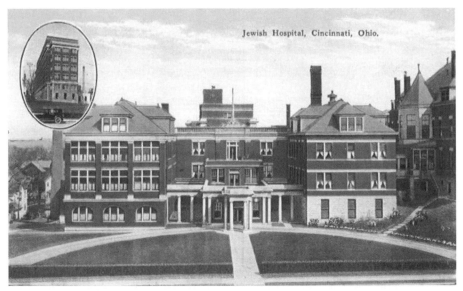

Cincinnati Jewish Hospital, founded in 1854. (*Wikimedia / Cincinnativiews.net*)

ond-generation immigrants from Eastern Europe, with the number of Jewish physicians growing even more than the rapidly increasing numbers of Jews in the overall population. However, from the beginning of the 20th century, medical schools and hospitals in the United States enforced restrictive quotas at all levels of education and practice. It was very difficult for Jews to be admitted to medical school, and those who managed to graduate had limited opportunity to secure an internship and even less chance to be offered a residency position. Once ready to practice, Jewish physicians faced the reality that large numbers of hospitals denied them staff privileges simply on the basis of their religious heritage. Even those fortunate enough to gain employment at non-Jewish hospitals were often the victims of physical harassment and various subtle and overt forms of written and verbal abuse. Therefore, Jewish hospitals became essential to provide training and employment opportunities for physicians who otherwise would have been virtually excluded from the medical profession.

Halperin estimates that, over the course of American history, there have been 113 "Jewish hospitals," of which 22 (19%) "are still operating independently under a name and with other characteristics that at least minimally connote a Jewish heritage."[31] However, almost all retain little of their Jewish roots. Their patients and physician staffs are no longer predominantly Jewish, their governing boards are no longer influenced

31. http://jewishweek.timesofisrael.com/jewish-hospitals-are-becoming-extinct/.

by the organized Jewish community, and some have even merged with non-Jewish hospitals.

The multiple reasons for the virtual disappearance of Jewish hospitals reflect underlying changes in the Jewish community. Since World War II, the percentage of self-identifying Jews in the population has decreased, as the rates of intermarriage and assimilation have increased. Jews have moved to the suburbs, far from traditional Jewish hospitals located in historically Jewish urban neighborhoods. Rather than support traditional Jewish charities such as hospitals, upwardly mobile Jews have been increasingly accepted into upper-class American society and are more likely to channel their philanthropic activities to general cultural organizations (symphony, opera, ballet) and even non-Jewish hospitals and medical schools.

Perhaps the most important reason for the decline of the Jewish hospitals in the United States is the waning of blatant anti-Semitism. Since the 1960s, quotas limiting access to medical schools and postgraduate training have become socially unacceptable and prohibited by law. Jews are now freely accepted in the medical schools of prestigious universities, and they have assumed major clinical and even high administrative positions at their associated hospitals. Jews are welcomed into specialty societies in all areas of medicine and have become editors of prestigious medical journals. No longer do Jews suffer any limitation in securing staff privileges at community hospitals throughout the country. Consequently, this basic reason for the rise of special Jewish hospitals no longer exists.

# THE AGE OF SPECIALIZATION

~: Basic Sciences :~

---

## BACTERIOLOGY, MICROBIOLOGY, INFECTIOUS DISEASE

---

Jewish bacteriologists showed that plant and animal vectors could spread contagious matter to humans and cause disease, but that heat-killed organisms could immunize animals against living organisms, the foundation for the development of the vaccine against typhus and polio. Cohn developed the classification of bacteria into four groups based on shape (sphericals, short rods, threads, and spirals), which is still in use today. Gruby described the *Trypanosoma* organism responsible for causing African sleeping sickness and the fungus *Candida albicans* (now a common form of infection in individuals who are immune suppressed). Neisser identified the causative agent of gonorrhea, a bacterium that was named *Neisseria gonorrhoeae* in his honor. Salmon documented the chain of transmission of *Salmonella* and made major contributions to veterinary medicine. Wasserman developed a complement fixation test for the diagnosis of syphilis, Schneerson produced a vaccine against bacterial meningitis, and Sterling developed a widely used classification for tuberculosis and introduced new methods for its diagnosis and treatment. Chain confirmed that, unlike other antibacterial drugs, penicillin did not produce any toxicity in humans, since its mechanism of action was to interfere with metabolic processes that are found only in the cell walls of bacteria. Waksman discovered the antibiotic streptomycin, and Finland later argued that the overuse of antibiotics had resulted in increased bacterial resistance to them. Kuvin founded the renowned Center for the Study of Infectious and Tropical Diseases at the Hebrew University of Jerusalem.

## Chain, Ernst Boris                                      (Germany, 1906–1979)

Born in Berlin, Ernst Chain obtained his chemistry degree from Friedrich Wilhelm University in 1930. Following graduation, Chain spent three years working on enzyme research at the Charité Hospital. However, after the Nazis took control, Chain left Germany for England because he was a Jew.

Chain spent several years at Cambridge University, where he earned a second Ph.D. working on phospholipids, a major component of biological membranes. He then was recruited to Oxford University by Australian Howard Florey, the new Chair of Pathology, who

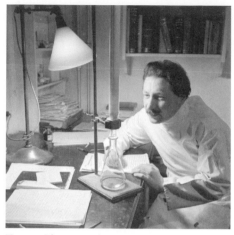

Ernst Chain undertaking an experiment in his office at the School of Pathology at Oxford University, 1944. (*Penicillin Past, Present and Future- the Development and Production of Penicillin, England, 1944*)

was attempting to attract scientists interested in studying the biochemical aspects of bacteriology. In 1939, Chain and Florey began investigating natural antibacterial agents produced by microorganisms. While revisiting the work of Alexander Fleming, who had described penicillin nine years previously, Chain and Florey proceeded to discover penicillin's therapeutic action and chemical composition. They developed a method for isolating and concentrating penicillin and also theorized its molecular structure, which later was confirmed by x-ray crystallography done by Dorothy Crowfoot Hodgkin. Chain and Florey showed that penicillin had dramatic effects on mice infected with such bacteria as streptococci, staphylococci, and clostridia (which causes tetanus, botulism, and gas gangrene), indicating its therapeutic potential in humans. They also confirmed that, unlike other antibacterial drugs, penicillin did not produce any toxicity in humans, since its mechanism of action was to interfere with metabolic processes that are found only in the cell walls of bacteria. For their research, Chain, Florey, and Fleming shared the 1945 Nobel Prize for Physiology or Medicine. All three were knighted, with Chain receiving this honor in 1969.

Chain was offered strong inducements to head a department at the new Weizmann Research Center in Rehovot, Israel. Although Chain decided that it would be better to remain in Europe to pursue his research activities in the development of new antibiotics, he agreed to join the Board of Governors and Executive Committee of the Weizmann Institute.

---

### Cohn, Ferdinand Julius (Germany, 1828–1898)

Born to a wealthy family in Breslau, in the Prussian province of Silesia, Ferdinand Cohn was such a precocious child that he felt socially isolated from his peers. This was exacerbated by a hearing impairment resulting from an accident at a young age. Although drawn to the study of medicine, he became fascinated by botany. However, because of his Jewish faith, Cohn was not permitted to sit for the final examinations for a doctorate in Breslau. Therefore, he was forced to move to the University of Berlin to receive his degree. While on a field trip outside the city, Cohn discovered a plant that was named after him, *Cohnia floribunda*.

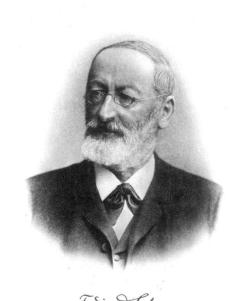

Portrait of Ferdinand Cohn. (*NLM / Bulletin of the Institute of History of Medicine, Johns Hopkins Press, Baltimore 1939, Volume VII*)

Although botany had traditionally focused on the visible morphology of plants, the faculty in Berlin was working with microscopy. In 1849, Cohn returned to the University of Breslau, where he served as a teacher and researcher for the rest of his career. His father bought him a large and expensive microscope, which Cohn used to study the growth and division of plant cells, writing papers on the sexuality of several species. In 1866, Cohn established the first institute for plant physiology. Soon afterwards, he shifted his focus and prolific writing to bacteria.

Cohn was the first to classify algae as plants and to define what distinguishes them from green plants. His classification of bacteria into four groups based on shape (sphericals, short rods, threads, and spirals) is still in use today. Cohn described the method by which bacteria reproduce, which was unlike that of animals. As he wrote, "The bacterium grows until it has reached perhaps double its original size, then constricts itself in the middle like a figure eight, and breaks into two new individuals."[32]

---

## Finland, Maxwell                                              (Ukraine, 1902–1987)

Born near Kiev, Maxwell Finland immigrated to the United States at age 4. He graduated from Harvard Medical School, specializing in infectious disease. For more than 50 years, Finland was associated with Harvard, working at Boston City Hospital and becoming Head of its Department of Medicine in 1963.

Finland worked with Chester Keefer on the first studies using penicillin to treat infectious diseases, demonstrating dramatic improvement in the mortality rate. His outspoken criticism of pharmaceutical companies for their marketing of fixed-dose antibiotics led to withdrawal of these drugs from the market. As an advisor to

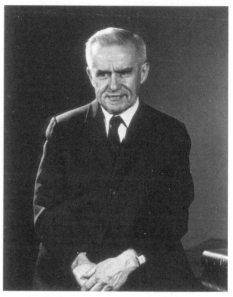

Maxwell Finland, 1976. (*NLM / Find a Grave*)

government agencies, Finland was a strong advocate of adequate testing of drugs. He was critical of medical practices leading to the indiscriminate use of antibiotics in both treatment and prevention of disease, which resulted in the growing resistance of some bacteria. Finland also identified the emergence of dangerous new infections in hospitalized patients.

---

## Gruby, David                                                  (Hungary, 1810–1898)

Considered the founder of medical microbiology, David Gruby was the son of a poor Jewish peasant and received his medical degree from the University of Vienna. Having difficulty finding a postgraduate academic position in Vienna because of his religion, Gruby turned to microscopy and moved to Paris to pursue a career in scientific research. Assisted by

---

32. Frank Heynick, *Jews in Medicine: An Epic Saga* (NJ: KTAV Publishing House, 2002), p. 261.

friends, he obtained a position in the Founding Hospital and began to give courses in microscopic anatomy and pathology.

From patients with a fungal infection of the scalp called favus, Gruby identified the causative organism and grew it on slices of potato (since agar media had not yet been developed). He showed that by inoculating the fungus on healthy tissue it was possible to produce the favus disease, the first demonstration that a microorganism was the cause of a human disease.

Soon afterward, Gruby discovered an animal parasite in the blood of the frog that he called *Trypanosoma* because the motion of the mobile organism reminded him of the action of a corkscrew.

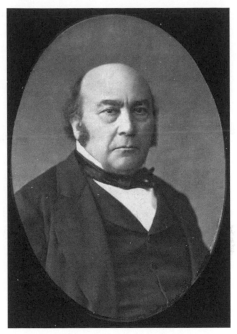

Portrait of David Gruby by Mathieu Deroche. (*Wikimedia / Israel National Library*)

This type of organism is responsible for causing African sleeping sickness. Gruby also described microfilia (the larval form of ringworm) in canine blood and the fungus *Candida albicans* (now a common form of infection in individuals who are immune suppressed). In the early days of general anesthesia administered by inhalation, Gruby performed valuable experiments on animals using ether and chloroform, which contributed to the knowledge of their effects on several bodily functions. Gruby was offered a professorship at the University of Vienna, but refused since this was conditioned on his first being baptized.

At the time of his death, Gruby was known primarily as a popular, though eccentric, medical practitioner in Paris, famous for the extravagant cures he prescribed for such distinguished patients as Frédéric Chopin, Alexandre Dumas père, Heinrich Heine, George Sand, and Franz Liszt. These prescriptions were actually clever applications of psychosomatic medicine. Only later did his original and important contributions to science become recognized – the founding of an important branch of modern medicine related to his discovery of the dermatomycoses, a group of skin diseases caused by parasitic fungi.

## Hannover, Adolph                                    (Denmark, 1814–1894)

Born in Copenhagen, Adolph Hannover studied medicine at the Borg-erdydskole. Known for his experimental studies in histology and micro-scopic technique, Hannover's detection of a plant parasite on the sala-mander was of vital importance to medicine because it proved for the first time the significance of vegetative contagious matter in the transmission of infectious diseases. Hannover's use of chromium acid as a hardening agent contributed to microscopic technique. *The Microscope* (1854) was his popular treatise on microscope building and use.

Hannover also engaged in research activities on a broad range of sub-jects, ranging from anatomy and physiology to pathologic anatomy and teratology, from diseases of the eye to medicines and medical statistics. A member of the Danish Academy of Sciences, Hannover received many awards and honorary memberships throughout Western Europe.

## Kuvin, Sanford                                         (USA, 1930–2015)

Sanford Kuvin received his medi-cal degree from Cambridge Uni-versity and a diploma from the London School of Tropical Med-icine. While at the National In-stitute of Allergy and Infectious Diseases, Kuvin was the first to demonstrate use of indirect fluo-rescent antibody tests for malaria. He was involved in malaria and infectious-tropical disease studies in countries in the Middle East, Central America, Africa, and Asia. Serving on the advisory board of the Americans for a Sound HIV/AIDS Policy in the early 1970's, Kuvin was an outspoken advocate to protect health care workers and patients alike against the threat of blood borne diseases including HIV/AIDS and hepatitis B. He

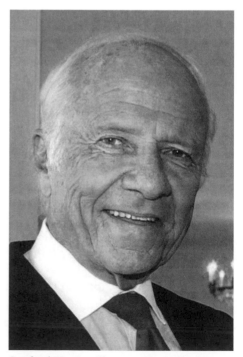

Sanford Kuvin. (*Jeanette Kuvin Oren*)

called for the universal reporting of HIV and routine HIV testing for all high-risk groups, including pregnant women.

Kuvin was the former Vice Chairman of the National Foundation for Infectious Diseases, and Founder and Chairman of the International Board of the renowned Sanford F. Kuvin Center for the Study of Infectious and Tropical Diseases at the Hebrew University of Jerusalem.

Retiring to Florida, Kuvin was a founding member of the Palm Beach Synagogue. An accomplished musician on flute and clarinet, Kuvin also helped found the Greater Palm Beach Symphony.

---

## Neisser, Albert Ludwig Sigesmund (Germany, 1855–1916)

Born in Silesia and the son of a physician, Albert Neisser was a schoolmate of Paul Ehrlich. Neisser studied medicine at the universities of Breslau and Erlangen. Initially planning to be an internist, Neisser was unable to find a suitable position and found work as an assistant to dermatologist Oskar Simon, focusing on sexually transmitted diseases and leprosy. In 1879, Neisser identified the causative agent of gonorrhea, a bacterium that was named *Neisseria gonorrhoeae* in his honor. Although an important scientific discovery, the identification of the gonorrhea pathogen was of little practical use until the discovery of penicillin.

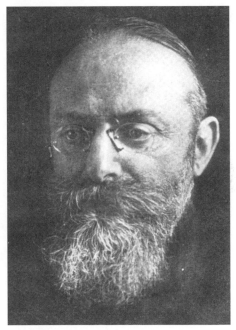

Albert Ludwig Sigesmund Neisser. (*NLM*)

Co-discoverer with Gerhard Armauer Hansen of the causative agent of leprosy, in 1882 Neisser was appointed Professor Extraordinarius at the University of Breslau and became Director of the Dermatology Department in the university hospital. Neisser published clinical trials on serum therapy in patients with syphilis, injecting cell free serum from patients with syphilis into those admitted for other medical conditions. Most of these patients were prostitutes, who were neither informed about the experiment nor asked for their consent. When some of them contracted syphilis Neisser argued that the women did not contract syphilis as a result of his serum injections, but rather from their occupations. To combat venereal disease, Neisser promoted preventive and educational measures to the public and the improved sanitary control of prostitutes. He was among the founders of the German Society for the Fight Against Venereal Diseases and the German Dermatological Society.

---

## Salmon, Daniel Elmer                                    (USA, 1850–1914)

Born in New Jersey and orphaned at age 8, Daniel Salmon attended Cornell University and earned the first Doctor of Veterinary Medicine degree awarded in the United States. As a veterinary surgeon, Salmon spent his career studying animal diseases for the U.S. Department of Agriculture. During his tenure as Chief of the Bureau of Animal Industry, Salmon made major contributions to veterinary medicine. Contagious pleural-pneumonia of cattle in the United States was eradicated and Texas fever was controlled after his associate, noted pathologist Theobald Smith, showed that ticks were responsible for the microbe causing it. Salmon inaugurated a number of significant public health pol-

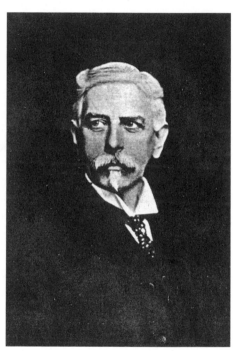

Daniel Elmer Salmon. (*Wikimedia / U.S. National Animal Parasite Collection Records*)

icies, including a nationwide system for meat inspection, a quarantine requirement for imported livestock, and the inspection of exported cattle and the ships in which they were transported. In 1906, Salmon established the Veterinary Department at the University of Montevideo in Uruguay, serving as its head for five years.

The *Salmonella* genus of bacteria was named in his honor. Although first isolated by Smith, Salmon documented the chain of transmission of *Salmonella cholera-suis*, which affects both pigs and humans. Salmon and Smith had a troubled relationship, because Salmon insisted on being the sole senior author of several research reports, even including the one on *Salmonella cholerae-suis*. Salmon made certain that he and other veterinarians undeservedly were credited with Smith's work on Texas cattle fever. Nevertheless, the pair collaborated in demonstrating that heat-killed organisms could immunize animals against living organisms, which was the foundation for the development of a vaccine against typhus and the polio vaccine of Jonas Salk. Salmon also showed that tuberculosis in cattle could be transmitted to humans, confirming the role of animal vectors in the spread of the disease.

---

**Salomonsen, Carl Julius**                                      (Denmark, 1849–1924)

---

Born in Copenhagen, Carl Salomonsen studied medicine at the university in his native city. After graduation, Salomonsen began his bacteriological investigations as an assistant at the Copenhagen Municipal Hospital. After studies with such luminaries in the field as Julius Friedrich Cohnheim, Robert Koch, and Louis Pasteur, Salomonsen succeeded in introducing bacteriology as a scientific discipline into Denmark. He was appointed Lecturer on Bacteriology at the University of Copenhagen, and later Professor of Pathology.

With the introduction of serotherapy and the discovery of diphtheria antitoxin, Salomonsen established a serotherapeutic laboratory in 1895, which served as the foundation of the well-known Danish State Serum Institute. He authored a large number of monographs on various branches of science, and published *Bacteriological Technology for Physicians* in 1890.

---

**Schneerson, Rachel**                                           (Poland, 1932–)

---

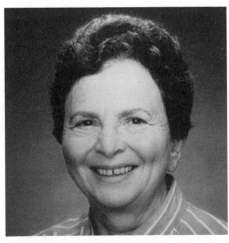

Born in Warsaw, Rachel Schneerson received her degree from Hadassah Medical School at the Hebrew University in Jerusalem. Specializing in pediatrics, Schneerson immigrated to the United States in 1969 and became a faculty member in the Department of Pediatrics and the Laboratory of

Rachel, Schneerson, circa 1996. (*NIH Photo Archives, Courtesy of Lasker Foundation*)

Immunology at Albert Einstein College of Medicine in New York. There she met John B. Robbins, and the two became an inseparable research team dedicated to developing vaccines to protect children from bacterial diseases. They later moved to the National Institute of Child Health and Human Development in 1970.

Schneerson is best known for her development with Robbins of the vaccine against bacterial meningitis caused by *Haemophilus influenzae* type b (Hib). Before the vaccine was developed, Hib infected 20,000 American children under age 5 each year, with 5% dying of the illness and one-third left with intellectual disability, deafness, or seizures. Indeed, bacterial meningitis was then the leading cause of acquired intellectual disability in the United States. After the vaccine became part of the standard immunization series for infants in 1987, Hib cases fell to fewer than 100 per year, and most pediatricians trained since 1995 have never seen a patient with this disease.

After the success of the Hib vaccine, Schneerson and Robbins continued their work, leading to the development and licensing of vaccines against pertussis (whooping cough), typhoid, Staphylococcus pneumonia, certain types of malaria, and anthrax. For all these efforts, Schneerson and Robbins shared the 1996 Lasker Award for Clinical Medical Research.

## Sterling, Seweryn                                    (Poland, 1864–1932)

Born in Tomaszów Mazowiecki, Seweryn Sterling studied medicine at the Imperial University of Warsaw. After graduation, Sterling worked as a factory physician. In 1894, Sterling moved to Lodz, where he established the first ward for chest disease patients in Poland and later the first tuberculosis outpatient clinic. In his scientific and clinical activity, Sterling preferred climatic and hygienic methods of therapy (exercise, sunlight, diet) and introduced new methods of pulse palpation and body temperature measurement for diagnosing tuberculosis.

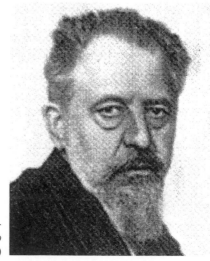

Seweryn Sterling. (*Wikimedia / Pamiętnik Wileńskiego Towarzystwa Lekarskiego 8 (4/5), 1932*)

Sterling developed a widely accepted classification of tuberculosis, based on anatomy and imaging and the dynamics of the disease process.

Sterling was one of the founders of the first anti-tuberculosis ward at the Jewish Hospital in Poland and initiated the Anti-Tuberculosis League. A prolific writer and author of two handbooks giving advice to patients with tuberculosis and characterizing the benefits of health resorts (sanitariums), Sterling was Professor and Head of the Department of Health School of the Free Polish University of Lodz.

## Waksman, Salman Abraham (Russia, 1888–1973)

Born in Podolia, now Ukraine, Salman Waksman immigrated to the United States in 1910 and began studies at Rutgers College (now University) in New Jersey. After receiving a doctorate in biochemistry from the University of California, Berkeley Waksman returned to Rutgers and remained on the faculty for more than 40 years.

As a biochemist and microbiologist, Waksman focused his research on soil organisms and their decomposition products. This led to his discovery of streptomycin (1943), neomycin (1948), and numerous other antibiotics (a word that he coined to describe compounds derived from other living organisms). The royalties earned from the licensing of his patents

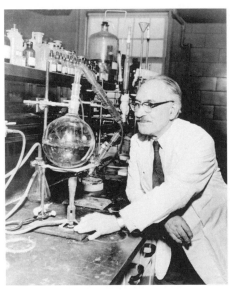

Photograph of Salman Abraham Waksman in his laboratory by Roger Higgins. (*Wikimedia / Library of Congress Prints and Photographs Division. New York World-Telegram and the Sun Newspaper*)

funded a foundation for microbiological research, which established the Waksman Institute of Microbiology on the Rutgers University campus in Piscataway. In 1952, Waksman was awarded the Nobel Prize in Physiology or Medicine for his discovery of streptomycin, the first antibiotic active against tuberculosis. In 1985, the American Chemical Society designated the research on antibiotics by Waksman as a National Historic Chemical Landmark.

A prolific author, among Waksman's multiple books are *Enzymes* (1926),

*Principles of Soil Microbiology* (1938), and an autobiography, *My Life with the Microbes* (1954).

---

### Wassermann, August Paul von                          (Germany, 1866–1925)

Born in Bamberg to a prominent Jewish banking family, August Wassermann received his medical degree from the University of Strasburg. Financially independent, in 1890 Wassermann began work under Robert Koch at the Institute for Infectious Diseases in Berlin, receiving no salary for a decade until he was appointed as Director of the Division for Experimental Therapy and Serum Research.

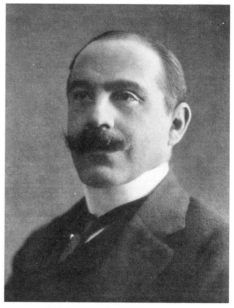

August Wasserman. (*Wikimedia*)

Wasserman is best known for his 1906 development of a complement fixation test for the diagnosis of syphilis, even in asymptomatic patients. Only one year previously, Fritz Schaudinn and Erich Hoffmann had identified the causative organism of this sexually transmitted disease (the spirochaete, *Treponema pallidum*). The "Wassermann test" is an antigen-antibody reaction in which a patient's blood sample is combined with an antigen – an alcoholic muscle extract, usually from the heart of a bull, which contains a lipid called cardiolipin that has nothing to do with syphilis. However, this antigen reacts with certain antibodies that commonly occur in the blood of patients with syphilis to prevent a component called *complement* from subsequently destroying red blood cells. Destruction of red blood cells results in clearing of the test solution, which is diagnostic for the absence of antibodies to *Treponema pallidum*. The results are categorized from 1–4, with the intensity of the reaction usually corresponding to the severity of the infection. The antibodies are not specific for syphilis and may occasionally occur in malaria and other diseases, but the Wassermann test can diagnose syphilis in about 95% of cases – allowing for its early detection and prevention of transmission. Over succeeding years, many modifications have been made to the Wassermann test, which today has been replaced by other methods to test for syphilis.

In 1913, Wassermann was elevated to the nobility by the German government, despite his Jewish origins, and named the head of the new Kaiser Wilhelm Institute of Experimental Studies in Dalheim, a position he held until his death.

## BIOCHEMISTRY, CELL BIOLOGY

Jewish researchers have greatly expanded the horizons in biochemistry and cell biology. Bloch, Brown, and Goldstein discovered how the body metabolizes and regulates cholesterol and fatty acids. Krebs described the citric acid cycle, a series of chemical reactions that produces energy in all living cells that utilize oxygen as part of cellular respiration, and the urea cycle in animal organisms that produce urea from ammonia. Fischer demonstrated the process whereby enzymes and receptors are switched "on" or "off." Levi-Montalcini discovered the existence of nerve growth factor, Cohen first noted epidermal growth factor, and Furchgott discovered endothelium-derived relaxing factor. Cori and Meyerhoff demonstrated the mechanism by which glycogen, a derivative of glucose, is broken down in muscle tissue into lactic acid and then resynthesized in the body and stored as a source of energy. At the cellular level, Benda discovered and coined the term "mitochondria" (containing the basic units of cellular activity), and Yonath unraveled the structure of the ribosome, which is responsible for synthesizing proteins according to instructions provided by the genetic code. De Hevesy co-discovered the chemical element hafnium, and he and Schoenheimer used radioactive isotopes to study the metabolic processes of plants and animals. Funk isolated the missing substance in beriberi, terming it a "vitamine," and correctly predicted that similar vitamin deficiencies were responsible for scurvy, pellagra, and rickets. Puck developed original methods for pure culture of living mammalian cells and successfully cloned a HeLa cell. Lipmann determined the active molecular structure of coenzyme A; and Puck showed that low levels of radiation can cause mutations in human cells.

## Baeyer, Adolf von                                    (Germany, 1835–1917)

Born in Berlin, the son of a Prussian general and a Jewess who
converted to Christianity in order to marry him, Adolf Baeyer
received a doctorate in chemistry
from the University of Berlin. In
1871, Baeyer became a professor in
Strasbourg; four years later, he was
appointed the Chemistry Professor
at the University of Munich.

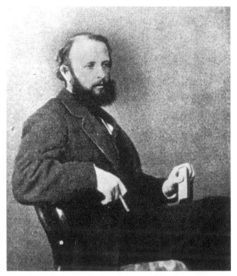

Baeyer derived barbituric acid,
the parent compound from which
the sedative drugs known as barbi-
turates were developed. His most
important work was defining the
chemical formula for indigo, the
deep blue dye produced from a

Adolf von Baeyer, 1872. (*NLM / Jerusalem Academy of Medicine*)

tropical shrub using a time-consuming and expensive extraction process.
Baeyer's success in developing synthetic indigo, which eventually displaced
the natural product, was the foundation of the German dyestuffs industry.

In 1885, on his 50th birthday, King Ludwig of Bavaria raised Baeyer to
the hereditary nobility, conferring on him the "von" distinction. Baeyer
was awarded the 1905 Nobel Prize in Chemistry "in recognition of his
services in the advancement of organic chemistry and the chemical industry, through his work on organic dyes and hydroaromatic compounds."

## Benda, Carl                                          (Germany, 1857–1932)

Born in Berlin, Carl Benda studied medicine in Berlin, Heidelberg, and Vienna
before receiving his degree from the University of Paris. Benda became Chief of
Pathology at the Urban Hospital, a city

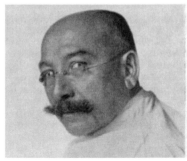

Carl Benda. (*Wikimedia / Jaffé R. Carl Benda†
Mit einem Bildnis. Anatomischer Anzeiger 76, Nr.
14/16, August 1933*)

facility in Berlin, and from 1908 until his retirement in 1925 was a staff member of the Institute of Pathology at the Moabit Hospital.

One of the first microbiologists to use a microscope to study the internal structure of cells, Benda became aware of the existence of hundreds of tiny bodies in the cytoplasm of nucleated cells, postulating that these structures were the basic units of cellular activity. Because of their tendency to form long chains, Benda coined the name *mitochondria* ("thread granules").

---

## Bloch, Konrad (Germany, 1912–2000)

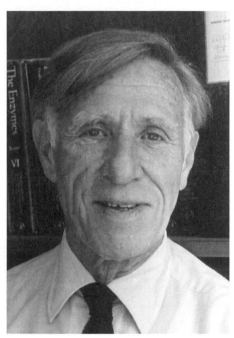

Born in Neisse in the Prussian Province of Silesia, Konrad Bloch obtained an undergraduate degree in chemistry at the Technical University of Munich. In 1934, Bloch fled to Switzerland to escape Nazi persecution of Jews and immigrated to the United States two years later. Bloch enrolled at Columbia University and received a doctoral degree in biochemistry, remaining on the faculty until 1946. Bloch then moved to the University of Chicago and finally to Harvard, where he was Professor of Biochemistry for almost 30 years until his retirement in 1982.

Bloch shared (with Feodor Lynen) the 1964 Nobel Prize in Physiology or Medicine for their discoveries of the mechanism and

Konrad Bloch. (*American Society for Biochemistry and Molecular Biology*)

regulation of the metabolism of cholesterol and fatty acids. By tracing all the carbon atoms in the process, they showed that the body first makes squalene from acetate in many steps before converting the squalene to cholesterol. Bloch also discovered that bile and a female sex hormone were made from cholesterol, which led to the understanding that cholesterol was the source of all steroids.

## Brown, Michael Stuart                    (USA, 1941–)

Born in Brooklyn, Michael Brown studied medicine at the University of Pennsylvania. After several years at the National Institutes of Health, Brown joined the Gastroenterology Unit at the University of Texas Southwestern in Dallas, where he ascended the academic ladder to become Professor of Medicine and Genetics and Director of the Center for Genetic Disease. There he developed a fruitful collaboration with Joseph Leonard Goldstein, a fellow researcher who had also worked at the NIH. They discovered that human cells have low-density lipoprotein (LDL) receptors that remove cholesterol from the blood. When these LDL receptors are not present in sufficient numbers, affected individuals develop excessive amounts of cholesterol in the blood and become at risk for such cholesterol-related diseases as heart attacks and stroke. Their studies, which led to the development of statin drugs, earned Brown and Goldstein the 1985 Nobel Prize in Physiology or Medicine for "discoveries concerning the regulation of cholesterol metabolism." In the same year, Brown and Goldstein shared the Lasker Award in Basic Medical Research for "receptors that control cholesterol."

## Ciechanover, Aaron                    (Israel, 1947–)

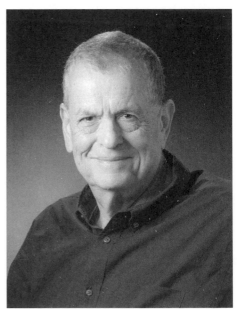

Born in Haifa, a year before the establishment of the State of Israel, to parents who had emigrated from Poland before World War II, Aaron Ciechanover received his medical degree from Hadassah Medical School at the Hebrew University in Jerusalem and his doctorate in biochemistry from the Technion–Israel Institute of Technology in Haifa.

Ciechanover shared (with colleague Avraham Hershko and Irwin Rose) the 2004 Nobel Prize in

Aaron Ciechanover. (*Courtesy of Dr. Ciechanover*)

Chemistry "for the discovery of ubiquitin-mediated protein degradation." The ubiquitin-proteasome pathway plays a critical role in maintaining the cell homeostasis and is believed to be involved in the development and progression of such conditions as cancer, muscular and neurological diseases, and immune and inflammatory responses. Ciechanover had shared (with Hershko and Alexander Varshavsky) the 2000 Lasker Award in Basic Medical Research for the "ubiquitin system for regulated protein degradation."

## Cohen, Stanley (USA, 1922–)

Born in Brooklyn, Stanley Cohen earned a doctorate in biochemistry at the University of Michigan. Cohen worked at Washington University in St. Louis in the 1950s with Rita Levi-Montalcini in isolating nerve growth factor (NGF). In 1959, Cohen moved to Vanderbilt University in Nashville, where he discovered epidermal growth factor (EGF). ·

Cohen shared with Levi-Montalcini the 1986 Nobel Prize in Physiology or Medicine for the discovery and isolation of nerve growth factor and epidermal growth factor. This led to improved understanding of many disease states, such as developmental malformations, degenerative changes in senile dementia and Alzheimer's disease, and delayed wound healing, paving the way for new therapeutic agents and treatments. Today, the EGF receptor is the target for a growing number of drugs against lung, breast, head and neck, and gastrointestinal malignancies, and the discovery of mutations in this receptor has revolutionized the care and outlook for many thousands of lung cancer patients worldwide. In the same year, Cohen and Levi-Montalcini also shared the Lasker Award in Basic Medical Research for "growth factors – NGF and EGF."

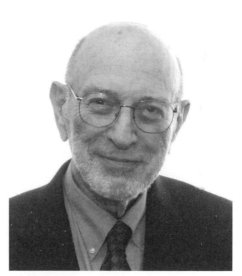

Stanley Cohen. (*NIH*)

## Cori, Gerty Theresa                    (Czechoslovakia, 1896–1957)

Born Gerty Radnitz in Prague, then a part of the Austro-Hungarian Empire, she studied medicine at the Karl-Ferdinands-Universität in her native city. There she met and married a non-Jewish fellow student, Carl Ferdinand Cori, and converted to Catholicism. After graduation, the Coris both accepted positions at the University of Vienna and decided to pursue careers in medical research, rather than practice. In 1922, they immigrated to the United States and joined the medical research faculty at the State Institute for the Study of Malignant Diseases (now the Roswell Park Memorial Institute) in Buffalo, New York. Reject-

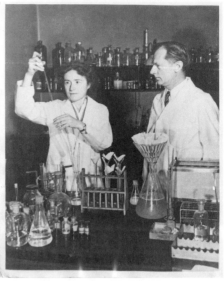

Gerty Theresa Cori (left) with her husband Carl Ferdinand Cori, 1947. (*Wikimedia / Smithsonian Institution Archives*)

ing advice that they work separately, they joined in investigating carbohydrate metabolism, especially how energy is produced and transmitted in the human body. The Coris published numerous papers, alternating first authorship depending on who had done the most research for that specific article.

In a 1929 publication, Gerty and Carl Cori proposed a theoretical cycle of the chemical reactions involved in carbohydrate metabolism, a process that is now known as the Cori cycle. This led to the Coris being awarded half of the 1947 Nobel Prize in Physiology or Medicine for their description of the mechanism by which glycogen, a derivative of glucose, is broken down in muscle tissue into lactic acid and then resynthesized in the body and stored as a source of energy. Gerty Cori became the third woman (after Marie Curie and Irène Joliot-Curie) and the first American woman awarded a Nobel Prize in science, and the first woman winner in the category of Physiology or Medicine. The Coris shared the award with Argentine physiologist Bernardo Houssay for his discovery of the part played by the hormone of the anterior pituitary lobe in the metabolism of sugar.

In 1931, Gerty and Carl Cori relocated to Washington University in St. Louis. They discovered and determined the structure of an intermediate compound (glucose 1-phosphate, now known as the Cori ester) that is the first step in the conversion of glycogen into glucose. While studying four glycogen storage diseases, Gerty Cori showed that each was due to a specific enzyme defect, thus being the first to prove that an enzymatic defect can be the cause of a human genetic disease.

## De Hevesy, George Charles (Hungary, 1885–1966)

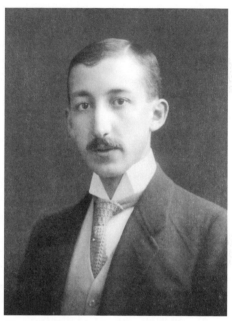

Born in Budapest, George de Hevesy received his doctorate in chemistry from the University of Freiburg. In 1919, he left for Copenhagen to discuss his future activities at the Niels Bohr Institute and settled in the capital of Denmark. Four years later, De Hevesy was a co-discoverer (with Dirk Coster) of the chemical element hafnium, named after Hafnia, the Latin name for Copenhagen.

De Hevesy concentrated his research on the use of radioactive isotopes to study the metabolic processes of plants and animals. This entailed tracing biologically important chemicals in the body by replacing part of stable isotopes (primarily phosphorus, so-

George Charles de Hevesy, circa 1913. (*Wikimedia*)

dium, and carbon) with small quantities of the radioactive isotopes of these same elements.

Working in Copenhagen at the Niels Bohr Institute when the Nazis occupied Denmark, De Hevesy was tasked with hiding the gold Nobel Prizes of Max von Laue and James Franck to prevent them from being used to support the German war effort. Rather than illegally sending the gold out of the country or hiding it, De Hevesy dissolved the medals in a mixture of nitric and hydrochloric acid (known as aqua regia) and placed the resulting solution on a shelf in his laboratory. After the war, De Hevesy returned to find the solution undisturbed and precipitated the gold out of the acid. The Nobel Society then recast the Nobel Prizes using the original gold.

With it no longer safe for a Jewish scientist to remain in Copenhagen, in 1943 De Hevesy followed Bohr by escaping on a fishing boat to Sweden, where he worked for almost 20 years at Stockholm University College. During this time, de Hevesy was awarded the 1943 Nobel Prize for Chemistry "for his work on the use of isotopes as tracers in the study of chemical processes."

---

## Eagle, Harry                                              (USA, 1905–1992)

Born in New York City, Harry Eagle received his medical degree from Johns Hopkins University. For more than a decade, Eagle was Director of the United States Public Health Service Venereal Disease Research Laboratory and Laboratory of Experimental Therapeutics at the Johns Hopkins School of Hygiene and Public Health. He then served as head of several sections at the National Institutes of Health before joining the faculty at the Albert Einstein College of Medicine in 1961 as the founding Professor and Chairman of the Department of Cell Biology.

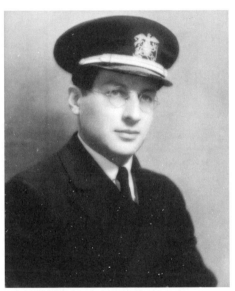

Harry Eagle, 1937. (*NLM*)

Eagle is best known for formulating the essential compounds needed to sustain the reproduction of human and other mammalian cells in a laboratory. Known as Eagle's minimum essential medium, this mixture was vital for subsequent research in viruses, genetic defects, and cancer. Other major contributions included his discovering that blood clotting is an enzymatic process; developing a treatment for arsenic poisoning; discovering the efficacy of penicillin to treat syphilis, and describing the metabolic differences between normal and malignant cells. Eagle also participated in a four-member team that employed freeze-drying for long-term storage of life-saving serums, which previously were perishable.

## Fischer, Edmond Henri (China, 1920–)

Born in the Shanghai International Settlement to a French mother and a Jewish Austrian father, Edmond Fischer was sent to a Swiss boarding school at age 7 and earned a doctorate in organic chemistry from the University of Geneva. Fischer moved to the University of Washington in Seattle for post-doctoral studies, remaining on the faculties of biochemistry and cell physiology throughout his academic career.

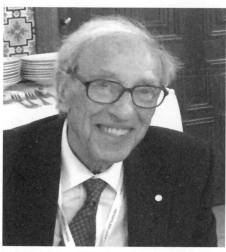

Edmond Henri Fischer, 2016. (*Wikimedia*)

Soon after arriving in Seattle, Fischer began a fruitful collaboration with Edwin G. Krebs, which led to them sharing the 1992 Nobel Prize in Physiology or Medicine "for their discoveries concerning reversible protein phosphorylation as a biological regulatory mechanism." This term refers to the process in which many enzymes and receptors are switched "on" or "off" by phosphorylation and dephosphorylation, respectively. This is accomplished by a conformational change in the structure of these enzymes and receptors, which causes them to become activated or deactivated.

## Fraenkel-Conrat, Heinz Ludwig (Germany, 1910–1999)

Born in Breslau, Heinz Fraenkel-Conrat received a degree in medicine from the University of Breslau in 1933. To escape the rise of Nazism, Franekel-Conrad left for Scotland to complete his doctorate in biochemistry at the University of Edinburg before immigrating to the United States. In 1952, Fraenkel-Conrat joined the research faculty at the University of California, Berkeley, where he remained for almost 30 years.

Fraenkel-Conrat helped to reveal the complementary roles of the structural components of viruses (a "core" of ribonucleic acid [RNA] enveloped by a protein "coat"). Working with tobacco mosaic virus, Fraenkel-Conrat discovered that the infectivity of the virus resided in its nucleic acid portion, which in the absence of the viral protein is broken down by RNA-splitting enzymes (nucleases). With biophysicist Robley Williams, Fraenkel-Conrat demonstrated that a functional virus could be created out of purified RNA and a protein coat, and he later accomplished the complete sequencing of the 158 amino acids in the virus. For his research, Fraenkel-Conrat received the 1958 Lasker Award in Basic Medical Research.

## Funk, Casimir                                          (Poland, 1884–1967)

Born in Warsaw, Casimir Funk studied at the University of Geneva before receiving a doctoral degree in biochemistry from the University of Bern. In 1910, Funk went to the Lister Institute in London to study beriberi, a disease of the peripheral nerves that causes pain and paralysis. Although the precise cause of beriberi was unclear, it was known that the disease occurred in areas of Asia where the population consumed polished rice. Those who ate brown rice were less affected. Determined to isolate the substance responsible, Funk succeeded in finding this material in the dark outer coating of rice, which is removed during polishing (also in yeast and milk). He called the substances "vitamines," with "vita" meaning vitality and "amines" meaning a chemical compound containing nitrogen. (The "e" was dropped in the 1920s, when it was found that vitamins were not necessarily nitrogen-containing amines.) Funk was convinced that there must at least four vitamins – with the others preventing the deficiency diseases of scurvy, pellagra, and rickets. In his 1914 book, *Vitamine* (*The Vitamins*, 1922), Funk hypothesized that these and other vitamins were essential to normal growth and development. This stimulated the work of other investigators in the field and laid the foundation for rational child nutrition and modern dietetics.

## Furchgott, Robert Francis                              (USA, 1916–2009)

Born in Charleston, South Carolina, Robert Furchgott earned a doctorate in biochemistry at Northwestern University. His academic posts included Cornell University Medical College, Washington University School of Medicine in St. Louis, and the State University of New York Downstate Medical Center, where he served as Professor of Pharmacology for more than 50 years (1956– 2009).

In 1978, Furchgott discovered a substance in the endothelium (the innermost layer of blood vessels) that causes the underlying smooth muscle to relax. Terming it endothelium-derived relaxing factor (EDRF), this was the first evidence of the crucial role that the endothelium plays in cardiovascular health and disease. Several years later, Furchgott discovered that EDRF was actually nitric oxide (NO), long known primarily as an air pollutant, which was the first indication that a gas produced by one cell could act as a signal molecule by penetrating through the membrane of another cell and regulating its functions. The release of EDRF was shown by others to interfere with the aggregation of platelets and their adhesion to blood vessel walls, thereby preventing the formation of small blood clots. When combined with the vasodilating effect of EDRF, this keeps blood vessels open and facilitates blood flow.

Furchgott shared (with Louis J. Ignarro and Farid Murad) the 1998 Nobel Prize for Physiology or Medicine "for their discoveries concerning nitric oxide as a signaling molecule in the cardiovascular system." Later research has shown that nitric oxide, or EDRF, mediates the control of blood pressure and blood flow, airway tone, gastrointestinal motility, penile erection, and the fighting of cancer and infection. In the brain, nitric oxide is an important and unusual neurotransmitter that may provide clues to an improved understanding of learning, memory, and emotion. Furchgott had shared (with Murad) the 1996 Lasker Award in Basic Medical Research for "nitrous oxide as a signaling molecule."

---

**Gilman, Alfred Goodman** (USA, 1941–2015)

---

Born in New Haven, CT, he was the son of Alfred Gilman, one of the authors of the classic textbook *The Pharmacological Basis of Therapeutics*, who gave his son a middle name honoring his co-author, Louis S. Goodman. The younger Alfred Gilman was one of the editors of the textbook from 1980–2000, initially collaborating with Goodman and his father and later succeeding them. He graduated from the MD-PhD program at Case Western Reserve University in Cleveland and then spent two years in postgraduate studies at the National Institutes of Health with Nobel laureate Marshall Nirenberg. In 1971, Gilman became a professor at the University of Virginia, and a decade later he was appointed Chairman of the Department of Pharmacology at the University of Texas Southwestern Medical Center in Dallas.

Gilman shared (with Martin Rodbell) the 1994 Nobel Prize in Physiology or Medicine for their discoveries regarding G-proteins. These represent a key intermediary between the activation of receptors on the cell membrane and actions within the cell. Rodbell initially demonstrated that GTP (guanosine triphosphate) was involved in cell signaling, while Gilman actually discovered the proteins that interacted with GTP to transmit and modulate signals within cells. Abnormal function of G-proteins can result in disease. For example, the direct action of cholera toxins on G-proteins causes a dramatic loss of salt and water, while altered transmission of signals through G-proteins has been implicated as producing symptoms in such common diseases as diabetes and alcoholism.

## Goldstein, Joseph Leonard                                (USA, 1940–)

Born in Kingstree, South Carolina, Joseph Goldstein received his medical degree from the University of Texas Southwestern Medical School in Dallas, After several years working in biochemical genetics at the National Institutes of Health, Goldstein returned to Southwestern Medical Center to become Head of the Division of Medical Genetics. There he developed a fruitful collaboration with Michael Stuart Brown, a fellow researcher who had also worked at the NIH. They discovered that human cells have low-density lipoprotein (LDL) receptors that remove cholesterol from the blood. When these LDL receptors are not present in sufficient numbers, affected individuals develop excessive amounts of cholesterol in the blood and become at risk for such cholesterol-related diseases as heart attacks and stroke. Their studies, which led to the development of statin drugs, earned Goldstein and Brown the 1985 Nobel Prize in Physiology or Medicine for "discoveries concerning the regulation of cholesterol metabolism." In the same year, Goldstein and Brown shared the Lasker Basic Medical Research Award for "receptors that control cholesterol."

## Hershko, Avram                                          (Hungary, 1937–)

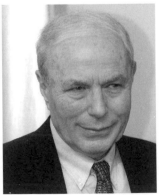

Born Herskó Ferenc in Karcag, Avram Hershko immigrated to Israel as a teenager. He received both a medical degree and a doctorate in chemistry from the Hadassah Medical School at the Hebrew University in Jerusalem. He is currently a Distinguished Professor at the Rappaport Faculty of Medicine at the Technion Institute of Technology in Haifa.

Photograph of Avram Hershko by Amos ben Gershom, 1994. (*Wikimedia / Government Press Office of Israel*)

Avram Hershko shared (with colleague Aaron Ciechanover and Irwin Rose) the 2004 Nobel Prize in Chemistry "for the discovery of ubiquitin-mediated protein degradation." The ubiquitin-proteasome pathway has a critical role in maintaining the homeostasis of cells and is believed to be involved in the development and progression of such diseases as cancer, muscular and neurological diseases, and immune and inflammatory responses. Hershko had shared (with Ciechanover and Alexander Varshavsky) the 2000 Lasker Award in Basic Medical Research for the "ubiquitin system for regulated protein degradation."

## Krebs, Hans Adolf

(Germany, 1900–1981)

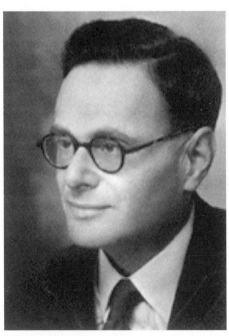

Born in Hildesheim, the son of an ear, nose, and throat surgeon, Hans Krebs studied medicine at the universities of Göttingen, Freiburg, and Berlin before receiving his medical degree from the University of Hamburg. In Berlin, Krebs became an assistant of Nobel Prize-winner Otto Warburg at the Kaiser Wilhelm Institute for Biology until 1930. Because of his Jewish heritage, Krebs was barred from practicing medicine in Germany. Consequently, he immigrated to England, where he eventually was appointed a Lecturer in Pharmacology and then Professor of Biochemistry at the University of Sheffield.

The pioneer in the study of cellular respiration, a biochemical

Hans Adolf Krebs. (*American Society for Biochemistry and Molecular Biology*)

pathway in cells for the production of energy, Krebs is best known for his discovery of two important metabolic reactions in the body. The urea cycle describes reactions in animal organisms that produce urea from ammonia. The citric acid cycle, often known as the Krebs cycle, is a series of chemical reactions that produces energy in all living cells that utilize oxygen as part of cellular respiration. For this latter discovery, Krebs shared (with Fritz Lipmann) the 1953 Nobel Prize in Physiology or Medicine. In collaboration with Hans Kornberg, Krebs also discovered the glyoxylate cycle, a slight variation of the citric acid cycle that is found in plants, bacteria, and fungi. In the same year, Krebs received the Lasker Award in Basic Medical Research for the "Krebs Cycle for converting food into energy."

## Lipmann, Fritz Albert                                    (Germany, 1899–1986)

Born in Königsberg, Fritz Lipmann studied medicine in his native city and in Munich before graduating from the University of Berlin. Lipmann joined Nobel Prize-winner Otto Meyerhof at the Kaiser Wilhelm Institute in Berlin for his doctoral thesis and then took academic positions in Heidelberg, New York, and Copenhagen. In 1939, Lipmann escaped the Nazi regime and immigrated to the United States, working first as a research associate in biochemistry at Cornell Medical School in New York and then as Head of Biochemistry Research at the Massachusetts General Hospital in Boston. Lipmann taught or conducted research at the Rockefeller Institute from 1957 until his death.

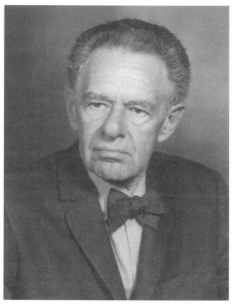

Portrait of Fritz Albert Lipmann. (*Wikimedia / Smithsonian Institution Libraries*)

Lipmann is best known for isolating (1947) and then determining the active molecular structure (1953) of coenzyme A, one of the most important substances in cellular metabolism. It helps in the conversion of amino acids, steroids, fatty acids, and hemoglobin into energy for bodily functions. For this discovery, Lipmann shared (with Hans Krebs) the 1953 Nobel Prize for Physiology or Medicine.

## Meyer, Karl                                              (Germany, 1899–1990)

After studying medicine at the University of Cologne and earning a doctorate in biochemistry from the University of Berlin, Karl Meyer specialized in connective tissue disease. He moved to the United States in 1930 to join the research staff at the University of California, Berkeley. Leaving

California for New York, Meyer taught and led research groups at Columbia University for 34 years and then was a Professor of Biochemistry for a decade at Yeshiva University. One of the first scientists to recognize the significance of bacterial enzymes as a tool in analyzing the structure of animal tissue components, Meyer received the 1956 Lasker Award in Basic Medical Research.

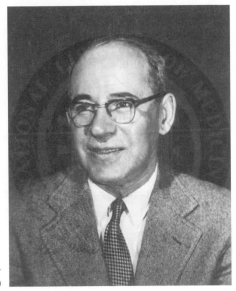

Karl Meyer. (*American Society for Biochemistry and Molecular Biology*)

## Meyerhof, Otto Fritz

(Germany, 1884–1951)

Born in Hannover, the son of a wealthy Jewish merchant, Otto Meyerhof spent most of his childhood in Berlin, where he started his study of medicine before continuing it in Strasbourg and Heidelberg. Moving to the University of Kiel, Meyerhof was passed over for the position of Chair of the Physiology, largely because of anti-Semitism.

Focusing on the chemical processes taking place within the living cell, Meyerhof made the first attempt to explain cell function in terms of physics and chemistry. His research into the chemical processes of muscle cells paved the way for full understanding of the breakdown of glucose to pro-

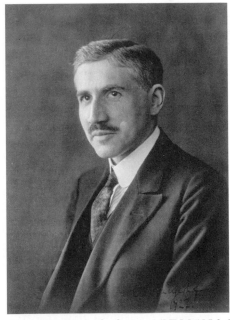

Otto Fritz Meyerhof, 1922. (*NLM / Nobel Foundation*)

vide body energy. He discovered the fixed relationship between the depletion of glycogen and the metabolism of lactic acid in muscle. Meyerhof demonstrated that when the muscle relaxes after work, molecular oxygen is consumed in oxidizing part of the lactic acid, but only about one-fifth of it. He concluded that the energy created by the oxidative process is used to convert the remaining lactic acid back to glycogen so that the cycle can begin again in the muscle cell. Thus, Meyerhof and his associates were able to reconstruct *in vitro* the main steps of the complicated chain of reactions leading from glycogen to lactic acid.

For his work on muscle metabolism, including glycolysis, Meyerhof shared (with Archibald Vivian Hill) the 1922 Nobel Prize in Physiology or Medicine. Seven years later, Meyerhof became one of the directors of the Kaiser Wilhelm Institute for Medical Research. However, he was forced to flee the Nazi regime in 1938, first to Paris and then to the United States.

---

## Puck, Theodore                                          (USA, 1916–2005)

Born in Chicago, Theodore Puck received his doctorate in physical chemistry from the University of Chicago. For six decades, Puck taught at the University of Colorado, serving as Chairman of the Department of Biophysics from 1948 to 1967. Puck also was the founding director of the Eleanor Roosevelt Institute, which studies cancer, diabetes, and other diseases.

Puck developed an efficient method for growing colonies of human cells, using a special incubator that he developed. With a ready source of cells, Puck performed groundbreaking experiments, exposing the cell colonies to different levels of radiation. In 1957, Puck suggested that earlier studies of radiation safety, based on research involving fruit flies and other subjects, had underestimated the dangers to humans, showing that low levels of radiation can cause mutations in human cells.

Puck and co-workers performed studies demonstrating that there were 46 (rather than 48) chromosomes in each human somatic cell, and he helped organize an international conference in 1960 that established this fact. Five years earlier, Puck and Phillip Marcus successfully cloned a HeLa cell, the oldest and most commonly used human cell line in scientific research.

In 1958, Puck received the Lasker Award for Basic Medical Research "for development of original methods for pure culture of living mammalian cells as a basis for new research in their nutrition, growth, genetics and mutation." As the Lasker Foundation noted, this permitted cells to be grown in "pure" colonies from nearly any organ, including normal and cancerous, adult and newborn tissue. Since each cell in the colony is an "identical twin" of the single parent cell, consistent and quantitative studies on individual mammalian cells could be made for the first time to demonstrate heritable differences that remain stable through innumerable successive generations. Moreover, this represented a new research tool for cellular research on the effects of carcinogens and other chemical agents, on the effects of foods and vitamins, the processes of growth and aging, and on the effects of the physical environment.

## Rodbell, Martin (1925–1998)

Born in Baltimore, Martin Rodbell received a doctorate in biochemistry from the University of Washington. After postgraduate work at the University of Illinois at Urbana-Champaign, Rodbell became a research biochemist at the National Heart Institute in Bethesda. In 1985, Rodbell became Scientific Director of the NIH's National Institute of Environmental Health Sciences in Research Triangle Park, North Carolina, where he remained for the rest of his career.

Rodbell shared (with Alfred G. Gilman) the 1994 Nobel Prize in Physiology or Medicine for their discoveries regarding G-proteins. These represent a key intermediary between the activation of receptors on the cell membrane and actions within the cell. Rodbell initially demonstrated that GTP (guanosine triphosphate) was involved in cell signaling, while Gilman actually discovered the proteins that interacted with GTP to transmit and modulate signals within cells. Abnormal function of G-proteins can result in disease. For example, the direct action of cholera toxins on G-proteins causes a dramatic loss of salt and water, while altered transmission of signals through G-proteins has been implicated as producing symptoms in such common disease as diabetes and alcoholism.

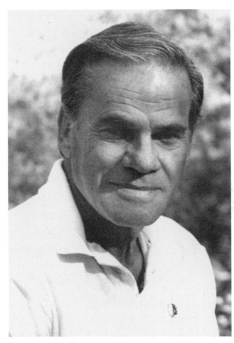

Martin Rodbell. (*Wikimedia / NIH*)

## Rose, Irwin Allan                                          (USA, 1926–2015)

Born in Brooklyn, Irwin Rose received his doctorate in biochemistry from the University of Chicago. After a decade on the biochemistry faculty at the Yale School of Medicine, Rose joined the Fox Chase Cancer Center in Philadelphia in 1963, remaining there until retiring in 1995. In the late 1970s, Rose collaborated with Avram Hershko of the Technion Institute of Technology in Israel and Aaron Ciechanover, a graduate student of Hershko, working together for a year at Fox Chase.

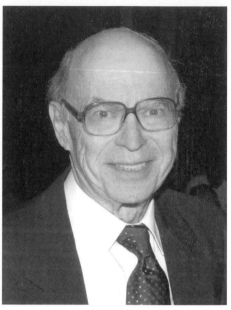

Irwin Rose shared (with Ciechanover and Hershko) the 2004 Nobel Prize in Chemistry "for the discovery of ubiquitin-mediated

Irwin Allan Rose. (*Fox Chase Cancer Center Archives*)

protein degradation." The ubiquitin-proteasome pathway has a critical role in maintaining the homeostasis of cells and is believed to be involved in the development and progression of such diseases as cancer, muscular and neurological diseases, and immune and inflammatory responses.

## Rothman, James Edward                                      (USA, 1950–)

Born in Haverhill, Massachusetts, James Rothman received his doctorate in biological chemistry from Harvard University. In addition to serving as Professor of Molecular Biology at Princeton University, in 1991 Rothman founded and headed the Department of Cellular Biochemistry and Biophysics at the Memorial Sloan-Kettering Cancer Center in New York. Since 2013, Rothman has been Director of the Nanobiology Institute and Chair of the Department of Cell Biology at Yale University.

Rothman shared (with Randy Schekman and Thomas Südhof) the 2013 Nobel Prize in Physiology or Medicine "for their discoveries of machinery regulating vesicle traffic, a major transport system in our cells." These vesicles are tiny sac-like structures that transport hormones, growth factors, and other molecules within cells. Rothman's research has concentrated on how these vesicles reach their correct destination, and where and when they release their contents. This cellular trafficking is essential for important physiological functions, including cellular division, communication between nerve cells in the brain, secretion of insulin and other hormones, and nutrient uptake. Abnormalities in this system can result in a broad spectrum of disorders, such as diabetes and infectious diseases. Rothman shared (with Schekman) the 2002 Lasker Award for Basic Medical Research for "membrane fusion and organelle formation."

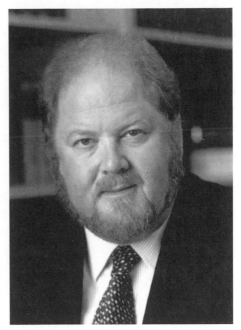

James Edward Rothman. (*Gairdner Foundation*)

## Schekman, Randy Wayne (USA, 1948–)

Born in St. Paul, Minnesota, Randy Schekman received a doctorate in molecular sciences from Stanford University for research on DNA replication. Schekman remained at Stanford for much of his career. A former Editor-in-Chief of the *Proceedings of the National Academy of Sciences*, in 2012 Rothman became the founding editor of *eLife*, a new high-profile, open-access journal. Schekman is currently a member of the Department of Molecular and Cell Biology at the University of California, Berkeley.

Schekman shared (with James Rothman and Thomas Südhof) the 2013 Nobel Prize for Physi-

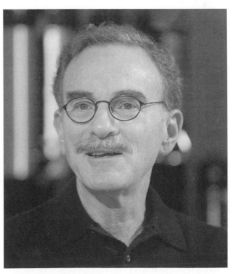

Photograph of Randy Wayne Schekman by James Kegley, 2012. (*Wikimedia / eLife Sciences Publications, Ltd.*)

ology or Medicine for their discoveries of machinery regulating vesicle traffic across and within cell membranes, a major transport process that affects how cells communicate with their environment. The vesicles contain proteins that are essential to neurotransmission, hormone secretion, cholesterol homeostasis, and metabolic regulation. Schekman shared (with Rothman) the 2002 Lasker Award for Basic Medical Research for "membrane fusion and organelle formation."

Schekman has championed publishing reform among academic journals and the development of open-access science publication, announcing that his laboratory would no longer submit to the prestigious closed-access journals *Nature*, *Cell*, and *Science*. He criticized these journals for artificially restricting the number of publications accepted to drive up demand, as well as preferentially accepting papers that will be cited often rather than those demonstrating important results.

## Schoenheimer, Rudolf                              (Germany, 1898–1941)

Born in Berlin, Rudolf Schoenheimer received his medical degree from the Friedrich Wilhelm University in his native city. Schoenheimer taught biochemistry in Leipzig and Freiburg until 1933, when the Nazi rise to power forced him to escape to the United States, where he joined the Department of Biological Chemistry at Columbia University.

Schoenheimer developed the technique of isotope tagging to label various foods fed to animals, which made it possible to trace the metabolic paths of organic substances through plants and animals and revolutionized metabolic studies. The results of his experiments led to a new view of metabolism and nutrition and the evolution of a concept of "continual regeneration" (continual release and uptake of substances by the cell and a "dynamic state of body constituents"). Schoenheimer also established that cholesterol is a risk factor in atherosclerosis.

## Sigal, Irving                                        (USA, 1953–1988)

Born in Indianapolis, Irving Sigal received a doctorate in biochemistry from Harvard University. He pursued postdoctoral training at MIT, Harvard, and the California Institute of Technology before joining E.I. DuPont, where he published a landmark paper on mutagenesis to study the structure and function of enzymes and proteins. An internationally recognized expert on recombinant DNA, Sigal became senior director of molecular biology at the Merck Sharp & Dohme Research Laboratories in Rahway, NJ, and a leader of their AIDS research team. Sigal played a major role in identifying the structure of the HIV protease enzyme and showing the efficacy of drugs that inhibit them, which was published in *Nature* shortly after his untimely death in the terrorist bombing of PanAm Flight 103 over Lockerbie, Scotland, while returning home from giving a lecture to the Royal Chemical Society in London.

## Varmus, Harold Eliot (USA, 1939–)

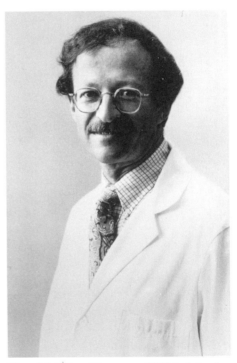

Harold Eliot Varmus. (*NLM / Lasker Award Archives*)

Born in Oceanside on Long Island, Harold Varmus earned a graduate degree in English at Harvard University before deciding to follow in his father's footsteps and become a physician. Twice rejected at Harvard, Varmus received his medical degree from Columbia University. After serving as a clinical associate at the National Institutes of Health, in 1970 Varmus began postdoctoral research in the laboratory of J. Michael Bishop at the University of California in San Francisco. Varmus soon joined the faculty in the Department of Microbiology and Immunology, rising to the rank of professor in 1979. From 1993 to 1999, Varmus served as Director of the National Institutes of Health, dramatically increasing its research budget. Varmus left the NIH to become the President of Memorial Sloan-Kettering Cancer Center in New York City. A decade letter, Varmus received a presidential appointment as the Director of the National Cancer Institute.

Varmus shared with Bishop the 1989 Nobel Prize in Physiology or Medicine for discovery of the cellular origin of retroviral oncogenes. These are a large family of genes that control the normal growth and division of cells. Disturbances in one or more of these oncogenes can lead to transformation of a normal cell into a tumor cell and result in cancer. Working with Rous virus, Varmus and Bishop discovered that the oncogene in the virus did not represent a true viral gene but instead was a normal cellular gene, which the virus had acquired during replication in the host cell and thereafter carried along. This gene was found to have a central function by controlling cellular growth and division. Varmus shared (with Bishop and others) the 1982 Lasker Award in Basic Medical Research for "oncogenes that transform normal cells into cancer cells."

## Varshavsky, Alexander Jacob                    (Russia, 1946–)

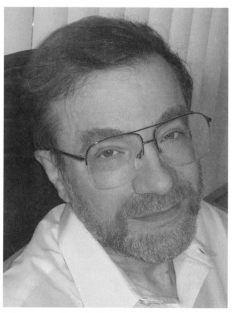

Born in Moscow, Alexander Varshavsky specialized in biochemistry and is currently a researcher at the California Institute of Technology. In collaboration with future Nobel Prize-winner Aaron Ciechanover, Varshavsky demonstrated that the ubiquitin system for protein degradation works not only in the test tube, but also in living cells, where it plays a key role in regulating cellular growth and division. He then discovered the first set of rules that dictates which proteins are destroyed. Rather than the previous concept of an unregulated protein incinerator within the cell, this work led to the current understanding that

Alexander Jacob Varshavsky. (*Courtesy of Dr. Varshavsky*)

protein destruction is a highly complex, temporally controlled, and tightly regular process that is critical to many basic cellular events and, when it malfunctions, causes disease. For this work, Varshavsky had shared (with Ciechanover and Hershko) the 2000 Lasker Award in Basic Medical Research for the "ubiquitin system for regulated protein degradation."

## Warburg, Otto Heinrich                    (Germany, 1883–1970)

Coming from a wealthy and prestigious Jewish family, it is unclear from various sources whether Otto Heinrich Warburg or his father converted to Christianity. Warburg received a doctorate in chemistry from the University of Berlin and a medical degree from the University of Heidelberg.

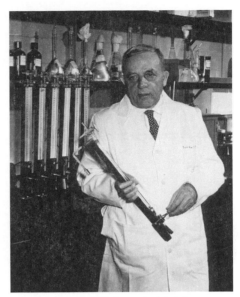

Otto Heinrich Warburg in his laboratory. (*NLM*)

In 1918, Warburg became a professor at the Kaiser Wilhelm Institute for cell physiology, where he investigated the metabolism of tumors and the respiration of cells – the chemical processes, involving oxygen and catalytic reactions, by which the cell absorbs oxygen from its surroundings and utilizes it for energy. Warburg demonstrated that abnormally growing cancer cells converted more glucose into lactose than normal cells. Expanding on studies of Otto Meyerhof, who had demonstrated that when muscle cells utilize oxygen, there is a mechanism to prevent all their glucose from being converted into lactose, Warburg concluded that a failure of this mechanism in cancer cells resulted in their unchecked growth. Considered one of the leading biochemists of the 20th century for his work in explaining these cellular processes in normal and cancer cells, Warburg was the sole recipient of the 1931 Nobel Prize in Physiology or Medicine. Today, it is thought that mutations in oncogenes and tumor suppressor genes are responsible for malignant transformation, and what has been called the "Warburg effect" is actually a result of these mutations rather than a cause.

When the Nazis came to power in Germany, physicians of Jewish descent were forced from their professional positions. It is believed that after Hitler had a vocal cord polyp removed, he feared developing a malignancy and wanted a recognized expert in cancer to be available to him. Consequently, he ordered Hermann Goring to search through Warburg's genealogy to find an excuse for this Jewish researcher to remain in Germany. It appeared than Warburg's father was actually half Aryan and, since he had a non-Jewish mother, Warburg became only a quarter Jewish and thus was exempt from most anti-Jewish legislation. Even though offered a position by the Rockefeller Foundation to move to the United States, Warburg refused, both because it would have meant breaking up his research team and facilities in Germany and he was convinced that a major breakthrough in cancer was imminent.

Warburg edited *The Metabolism of Tumours* (1931), which contains much of his original work, and wrote *New Methods of Cell Physiology* (1962).

---

**Yonath, Ada E.**                                                    (Israel, 1930–)

---

Born Ada Livshitz in Jerusalem to a rabbinical family of Polish immigrants before the founding of the State of Israel, Ada Yonath earned bachelor's and master's degrees from the Hebrew University and a doctoral degree in chemistry from the Weizmann Institute of Science in Rehovot. Yonath joined the faculty of the Chemistry Department in 1970, establishing the only protein-crystallography laboratory in Israel, and she continued to ascend the academic ladder to become Head of the Departments of Structural Chemistry and later Structural Biology.

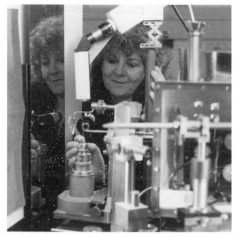

Ada E. Yonath. (*Courtesy of Dr. Yonath / Weizmann Institute of Science*)

Yonath is best known for her pioneering work unravelling the structure of the ribosome, the "protein factory" of the cell responsible for synthesizing proteins according to instructions provided by the genetic code. Her technical advances in ribosomal crystallography revolutionized structural biology worldwide, allowing her to determine the structures of the two ribosomal subunits. Moreover, Yonath demonstrated the modes of action of more than 20 antibiotics targeting the ribosome, illuminating mechanisms of drug resistance and synergism and the structural basis for antibiotic selectivity, all of which has paved the way for the design of structure-based drugs.

Yonath shared (with Venkatraman Ramakrishnan and Thomas Steitz) the 2009 Nobel Prize in Chemistry "for studies on the structure and function of the ribosome," becoming the first Israeli woman (of ten laureates) to win the Nobel Prize. Yonath has the distinction of being the first woman from the Middle East to win a Nobel Prize in the sciences, and the first woman from any country to receive the chemistry award in 45 years.

## DNA-RNA RESEARCH

Jewish scientists have been at the forefront of DNA and RNA research and won at least 16 Nobel Prizes for discoveries in the field. Chargaff established the basic rules for how DNA is constructed, and Franklin and Klug used X-ray diffraction, microscopy, and structural modelling to develop two- and later three-dimensional images that revealed the internal structure of transfer RNA, the DNA-protein complex, and several viruses. Arthur Kornberg isolated the polymerizing enzyme essential for the biological synthesis of DNA, and Nathans designed "chemical knives" that cut genes into defined fragments to determine their order on chromosomes, analyze their chemical structure and sites that regulate specific function of genes, and create new combinations of genes by chemical means. Gilbert created sophisticated techniques for the rapid sequencing of DNA, thus permitting the information in hundreds of links in the DNA chain to be "read" at one time and paving the way for the human genome project. Roger Kornberg described transcription, the process in which a copy of the information stored in genes is made so that the information can be transferred to the outer parts of the cells as an instruction for protein production.

Axel, Berg, Cohen, and Lederberg pioneered the field of recombinant DNA and genetic engineering, the artificial introduction of genetic material from one organism into the genome of another organism (transduction), which is then replicated and expressed by that other organism. Nirenberg discovered the importance of messenger RNA to provide genetic instructions in the cell nucleus to control protein synthesis. Baltimore and Temin identified that certain tumor viruses carried the enzymatic ability to reverse the flow of information from RNA back to DNA using reverse transcriptase. This was a revolutionary discovery in modern medicine, because reverse transcriptase is the central enzyme in such widespread human diseases as HIV (the virus that causes AIDS) and hepatitis. Milstein discovered the principles for the production of monoclonal antibodies, which can be used for safer and more powerful cancer chemotherapy, and Witkin described the concept of DNA-damage response, a fundamental mechanism that protects the genomes of all living organisms from a variety of insults by external agents, such as chemicals and radiation, and errors in normal physiological processes.

## Altman, Sidney                                    (Canada, 1939–)

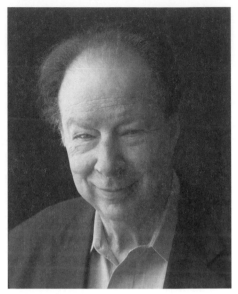

Sidney Altman. (*Courtesy of Dr. Altman*)

Born in Montreal to immigrants from Eastern Europe, Sidney Altman received his doctorate in biophysics from the University of Colorado. After research fellowships at Harvard University and the MRC Laboratory of Molecular Biology in Cambridge, England, Altman joined the faculty at Yale University, where he ascended the academic ladder and was promoted to Professor in 1980. Chair of his department from 1983 to 1985, for the next four years Altman served as Dean of Yale College. Altman currently is the Sterling Professor of Molecular, Cellular, and Developmental Biology and Chemistry at Yale University.

Altman analyzed the catalytic properties of the ribozyme RNase P, a ribonucleoprotein particle consisting of both a structural RNA molecule and one or more proteins. At the time, it was believed that, in the bacterial RNase P complex, the protein subunit was responsible for the catalytic activity of the complex, which is involved in the maturation of tRNAs. However, a series of experiments in which the complex was reconstituted in test tubes proved that the RNA component, in isolation, was sufficient for the observed catalytic activity of the enzyme. The discovery indicating that the RNA itself had catalytic properties, resulted in Altman sharing the 1989 Nobel Prize for Chemistry with Thomas Cech, who showed that RNA molecules could reorganize themselves without enzymes and directly affect chemical reactions within cells.

Altman's later work on eukaryotic organisms, which unlike bacteria, have cells that contain a nucleus and other organelles enclosed within membranes, showed that the protein subunits of the RNaseP complex are essential to the catalytic activity. Thus, Altman improved understanding of how genetic data is transferred and how the defenses of the body can be strengthened in the face of a viral attack.

## Axel, Richard (USA, 1946–)

Born in New York City, Richard Axel received a medical degree from Johns Hopkins University and joined the faculty at Columbia University, becoming a Professor in the Department of Neuroscience in 1978.

Axel focused his major research interest in how the brain interprets the sense of smell, mapping the parts of the brain that are sensitive to specific olfactory receptors. Collaborating with Linda Buck, a former postdoctoral research scientist in his laboratory, Axel published a seminal 1991 paper describing the almost 1,000 different genes that constitute the olfactory receptors in the mammalian genome. In later work performed independently, they showed that each olfactory receptor neuron expresses only one kind of olfactory protein. The input from all neurons expressing the same receptor is collected by a dedicated glomerulus of the olfactory bulb. In 2004, Axel and Buck shared the Nobel Prize in Physiology or Medicine "for their discoveries of odorant receptors and the organization of the olfactory system."

During the late 1970s, Axel joined microbiologist Saul J. Silverstein and geneticist Michael H. Wigler in the discovery of a technique of cotransformation, a process in which foreign DNA can be inserted into a host cell to produce certain proteins. Patents for this fundamental process in recombinant DNA research (known colloquially as "Axel patents") used widely by pharmaceutical and biotech companies earned huge amounts for Columbia University until they expired in 2000.

## Baltimore, David (USA, 1938–)

Born in New York City, David Baltimore received his doctoral degree from Rockefeller University. After several years at the Salk Institute for Biological Studies in La Jolla, California, in 1968 Baltimore joined the faculty of the Massachusetts Institute of Technology. Five years later, he became the American Cancer Society Professor of Microbiology. Baltimore served as the President of Rockefeller University (1990–1991) and the California Institute of Technology (1997–2006).

Baltimore exerted a major influence in such varied scientific fields as immunology, virology, cancer research, biotechnology, and recombinant DNA research. In 1975, Baltimore shared (with Howard Temin and Renato Dulbecco) the Nobel Prize in Physiology or Medicine "for their discoveries concerning the interaction between tumor viruses and the genetic material of the cell." Baltimore was recognized for his discovery of reverse transcriptase, which transcribes RNA into DNA, reversing the traditional belief that DNA led to RNA, which in turn led solely to proteins. Reverse transcriptase is an essential factor in the reproduction of retroviruses, such as HIV.

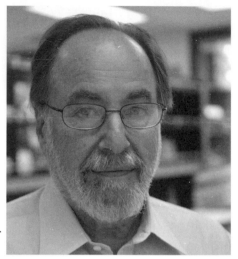

David Baltimore. (*California Institute of Technology*)

## Berg, Paul                                                            (USA, 1926–)

Born in Brooklyn, Paul Berg received a doctorate in biochemistry from Case Western Reserve University. After several years as a Professor of Medicine at Washington University in St. Louis, in 1959 Berg moved to the Stanford University School of Medicine, where he taught biochemistry for 40 years and served as Director of the Beckman Center for Molecular and Genetic Medicine from 1985–2000.

Berg is most famous for being the first to construct a recombinant-DNA molecule, which contains parts of DNA from a different species. In his pioneering work, Berg combined a chromosome

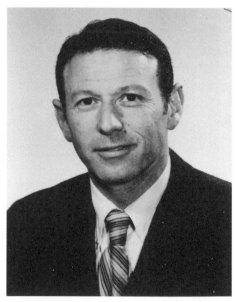

Paul Berg, 1980. (*NLM / Lasker Award Archives*)

from a virus with genes from a bacterial chromosome – a process that has led to the development of modern genetic engineering. In 1980, Berg was awarded half of the Nobel Prize in Chemistry (the other half shared by Walter Gilbert and Frederick Sanger) "for their fundamental studies of the biochemistry of nucleic acids, with particular regard to recombinant DNA." In the same year, Berg shared (with Herbert Boyer, Dale Kaiser, and Stanley N. Cohen) the Lasker Award in Basic Medical Research Award for "cloning genes by recombinant DNA technology."

---

## Chargaff, Erwin (Austria, 1905–2002)

Born in Czernowitz, now in the Ukraine, Erwin Chargaff earned a doctorate in analytic chemistry from the University of Vienna. Serving as the assistant in charge of chemistry for the Department of Bacteriology and Public Health at the University of Berlin, Chargaff was forced to resign his position in Germany as a result of Nazi policies against the Jews. In 1935, Chargaff immigrated to the United States, becoming a research associate and eventually a Professor of Biochemistry at Columbia University in New York, where he remained for most of his career. Chargaff focused his research on the study of nucleic acids using chromatographic techniques, proposing two main rules (Chargaff's rules) dealing with DNA.

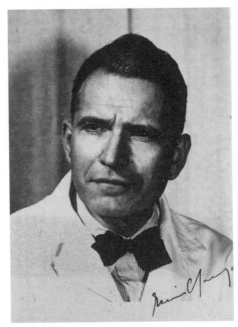

Erwin Chargaff, 1953. (*NLM / Lasker Award Archives*)

The first rule is that in DNA, the number of guanine units equals the number of cytosine units and the number of adenine units equals the number of thymine units. This strongly hinted at the base pair makeup of DNA, though Chargaff did not explicitly state this connection. The second rule is that the relative amounts of guanine, cytosine, adenine, and thymine bases varies from one species to another, suggesting that DNA rather than protein is the genetic material.

Despite not getting along well with James Watson and Francis Crick, in 1952 Chargaff explained his findings to them at Cambridge. Watson and Crick soon were able to deduce the double-helix structure of DNA, for which they were awarded the Nobel Prize in Physiology or Medicine ten years later.

## Cohen, Stanley Norman    (USA, 1935–)

Born in Perth Amboy, New Jersey, Stanley Norman Cohen studied medicine at the University of Pennsylvania. After postgraduate training at several institutions, including the National Institutes of Health, Cohen joined the faculty of Stanford University in 1968, where he is now a Professor of Genetics and Medicine.

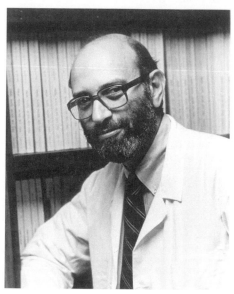

In collaboration with Paul Berg and Herbert Boyer, in 1983 Cohen performed one of the first genetic engineering experiments, in which they showed that the gene for frog ribosomal RNA could be transferred into bacterial cells and expressed by them. This eventually

Stanley Norman Cohen. (*NLM / Lasker Award Archives*)

led to the invention of recombinant DNA technology – the artificial introduction of genetic material from one organism into the genome of another organism, which is then replicated and expressed by that other organism.

In 1988, Cohen and Boyer were honored with the National Medal of Science "for their fundamental discovery of gene splicing, techniques allowing replication in quantity of biochemically important, new products, and beneficially transformed plant materials. This discovery of recombinant DNA technology has transformed the basic science of molecular biology and the biotechnology industry."

## Fire, Andrew Zachary    (USA, 1959–)

Born in Palo Alto, Richard Fire received a doctorate in biology from the Massachusetts Institute of Technology. Fire served as a staff member of the Department of Embryology at the Carnegie Institution of Washington in Baltimore (1986–2003) before becoming Professor of Pathology and Genetics at the Stanford University School of Medicine.

Fire shared (with Craig Mello) the 2006 Nobel Prize for Physiology or Medicine for the discovery of RNA interference (RNAi) as a "fundamental mechanism for controlling the flow of genetic information." This work was first published in a 1998 article, in which Fire and Mello showed that tiny pieces of double-stranded RNA (dsRNA) effectively shut down specific genes by preventing the messenger RNA (mRNA) with sequences matching the dsRNA from being translated into protein. They demonstrated that gene silencing by double-stranded RNA was much more effective than the previously described method of RNA interference with single-stranded RNA.

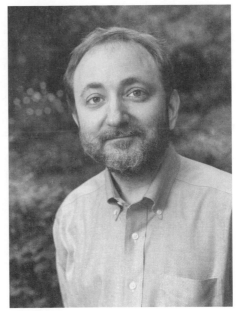

Photograph of Andrew Zachary Fire by Linda A. Cicero, 2008. (*Wikimedia / Stanford News Service*)

## Franklin, Rosalind Elsie                    (England, 1920–1958)

Born to a prominent British Jewish family, Rosalind Franklin earned her doctorate in physical chemistry from Cambridge. In 1951, Franklin began working as a research associate at the biophysics unit at King's College, London. Studying the structure of DNA using X-ray diffraction techniques to create images of crystalized solids, Franklin took pictures of DNA and discovered that there were two forms depending on the degree of hydration – a dry "A" form and a

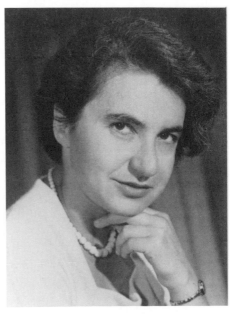

Rosalind Elsie Franklin. (*NLM / Courtesy of Jenifer Glynn*)

wet "B" form. One of her X-ray diffraction pictures of the "B" form of DNA, known as Photograph 51, became famous as critical evidence in identifying the structure of DNA. Without her knowledge, a superior in her laboratory shared her data with Watson and Crick at Cambridge University, which proved to be the key to their discovery of the double helix of DNA and winning the 1962 Nobel Prize for Physiology or Medicine. Many believed that Franklin would have received the Nobel Prize for Chemistry if still alive, but the Nobel Committee is not permitted to make posthumous awards.

---

## Gilbert, Walter                                                    (USA, 1932–)

Born in Boston, Massachusetts, Walter Gilbert received his doctorate in physics at the University of Cambridge in the United Kingdom. Gilbert then became a member of the faculty of Harvard University, his undergraduate alma mater.

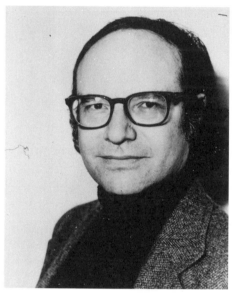

Gilbert shared (with Frederick Sanger) half of the 1980 Nobel Prize for Chemistry "for their contributions concerning the determination of base sequences in nucleic acids," which advanced the science of genetic engineering. Gilbert created a new technique for the rapid sequencing of DNA, the genetic material in the

Walter Gilbert. (*NLM / Lasker Award Archives*)

cells of all living things and the chemical blueprint for all life processes. He utilized chemical reagents to break the DNA molecules into fragments in such a way as to determine their sequence. By enabling several hundred links in the DNA chain to be "read" at a time, scientists could gain specific knowledge regarding the structure of genes and to discover a basic DNA defect that results in a specific genetic disease, thus offering the ability to eventually restructure the abnormal gene and eliminate the particular condition. Gilbert and Sanger had shared the 1979 Lasker Award in Basic Medical Research for "technology for sequencing DNA."

While retaining his affiliation with Harvard University, in 1979 Gilbert joined a group of other scientists and businessmen to form Biogen, a commercial genetic-engineering research corporation. He later became a chief proponent of the Human Genome Project, the government-funded effort to compile a complete map of the gene sequence in human DNA.

## Jacob, François (France, 1920–2013)

Born in Nancy, François Jacob began studying medicine at the Faculty of Paris before leaving for Great Britain to join the Free French Forces. Sent as a medical officer to several locations in Africa and Europe, though he had only completed his second year of medical studies, Jacob was severely wounded at Normandy in 1944 and was awarded the Croix de la Libération, the highest French military decoration of World War II. After his recovery, Jacob returned to complete medical school, but was unable to practice surgery

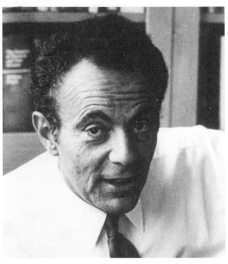

François Jacob. (*NLM / Gift of Dr. Jacob*)

because of his injuries. Jacob joined the research team at the Pasteur Institute under the guidance of André Lwoff and earned a doctoral degree in biology at the Sorbonne in 1954. Appointed Laboratory Director at the Institute and then Head of the Department of Cell Genetics, ten years later Jacob was named Professor at the Collège de France, where a Chair of Cell Genetics was created for him.

Jacob shared (with Jacques Monod and André Lwoff) the 1965 Nobel Prize for Medicine for their research on the concept that control of enzyme levels in all cells happens through feedback on the transcription of DNA sequences. This work spurred the emerging field of molecular developmental biology, especially the idea of transcriptional regulation.

## Klug, Aaron (Lithuania, 1926–)

Born in Zelvas, at age two Aaron Klug moved with his family to Durban, South Africa. After earning his medical degree at the University of Witwatersrand in Johannesburg, Klug joined the University of Cape Town as a researcher in physics and crystallography, the experimental science of determining the arrangement of atoms in solids. In 1949, Klug moved to England to study at Trinity College in Cambridge, where he received his doctorate four years later. Klug joined Rosalind Franklin at Birkberk College in London to investigate the molecular structure of the (RNA) tobacco mosaic virus.

In 1962, Klug returned to Cambridge to the newly built Medical Research Council Laboratory of Molecular Biology, where he used

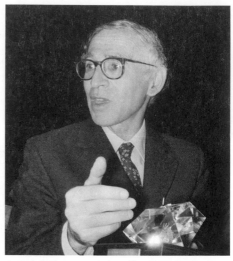

Aaron Klug receiving the H.P. Heineken prize from Prince Claus, 1979. Photograph by Rob Bogaerts. (*Wikimedia / Dutch National Archives, The Hague*)

X-ray diffraction, microscopy, and structural modelling to develop crystallographic electron microscopy. This type of microscopy entails combining a sequence of two-dimensional images of crystals taken from different angles to produce three-dimensional images of the target. Using this technique to study biologically functional molecular aggregates, Klug revealed the internal structure of transfer RNA; the DNA-protein complex, chromatin; and several viruses. In recognition of this work, Klug was awarded the 1982 Nobel Prize in Chemistry "for his development of crystallographic electron microscopy and his structural elucidation of biologically important nucleic acid-protein complexes." In 1988, Klug was knighted by Queen Elizabeth.

---

## Kornberg, Arthur                                          (USA, 1918–2007)

---

Born in Brooklyn, the son of immigrant parents from what is now Poland, Arthur Kornberg studied medicine at the University of Rochester. After serving for ten years as a research scientist at the National Institutes of Health and a commissioned officer in the U.S. Public Health Service, in 1953 Kornberg became Chair of the Department of Microbiology at the Washington University of Medicine in Saint Louis. Six years later, Kornberg moved to the Stanford University School of Medicine to organize its Department of Biochemistry, remaining there for the rest of his academic career.

Kornberg's major research interests were in enzyme chemistry, deoxyribonucleic acid synthesis (DNA replication), and studying the nucleic acids that control heredity in animals, plants, bacteria, and viruses. For his discovery of the mechanisms in the biological synthesis of DNA and isolating the first DNA polymerizing enzyme, now known as DNA polymerase, Kornberg shared (with his teacher, Severo Ochoa) the 1959 Nobel Prize in Physiology or Medicine.

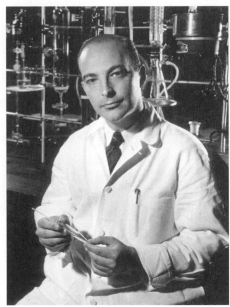

Arthur Kornberg in his laboratory. Photograph by Arthur Hulic. (*NLM*)

## Kornberg, Roger David

(USA, 1947–)

Born in St. Louis and the son of 1959 Nobel Prize-winner Arthur Kornberg, Roger Kornberg received his doctorate in chemical physics from Stanford University, where he now is a Professor of Structural Biology. He and his Israeli wife, also a Professor of Structural Biology, spend almost half the year in Jerusalem, where Kornberg serves as a visiting professor at the Hebrew University and advises his research team over the Internet.

Kornberg was awarded the 2006 Nobel Prize for Chemistry "for his studies of the molecular basis of eukaryotic transcription." As the Nobel press release notes, for the

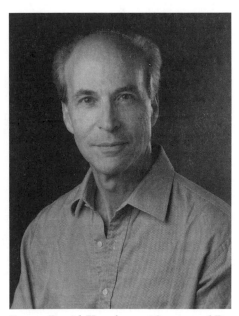

Roger David Kornberg. (*Courtesy of Dr. Kornberg*)

body to make use of the information stored in the genes, a copy must first be made and transferred to the outer parts of the cells as an instruction for protein production. This copying process is known as transcription, and Kornberg was the first to create an actual picture of how transcription works at a molecular level in the important group of organisms called eukaryotes (organisms whose cells have a well-defined nucleus, from ordinary yeast to human beings). If transcription stops, genetic information is no longer transferred into the different parts of the body and the organism dies within a few days. This is the result in cases of poisoning by certain toadstools, like the death cap, since the toxin stops the transcription process. Understanding of the working of the transcription process has fundamental medical importance, since disturbances in its proper functioning are involved in such human illnesses as cancer, heart disease, and various kinds of inflammation.

---

## Lederberg, Joshua                                    (USA, 1925–2008)

---

Born in Montclair, New Jersey, and the son of a rabbi, Joshua Lederberg was a pre-medical student at Columbia University when he enlisted as a hospital corpsman in World War II. Returning to civilian life, Lederberg began medical school but took two years off to earn a doctorate at Yale University under Edward Tatum. Instead of finishing medical school, in 1947 Lederberg accepted a position in the genetics department at the University of Wisconsin in Madison, where his wife received her doctorate three years later.

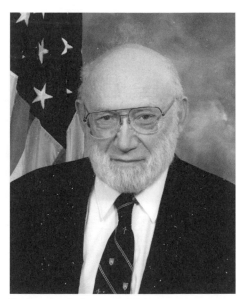

Joshua Lederberg. (*NLM*)

Following the discovery of the importance of DNA, Lederberg questioned the prevailing hypothesis that bacteria simply split into two to pass down exact copies of genetic information, so that all cells in a lineage were essentially clones. Collaborating with Tatum, Lederberg showed that the bacterium *Escherichia coli* entered a sexual phase during which two different strains could share genetic information through recombination, thus leading to a new, crossbred strain of the bacterium. Later, Lederberg and student Norton Zinder demonstrated that certain bacteriophages (bacteria-infecting viruses) could carry genetic material from one strain of the bacterium *Salmonella typhimurium* to another, a process known as transduction. The concept that the genetic material of living things could be inserted into cells eventually led to the development of the field of genetic engineering, or recombinant DNA technology. For discovering the mechanisms of genetic recombination in bacteria, Lederberg shared (with Edward Tamm and George Beadle) the 1958 Nobel Prize for Physiology or Medicine.

After receiving this award, Lederberg became the founder and Chairman of the Department of Genetics at Stanford University. With the launching of *Sputnik* in 1957, Lederberg became concerned about the biological impact of space exploration. In a letter to the National Academies of Sciences, he outlined his fear that extraterrestrial microbes might gain entry to Earth onboard spacecraft and cause catastrophic diseases. Conversely, he argued that microbial contamination of manmade satellites and probes could make it much more difficult to search for extraterrestrial life. Consequently, Lederberg recommended that returning astronauts and equipment be quarantined, and that equipment should be sterilized before being launched into space. With Carl Sagan, Lederberg advocated for NASA to expand the role of biology in searching for extraterrestrial life and the effects of extraterrestrial environments on living organisms. In conjunction with Edward Feigenbaum, Lederberg pioneered a project on artificial intelligence in the computer science program at Stanford. Lederberg became the President of Rockefeller University in 1978, serving in this capacity until his retirement in 1990.

---

**Levene, Phoebus Aaron Theodore**　　　　　　　　(Lithuania, 1863–1940)

---

Born Fishel Aaronovich Levin in Žagarė, Phoebus Levene studied medicine at the Imperial Military Medical Academy in St. Petersburg, Russia. In the wake of the 1893 anti-Semitic pogroms, Levene and his family immigrated to the United States and settled in New York City. After studying chemistry at Columbia University, Levene decided to devote his life to chemical research. In 1905, Levene was appointed as Head of the Biochemical Laboratory at the Rockefeller Institute of Medical Research, where he spent the rest of his career.

Levene's research focused on the structure and function of nucleic acids. He found that DNA consisted of four purine or pyrimidine bases (adenine, guanine, thymine, cytosine), a sugar called deoxyribose, and a phosphate group. In addition to identifying the components of DNA, Levene also showed that the components were linked together in the order *phosphate-sugar-base* to form units, which he called "nucle-otides." Thus the DNA molecule consisted of a string of nucleotide units linked together through the phosphate groups, which consti-tute the "backbone" of the mole-cule. Although Levene's concept of the structure of DNA was incor-rect, as was his conclusion that it was chemically too simple to store the genetic code, his work was the basis for later studies that deter-mined the structure of DNA.

Levene is known for his "tetra-nucleotide hypothesis," in which he was the first to propose that DNA was composed of *equal* amounts of adenine, guanine, cyto-

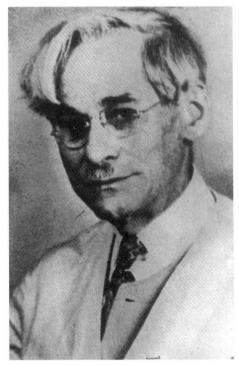

Phoebus Aaron Theodore Levene. (*NLM / Jerusalem Academy of Medicine*)

sine, and thymine. Before the later work of Erwin Chargaff, which showed that, within a species, the amount of adenine was similar to cytosine, the general consensus was that DNA was organized into repeating "tetranu-cleotides" that could not carry genetic information. Instead, the basis of hereditary was thought to be the protein component of chromosomes.

---

**Milstein, César**                                    (Argentina, 1927–2002)

Born to an immigrant Jewish family from Lithuania, César Milstein grad-uated from the University of Buenos Aires and earned a doctoral degree in biochemistry from Cambridge University.

Milstein shared (with Niels Kaj Jerne and Georges J. F. Köhler) the 1984 Nobel Prize in Physiology or Medicine "for theories concerning the specificity in development and control of the immune system and the discovery of the principle for production of monoclonal antibodies." By merging cells that produce natural antibodies with those of a tumor that multiplies indefinitely, Milstein was able to create a new combined cell that generates a large quantity of specific antibody to target single disease organisms invading the body, unlike the generalized attack of most antibodies. Monoclonal antibodies can produce markers that allow distinction among different cell types, as well as for the investigation of the pathological pathways in neurological disorders and many other diseases. Applying recombinant DNA technology to monoclonal antibodies inspired the field of antibody engineering, which has resulted in safer and more powerful monoclonal antibodies for use as therapeutics. In the same year, Milstein had shared (with Georges Kohler and Michael Potter) the Lasker Award in Basic Medical Research for "monoclonal antibody technology."

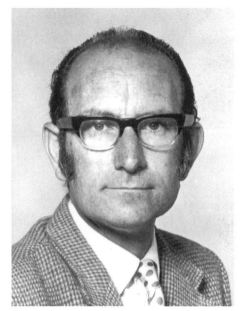

César Milstein. (*Gairdner Foundation*)

Milstein did not patent his enormous discovery, convinced that this was an essential part of the intellectual property of mankind, which therefore should have only scientific and no economic value.

---

**Nathans, Daniel**　　　　　　　　　　　　　　　　　　　(USA, 1928–1999)

---

Born to Russian immigrant parents in Wilmington, Delaware, Daniel Nathans received his medical degree from Washington University in St. Louis. In 1962, Nathans accepted a position at Johns Hopkins University School of Medicine in the Department of Microbiology, becoming Professor and Director of the section ten years later.

Nathans shared (with Werner Arber and Hamilton Smith) the 1978 Nobel Prize in Physiology or Medicine for the discovery of restriction enzymes. These are "chemical knives" that cut chains of DNA (genes) into defined fragments, which can be used to determine the order of genes on chromosomes, analyze their chemical structure and sites that regulate specific function of genes, and create new combinations of genes by chemical means. Nathans' work paved the way for the preparation of recombinant DNA, the production of gene therapy, and the Human Genome Project.

## Nirenberg, Marshall Warren                    (USA, 1927–2010)

Born in New York City, Marshall Nirenberg received his doctoral degree in biochemistry from the University of Michigan. Nirenberg began his postdoctoral work at the National Institutes of Health in 1957, advancing within five years to become Head of the Section of Biochemical Genetics at the National Heart Institute (now the National Heart, Lung, and Blood Institute), where he remained a laboratory chief until his death.

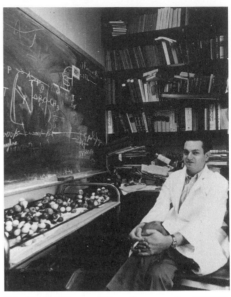

Marshall Warren Nirenberg, 1962. (*NLM*)

When Nirenberg began his research, multiple studies had shown that DNA was the molecule of genetic information, but it was not known how DNA directed the expression of proteins and the role of RNA in this process. Collaborating with Heinrich Matthaei, Nirenberg succeeded in deciphering the genetic code for multiple amino acids and showed that messenger RNA is required to provide genetic instructions in the cell nucleus to control protein synthesis. For this work, Nirenberg shared (with Robert W. Holley and H. Gobind Khorana) the 1968 Nobel Prize in Physiology or Medicine. In the same year, Nirenberg shared (with Khorana) the Lasker Award in Basic Medical Research for "deciphering the genetic code."

## Ruvkun, Gary Bruce                              (USA, 1952–)

Born in Berkeley, California, Gary Ruvkun received his doctorate in biophysics at Harvard University. Ruvkun is currently a molecular biologist at Massachusetts General Hospital and Professor of Genetics at Harvard Medical School in Boston.

In 2008, Ruvkun shared (with Victor Ambros and David Baulcombe) the Lasker Award for Basic Medical Research "for discoveries that revealed an unanticipated world of tiny RNAs that regulate gene function in plants and animals." As the Lasker foundation noted, recent studies have indicated that there may be as many as 1,000 mini-RNAs that collectively control a third of all of our protein-producing genes. This unforeseen universe of potent molecules not only plays a role in embryonic development, but also in blood-cell specialization, cancer, muscle function, heart disease, viral infections, and possibly neurological signaling and stem-cell behavior. Researchers are exploring the possibility of using mini-RNAs "signatures" for diagnosis and prognosis and even the possibility of manipulating their quantities for therapeutic purposes.

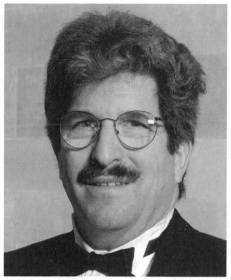

Gary Bruce Ruvkun. (*Gairdner Foundation*)

## Spiegelman, Sol                            (USA, 1914–1983)

Born in New York City, Sol Spiegelman received a doctorate in cellular physiology from Washington University in St. Louis. While an undergraduate majoring in mathematics at City College of New York, Spiegelman began studying bacteria in order to understand cell genetics. This flew into the face of the conventional belief of leading geneticists, who were convinced that bacteria have no nucleus and therefore can have no genetics. However, after discovering mutations in bacteria, Spiegelman concluded that bacteria are genetically quite similar to higher forms of life. He asserted

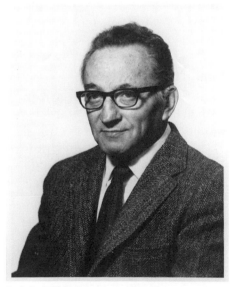

Sol Spiegelman, 1974. (*Lasker Award Archives, NLM*)

that bacteria could be an ideal model for studies of cell genetics and cancer, since cancer is involved with cell-population genetics. After postgraduate studies, Spiegelman joined the faculty of the University of Illinois, rising in academic rank to become Professor of Microbiology. In 1969, Spiegelman became Director of the Institute of Cancer Research and the Comprehensive Cancer Center at Columbia University.

Spiegelman is best known for his discovery that, of the two strands of molecules that make up DNA (the transmitter of hereditary patterns), only one carried the message that generated genetic information for the production of new substances. The carrier was another form of nucleic acid called ribonucleic acid. In 1962, Spiegelman developed a technique to detect specific DNA and RNA molecules in cells. Known as nucleic acid hybridization, this procedure is credited with helping to lay the groundwork for advances in recombinant DNA technology.

Spiegelman later turned his attention to the molecular basis of cancer. Working with tumors of viral origin (leukemia and human breast cancer), Spiegelman showed that RNA molecules similar to those present in tumors of viral origin in mice could be found in comparable human malignancies. Just before his death, Spiegelman was working on perfecting a blood test for the diagnosis of breast cancer, based on his earlier discovery that women with a family history of such cancer carry particles in their milk indistinguishable from the viruses that cause breast cancer in mice.

Spiegelman received the 1974 Lasker Award in Basic Medical Research "for his contributions to molecular biology, including techniques of molecular hybridization and the first synthesis of an infectious nucleic acid."

---

## Temin, Howard Martin                                    (USA, 1934–1994)

Born in Philadelphia, Howard Temin earned a doctorate in animal virology from the California Institute of Technology. In 1960, Temin joined the faculty at the University of Wisconsin in Madison, rising through the academic ranks to become Professor of Viral Oncology and Cell Biology.

Temin shared (with David Baltimore, who made an independent discovery at the Massachusetts In-

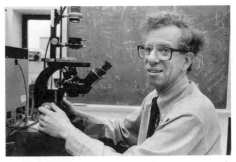

Howard Martin Temin in laboratory with microsope, 1987. (*University of Wisconsin-Madison Archives, ID S00158*)

stitute of Technology, and Renato Dulbecco) the 1975 Nobel Prize in Physiology or Medicine for his discovery of reverse transcriptase. Contrary to the general belief that genetic information flowed exclusively from DNA to RNA to protein. Temin showed that certain tumor viruses carried the enzymatic ability to reverse the flow of information from RNA back to DNA using reverse transcriptase. This was a revolutionary discovery of major value to modern medicine, because reverse transcriptase is the central enzyme in several widespread human diseases, such as HIV (the virus that causes AIDS) and hepatitis B. Reverse transcriptase is also a component of important techniques in molecular biology and diagnostic medicine, such as the polymerase chain reaction that is used to amplify a single copy or a few copies of a piece of DNA across several orders of magnitude to generate thousands or even millions of copies of a particular DNA sequence. Temin had received the 1974 Lasker Award in Basic Medical Research for "reverse transcriptase."

## Witkin, Evelyn M. (USA, 1921–)

Born Evelyn Maisel in New York City, Evelyn Witkin received a doctoral degree in genetics from Columbia University. During a summer studying bacterial genetics at Cold Spring Harbor Laboratory (CSHL), Witkin induced mutations in *Escherichia coli* bacteria using ultraviolet (UV) light and performed the first successful isolation of UV-resistant *E. coli* mutants. After graduation, Witkin remained at CSHL until 1955, when she moved to SUNY Downstate, and in 1971 she was appointed a Professor of Biological Sciences at Rutgers University.

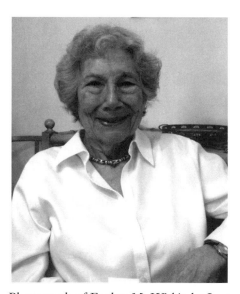

Photograph of Evelyn M. Witkin by Jane Gitschier during interview for PLOS Genetics, 2012. (*NLM*)

Witkin's groundbreaking research on mutagenesis in bacteria provided valuable insight into mechanisms of DNA repair, the fundamental process by which living organisms maintain their genetic integrity in order to survive. Witkin shared (with Stephen J. Elledge) the 2015 Lasker Award for Basic Medical Research "for discoveries concerning the DNA-damage response – a fundamental mechanism that protects the genomes of all living organisms." As the Lasker Foundation observed, throughout their lives, cells withstand an onslaught of insults to their DNA from external agents such as chemicals and radiation and errors in normal physiological processes. This incites cells to implement a multi-faceted strategic response to ensure survival. Like bacteria, mammalian cells construct DNA-repair equipment and arrest division when they detect genetic peril. When the extent of injury overwhelms DNA-re-storative capacities, as in the unbridled duplication of cells caused by cancer, the DNA-damage response sparks cell suicide to maintain the overall integrity of the entire organism. She also noted that UV awakens bacterial viruses (phages), whose DNA has settled silently into the bacterial genome, by destroying a protein that normally restrains these foreign genes.

To divide successfully, a bacterium must create a partition that separates the two daughter cells, and UV exposure temporarily impedes this process. Witkin discovered that in the parental strain of *E. coli* that she used, tiny amounts of UV light demolished the ability of the bacteria to create the partition, and the creature never recovered. However, the UV-resistant strain resumed division after a short lag. In the 1960's, Witkin discovered that UV treatment of the parent *E. coli* strain stimulated production of a substance that hinders cell separation. She speculated that this substance is normally inhibited by another molecule (repressor), which resembles the one that hampers phage gene activation. This concept gained support from the observation by another group that cells with a single genetic defect spur both processes via a common pathway.

Witkin then noted that, rather than causing inherited genetic changes, UV light triggers chemical reactions within DNA molecules that disrupt its structure and render the genetic code uninterpretable at those spots. Unless the original DNA letter is restored, a random, and often incorrect, DNA building block is inserted. Witkin predicted accurately that DNA damage stirs production of an error-prone copying enzyme that fosters mutagenesis long before there was direct evidence for it. Thus, Witkin (and Elledge) "laid the conceptual and experimental foundation for our understanding of these intricately organized systems, which ensure genetic fidelity and safeguard organismal vitality."[33]

---

33. http://www.laskerfoundation.org/awards/show/discoveries-concerning-dna-damage-response/.

## Yanofsky, Charles (USA, 1925–)

Born in New York, Charles Yanofsky earned a doctorate in chemistry and microbiology at Yale University. After several years at Western Reserve University School of Medicine, Yanofsky joined the faculty at Stanford University. Working with the bacterium *Escherichia coli*, Yanofsky showed that the sequence of the nitrogen-containing bases forming part of the structure of the genetic material has a linear correspondence to the amino acid sequence of proteins. This means that changes in DNA sequence can produce changes in protein sequence at corresponding positions. Yanofsky's work revealed how controlled alterations in its structure allow RNA to serve as a regulatory molecule in both bacterial and animal cells.

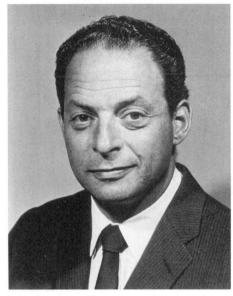

Charles Yanofsky, 1971. (*Gairdner Foundation*)

---

### GENETICS

Benzer proved that genes are structured like words from small units of DNA and are responsible for memory, internal body clocks, and differences in behavior. Brenner and Horwitz investigated the genetic regulation of organ development and programmed cell death. Ptashne demonstrated the existence of a genetic switch that turns on and off a mechanism for making specific enzymes and proteins, while Friedman discovered the gene that produces leptin, the hormone regulating appetite and body weight. Leder proved that an otherwise normal gene can permit cancer to develop if it is stripped of its regulatory sequences and received the first patent for a genetically engineered animal. Bernstein performed statistical analysis of population genetics to show that the A, B, and O blood groups are inherited on the basis of a set of triple alleles found in a single gene. Muller demonstrated that x-rays striking the genes and chromosomes of living cells can cause mutations and hereditary changes, with these artificially induced genetic mutations having the potential for far-reaching consequences.

---

## Benzer, Seymour

(USA, 1921–2007)

Born in Brooklyn to immigrants from Poland, Seymour Benzer received a doctorate in solid state physics from Purdue University. During World War II, Benzer was recruited for a secret military project to develop germanium semiconductors for use in radar devices. Silicon semiconductors, which were being used at that time, tended to burn out when subjected to high voltages. Benzer discovered a crystal form of germanium that withstood such voltages. He and his supervisor in the lab, Karl

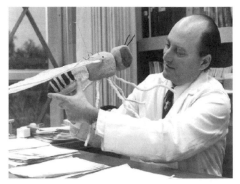

Seymour Benzer in his office at Caltech with a big model of Drosophila, 1974. Photograph by WA Harris. (*Wikimedia / The Man Who Took Us from Genes to Behaviour.* PLoS Biology Vol. 6, No. 2.)

Lark-Horovitz, were ultimately awarded six patents for their research discoveries, and the crystal form of germanium was later used at Bell Labs to develop the first transistor.

Turning to the field of molecular and behavioral genetics, in the early 1950s Benzer addressed the controversial issue of whether genes were indivisible units or composed of smaller parts. He experimented with viruses that infected the bacterium *Escherichia coli*, selecting those that were unable to infect a particular strain (called K) because they had defective versions of a gene. Knowing that two viruses infecting the same host sometimes have their genetic material blended in their offspring, Benzer discovered that some of the resulting viruses could infect the K strain. He was able to show that the viruses had swapped pieces of the same gene, which in some cases resulted in a working version of the gene. In effect, Benzer's experiments proved that genes are structured like words from smaller units of DNA. The mutant viruses had misspelled genes, which could be combined into the correct sequence.

Moving to the California Institute of Technology in 1967, Benzer began investigating the relationship between genes and behavior. Using mutants of a strain of *Drosophila* flies, he analyzed a simple behavior – the attraction of flies to light. After exposing flies to toxins to trigger mutations, Benzer and his colleagues sorted through the offspring of the mutant flies to find those that behaved strangely, such as not responding to light or flying away from it. By breeding these mutant flies, Benzer was able to pinpoint the location of some of the genes responsible for the differences in behavior. These experiments were replicated in other animal models, forming the foundation for the field of molecular biology of behavior. Benzer and colleagues also discovered genes in flies linked to memory and their internal body clocks.

Benzer shared (with Charles Yanovsky and Sydney Brenner) the 1971 Lasker Basic Medical Research Award for "nonsense and suppressor mutations."

## Bernstein, Felix                                    (Germany, 1878–1956)

Born in Halle and receiving his doctorate after studies in Munich and Berlin, Felix Bernstein became a Professor of Mathematics and Biostatistics at the University of Göttingen. He was renowned for having proven as a teenager the Schröder–Bernstein theorem of set theory, which states that if each of two sets A and B are equivalent to a subset of the other, then A is equivalent to B.

In the 1920's, Bernstein turned his attention to the development of population genetics in the analysis of modes of inheritance. With the discovery of human blood groups, in 1924 Bernstein applied statistical analysis of population genetics to show that the A, B, and O blood groups are inherited on the basis of a set of triple alleles found in a single gene, rather than the previous theory that they reflected two pairs of genes.

With the rise of the Nazis to power, Bernstein was removed from his position while lecturing in the United States, remaining there for the rest of his teaching career.

## Brenner, Sydney                                    (South Africa, 1927–)

Born in Germiston to Jewish immigrants from Lithuania and Latvia, Sydney Brenner studied medicine at the University of Witwatersrand in Johannesburg and received a doctorate in physical chemistry from Oxford University. In 1956, Brenner joined the Medical Research Council Unit in Cambridge, where he made significant contributions to work on the genetic code and other areas of molecular biology. In 1976, Brenner joined the Salk Institute to pursue a new career in neuroscience, and in 1996 he founded the Molecular Sciences Institute in Berkeley.

In the early 1960s, Brenner focused his research on the problem of studying organ development and related processes in higher animals, which is very difficult because they have enormous numbers of cells. His search for a simple organism with many of the basic biological characteristics of humans led to the nematode *Caenorhabditis elegans*, a near-microscopic soil worm that begins life with just 1,090 cells. In addition, the animal is transparent

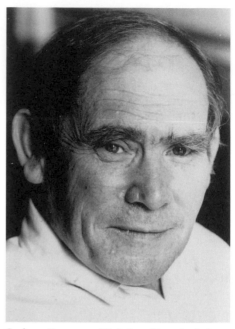

Sydney Brenner. (*Gairdner Foundation*)

(permitting scientists to follow cell divisions under a microscope), reproduces quickly, and is inexpensive to maintain. Researchers later learned that programmed cell death eliminates 131 cells in the organism, so that adults end up with 959 body cells. Brenner also showed that a chemical compound could induce genetic mutations in the worm, which had specific effects on organ development.

Brenner's work laid the foundation for future research by John E. Sulston and H. Robert Horvitz, which led to all three sharing the 2002 Nobel Prize for Physiology or Medicine "for their discoveries concerning genetic regulation of organ development and programmed cell death." Brenner's Nobel lecture, entitled "Nature's Gift to Science," was a paean to *Caenorhabditis elegans*, which he had established as a model organism for the investigation of neural development and genetic analysis.

## Friedman, Jeffrey (USA, 1954–)

Born in Orlando, Florida, Jeffrey Friedman studied medicine at Albany Medical College and received a doctorate from Rockefeller University. Joining the staff in molecular genetics, Friedman focused his efforts on weight regulation, using a special strain of mice to identify the hormone that normal animals use to control their appetite, and which was missing in the plump rodents. After eight years, Friedman discovered the gene that produces this hormone, which he called "leptin" from the Greek word for "thin." By injecting the encoded protein, Friedman showed that as fat accumulates it exudes leptin, which binds to a receptor in the brain that quells the desire to eat. This decreases the body weight of mice by reducing food intake as well

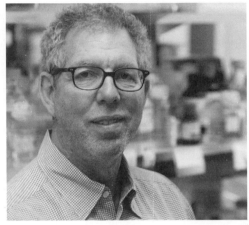

Jeffrey Friedman. (*Zach Veilleux /The Rockefeller University*)

as increasing energy expenditure. As Professor and Head of the Laboratory of Molecular Genetics at Rockefeller University, Friedman's current research seeks to understand the genetic basis of obesity in humans and the mechanisms by which leptin transmits its weight-reducing signal.

Friedman shared (with Douglas Coleman) the 2010 Lasker Award for Basic Medical Research "for the discovery of leptin, a hormone that regulates appetite and body weight—a breakthrough that opened obesity research to molecular exploration." As the Lasker Foundation noted, their work has "fostered an explosion in our knowledge about how the body manages hunger and weight control. Leptin presides over a network that plays a crucial role in normal physiology and disease, and scientists have only begun to explore the myriad ways that we might manipulate this system to enhance people's health and well-being."[34]

## Horwitz, H. (Howard) Robert  (USA, 1947–)

Born in Chicago, Robert Horwitz received a doctorate in biology from Harvard University. Horwitz joined the faculty of the Department of Biology at the Massachusetts Institute of Technology and soon was promoted to professor.

Horwitz shared (with Sydney Brenner and John E. Sulston) the 2002 Nobel Prize for Physiology or Medicine for his research on the nematode

---

34. http://www.laskerfoundation.org/awards/show/leptin-a-hormone-that-regulates-appetite-and -body-weight/.

*Caenorhabditis elegans.* He discovered and characterized key genes, demonstrating how these genes interact with each other in the process of cell death and that corresponding genes exist in humans.

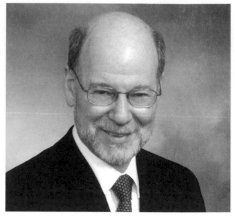

H. Robert Horwitz.
(*Courtesy of Dr. Horwitz*)

## Leder, Philip                                                    (USA, 1934–)

Born in Washington, D.C., Philip Leder studied medicine at Harvard University and specialized in internal medicine. In 1968, Leder was appointed as Head of the Biochemistry Department of the Graduate Program of the Foundation for Advanced Education in the Sciences at the National Institute of Health. Four years later, he was appointed Director of the Laboratory for Molecular Genetics at the NIH, remaining in that post until 1980, when he returned to Harvard Medical School as the founder of its newly formed Department of Genetics.

In collaboration with Nobel laureate Marshall Nirenberg, Leder demonstrated the triplet nature of the genetic code. Leder was the first to define the base sequence of a complete mammalian gene (the gene for beta globin), which enabled him to determine its organization in detail, including its associated control signals. In his pioneering research into the structure of genes that carry the code for antibody molecules, Leder showed that the enormous diversity of antibody molecules is formed by a limited number of encoded genes. He extended this work to investigate Burkitt's lymphoma, a tumor of antibody-producing cells that involves the oncogene c-myc. Stripping this gene of its regulatory sequences and introducing the deregulated gene into laboratory mice, Leder showed that these transgenic mice produced offspring with an inherited tendency to develop cancers involving c-myc, thus proving that the deregulation of an otherwise normal gene can permit cancer to develop. Leder received the 1987 Lasker Award for Basic Medical Research "for his elegant studies of the genetic basis of antibody diversity and the role of genetic rearrangement in carcinogenesis."

In 1988, Leder and Timothy Stewart were granted the first patent for a genetically engineered animal. After isolating a gene that causes cancer in many mammals, including humans, they injected it into fertilized mouse eggs and developed a new breed of genetically altered mice. Because half the females develop cancer, the altered breed serves as a more effective model for studying how genes contribute to cancer, particularly breast cancer. Moreover, the genetically engineered mouse offers scientists a more efficient biological system for testing new drugs and therapies to treat cancer, as well as for determining whether chemicals and other toxic substances found in food or the environment are harmful.

## Muller, Hermann Joseph                                    (USA, 1890–1967)

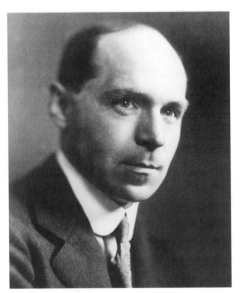

Born in New York City, Hermann Muller attended Columbia University, where he became interested in genetics under the influence of E.B. Wilson, the founder of the cellular approach to heredity, and T. H. Morgan, who introduced the fruit fly *Drosophila* as a tool in experimental genetics. Muller was fascinated by the concepts of genetic mutations and natural selection as the basis for evolution, and the possibility of his scientific endeavors consciously guiding the evolution of human beings. At Columbia, he became a proponent of eugenics and was always concerned with how developments in biology could impact on society. After completing his doctorate, Muller was recruited to Houston to join the newly founded William Marsh Rice Institute, now Rice University.

Hermann Muller. (*The Lilly Library, Indiana University, Bloomington, Indiana*)

Muller is best known for his work on the physiologic and genetic effects of radiation, He demonstrated that x-rays striking the genes and chromosomes of living cells can cause mutations and hereditary changes, with these artificially induced genetic mutations having the potential for far-reaching consequences. For these discoveries, Muller was awarded the 1946 Nobel Prize for Physiology or Medicine.

Muller was an outspoken critic of nuclear testing, issuing stern warnings and raising public awareness about the long-term dangers of radioactive fallout related to nuclear testing and war. This was accentuated by the timing of the Nobel Prize, not long after the atomic bombings of Hiroshima and Nagasaki. Regarding the processes of natural selection operating in modern society, Muller made the controversial suggestion that the sperm of gifted men be frozen and preserved as part of a purposeful program of eugenics for future generations.

## Ptashne, Mark                                                    (USA, 1940–)

Born in Chicago, Mark Ptashne received a doctorate in molecular biology from Harvard University. Ptashne currently is the Chair of Molecular Biology at Memorial Sloan–Kettering Cancer Center in New York.

In the early 1960s, three French scientists (François Jacob, Jacques Monod, and André Lwoff) were awarded the Nobel Prize for providing the theoretical basis for the existence of genetic switches. This set off an international search to find an actual gene switch in living creatures. The race ended in a virtual dead heat, with Ptashne describing a genetic switch that turned on and off a virus called

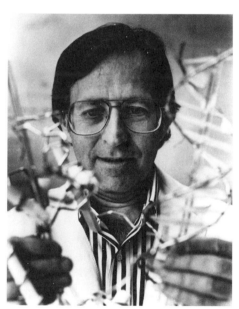

Mark Ptashne. (*Wikipedia / National Cancer Institute*)

lambda, while Walter Gilbert demonstrated a switch that turned on and off the ability of a cell to digest a milk sugar.

Of the approximately 75,000 genes in the genetic makeup of a person, only a small fraction operates at any given moment. Different sets of genes are turned on in each type of cell, which enables differentiation in function between liver and skin cells. Ptashne showed that when a lambda virus enters an *E. coli* bacterium, it inserts itself into the bacterial DNA and then turns itself off, remaining dormant for long periods. When an infected bacterium is injured by a flash of ultraviolet light, the virus is awakened and multiplies rapidly. Eventually, the bacterium bursts and virus particles escape to other bacteria. After discovering the molecule that kept the virus dormant, Ptashne showed that similar gene switches exist in higher organisms. In further experiments, Ptashne determined that as long as a control spot on the DNA at the front of a gene is empty, the gene is inactive. When an activator protein settles onto a control spot, the gene with the blueprints to make an enzyme or another kind of protein can be read and its commands carried out. This is performed by a huge composite of molecules called the transcription complex, which requires up to 10 activators to begin its task. For this body of work, Ptashne was awarded the 1997 Lasker Award for Basic Medical Research.

## Weinberg, Wilhelm (Germany, 1862–1937)

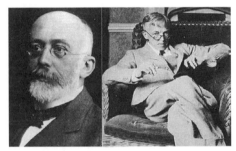

Born in Stuttgart, Wilhelm Weinberg studied medicine in Tübingen, Berlin, and Munich, specializing in obstetrics and gynecology. Establishing a highly successful practice in his native city, Weinberg spent most of his academic life studying genetics, especially on how the laws of inheritance apply to populations. Based on an analysis of a large number of identical

Wilhelm Weinberg (left) and G.H. Hardy. (*Courtesy of the Genetics Society of America*)

and fraternal twins, Weinberg developed the principle of genetic equilibrium. This describes a condition in which an allele or genotype in a gene pool (such as a population) does not change in frequency from one generation to another if a series of assumptions are met. Later models have been developed to describe conditions in which one or more of these assumptions are violated, assuming instead a balance between the diversifying effects of genetic drift and the homogenizing effects of migration between populations.

In England, mathematician G. H Hardy made similar, but less comprehensive, observations that were published a few months after Weinberg's. However, Weinberg's work remained largely unknown in the English-speaking world for decades, and his discovery is now generally known as the Hardy-Weinberg principle.

## IMMUNOLOGY

Jewish research scientists have played major roles in understanding the mechanisms of the immune system and developing vaccines and medications against a broad spectrum of diseases. Ehrlich proposed that cells under threat from toxins grow side-chains that break off to become antibodies, which circulate through the body and bind with infectious agents to inactivate them. In a search for a "magic bullet" against syphilis, Ehrlich discovered Salvarsan, the first effective treatment that resulted in dramatic cures. Edelman deciphered the chemical structure of antibodies, also known as immunoglobulins. Feldman proposed cytokines as stimulating the movement of cells toward sites of inflammation, infection, and trauma and a mechanism for the induction of autoimmune diseases. Doniach showed that in the autoimmune disease known as Hashimoto's disease, antibodies were not directed against the expected external microbes (bacteria and viruses), but rather against the thyroid gland. Metchnikoff established the concept of cell-based immunity by identifying the process of phagocytosis, in which a specific type of white blood cells (macrophages) surround, engulf, and then destroy harmful bacterial invaders. Heidelberger discovered that the powerful antigens of pneumococcus bacteria are polysaccharides, establishing a relationship between chemical constitution and immunological specificity of antigens and disproving the prevailing assumption that only proteins could act as antigens. Bencerraf and Strominger showed the structure and function of human histocompatibility proteins and their role in disease. Sela and Arnon discovered the genetic control of the immune response and designed vaccines based on synthetic molecules.

Yalow and Berson developed radioimmunoassay to measure the small amount of insulin in the blood of adult diabetics, a technique subsequently used to measure hormones, vitamins, and enzymes, which were too small to be detected previously.

Haffkine developed an attenuated vaccine against cholera and one using killed bacteria against plague. Freund strengthened immunization procedures against such diseases as tuberculosis, malaria, rabies, and poliomyelitis, while Besredka made important contributions to the development of vaccinations against cholera, dysentery, typhus, paratyphus, and anthrax.

Sela and Arnon co-developed copaxone, a drug to combat multiple sclerosis, and Feldman demonstrated that medications blocking Tumor Necrosis Factor Alpha (TNFα) could stop the inflammatory and tissue-destructive pathways of rheumatoid arthritis and other autoimmune diseases.

Rose discovered the rheumatoid factor and developed an agglutination test to accurately diagnose rheumatoid arthritis, while Gutman elucidated the metabolic defects present in gout.

## Arnon, Ruth (Israel, 1933–)

Born in Tel Aviv, Ruth Arnon earned her doctoral degree in biochemistry at the Weizmann Institute of Science in Rehovot. Arnon has held multiple academic posts at the Weizmann Institute, including Dean of the Department of Clinical Immmunology and Dean of the Faculty of Biology. She is currently a Professor of Immunology and involved in researching a universal, recombinant influenza vaccination and a vaccine against cancer.

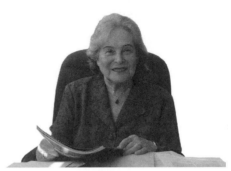

Ruth Arnon. (*Wikimedia / Weizmann Institute of Science*)

Arnon is best known as a co-developer (with her teacher, Michael Sela) of copaxone, a drug to combat multiple sclerosis. This leads to neuroprotection and neurogeneration and prevents demyelination, the process in which the myelin sheath of neurons is damaged. Therefore, in addition to treating multiple sclerosis, copaxone can be used for other demyelinating diseases, such as optic neuritis (inflammation of the optic nerve) and vitamin B12 deficiency. In 2001, Arnon was awarded the Israel Prize in the Natural Sciences.

## Benacerraf, Baruj (Venezuela, 1920–2011)

Born in Caracas to Sephardic Jewish parents from Morocco and Algiers, Baruj Benacerraf moved with his parents to Paris at a young age. After returning to Venezuela, Benacerraf immigrated to the United States in 1940 and attended the Medical College of Virginia, the only medical school to which he was accepted. Eventually, Benacerraf became the Director of the Laboratory of Immunology of the National Institute of Allergy and Infectious Disease, before accepting the Chair of Pathology at Harvard Medical School in 1970.

Focusing his research in the study of allergy and immunology, Benacerraf shared (with Jean Dausset and George Davis Snell) the 1980 Nobel

Prize in Physiology or Medicine for what the Nobel Committee described as the "discovery of the major histocompatibility complex genes which encode cell surface protein molecules important for the immune system's distinction between self and non-self" – the genes that govern transplant rejection.

Benacerraf had observed that if antigens were injected into animals with a similar heredity, some responded while others did not. Further studies showed that the dominant autosomal genes, termed the immune response genes, determined the response to certain antigens. Since Benacerraf's initial discovery, more than 30 genes have

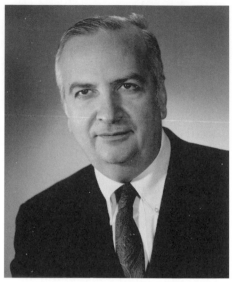

Baruj Benacerraf as President of the American Association of Immunologists, 1973–4. (*Federation of American Societies for Experimental Biology Archive*)

been discovered in what has been termed the major histocompatibility complex, the part of DNA that controls the immune response. In addition to its value in the body's response to transplantation, Benacerraf's research has enabled better understanding of auto-immune diseases such as multiple sclerosis and rheumatoid arthritis. In 1972, Benacerraf demonstrated the existence of T- and B-cell lymphocytes.

## Berson, Solomon Aaron                                    (USA, 1918–1972)

Born in New York City, Solomon Berson graduated from the City College of New York but was not admitted to medical school. Berson pursued graduate work and served as an anatomy instructor at New York University before finally securing a place at the NYU Medical School three years later. After earning his medical degree and two years of military service, Berson completed an internal medicine residency at the Bronx VA Hospital.

In 1950, Berson became a member of the Radioisotope Service of the hospital, where he teamed with Rosalyn Yalow in what developed into an extremely rewarding research partnership. Their early laboratory work concerned iodine and human serum albumin metabolism, but they then turned their attention to insulin, a hormone that was difficult to measure in the blood. Berson and Yalow developed the technique of radioimmuno-assay (RIA), the use of radioisotope tracers to measure the concentration of a wide array of pharmacologic and biologic substances in the blood and other fluids of the human body, animals, and plants. In addition to detecting and measuring insulin, they extended their success to other hormones, such as corticotropin, gastrin, parathyroid hormone, and growth hormone. In 1968, Berson was appointed as the Chair of Medicine at Mount Sinai School of Medicine.

Berson and Yalow shared many prestigious scientific awards. However, Berson died in 1972, three years before Yalow received the 1975 Nobel Prize for Physiology or Medicine for their joint work in developing the technique of radioimmunoassay technique (Nobel Prizes cannot be awarded posthumously).

## Besredka, Alexandre Mikhailovich (Russia, 1870–1940)

Born in Odessa, Alexandre Besredka studied biology in his native city before moving to Paris in 1893 to become an assistant to Elie Metchnikov at the Pasteur Institute, where he obtained his medical education. Besredka co-founded the *Bulletin de l'Institut Pasteur*, and for a decade he directed the laboratory at the Pasteur Institute, focusing his research on immunology, cellular self-defense mechanisms and phagocytosis, antiviral therapy, and the development of vaccines against various infectious diseases. Besredka is best known for his fundamental research on anaphylaxis, and his name is associated with a type of vaccination he proposed for avoiding anaphylactic shock ("Besredka's method") and the use of serotherapy ("Besredka's desensitization") for those who had developed an allergic sensitivity. He also made important contributions to the development of vaccinations against various infectious diseases, such as cholera, dysentery, typhus, paratyphus, and anthrax.

A prominent advocate for Jewish public health, Besredka established a preventive medicine service for the families of Jewish immigrants to the Paris area and organized a welcome reception for the first 300 German, Austrian, and Czech Jewish children arriving after Kristallnacht in 1938.

## Doniach, Deborah (UK, 1912–2004)

Born in Geneva and the daughter of a concert pianist who accompanied violinist Josef Szigeti and later became a Professor of Music at the Jerusalem Conservatory, Deborah Doniach was a medical student at the Sorbonne in Paris. Interrupting her studies to marry Sonny Doniach, later Professor of Pathology at the London Hospital, she moved to London and enrolled at the Royal Free Medical School. After graduation, she became an endocrinologist at the Middlesex Hospital.

In the 1960s, Doniach joined the newly formed Department of Immunology and became a Professor of Clinical Immunology in 1974. In collaboration with fellow Jewish scientist Ivan Roitt, Doniach showed that patients with Hashimoto's disease, an inflammation of the thyroid, had raised levels of immune proteins in their blood, which returned to normal after the thyroid was surgically removed. She also noted that the thyroid contained many plasma cells, which produce the serum proteins (antibodies) that normally protect against infection. From this information, Doniach deduced that in Hashimoto's disease, the antibodies were not directed against the expected external microbes (bacteria and viruses), but rather against the thyroid gland itself. This discovery led to the wider concept of organ-specific autoimmunity. Doniach and Roitt later showed that the same immunological mechanism damaged the stomach in pernicious anemia, the liver in primary biliary cirrhosis, and the pancreas in type 1 diabetes.

---

**Edelman, Gerald Maurice**                              (USA, 1929–2014)

Born in New York City, Gerald Edelman attended medical school at the University of Pennsylvania. In 1960, Edelman received his doctoral degree in biology from the Rockefeller Institute, where he remained for the next three decades.

Edelman shared (with Rodney Robert Porter) the 1972 Nobel Prize in Physiology or Medicine for his work on the immune system, specifically deciphering the

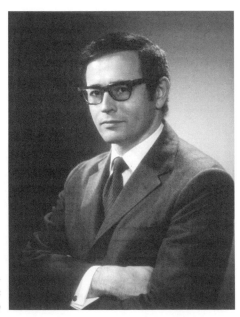

Photograph of Gerald Edelman by Fabian Bachrach. (*Federation of American Societies for Experimental Biology Archive*)

chemical structure of antibodies, also known as immunoglobulins. He discovered that antibodies were not constructed in the shape of one long peptide chain, as previously thought, but rather composed on two different chains, one heavy and one light, which were linked. As the Nobel Committee observed, the advances of Edelman and Porter "incited a fervent research activity the whole world over, in all fields of immunological science, yielding results of practical value for clinical diagnostics and therapy."[35]

After winning the Nobel Prize, Edelman turned his attention to neuroscience and philosophy of the mind, authoring a trilogy of technical books. In *The Mindful Brain* (1978), Edelman developed his theory of Neural Darwinism, related to the concept of plasticity in the neural network in response to the environment. In *Topobiology* (1988), Edelman proposed a theory of how the neuronal network of the newborn brain is established during development of the embryo. The final book in the series, *The Remembered Present* (1990), deals with Edelman's theory of consciousness. In 1992, Edelman moved to La Jolla, California, to become the founder and Director of Neurosciences at the Scripps Institute, which studies the biological basis of higher brain function in humans.

---

## Ehrlich, Paul                                    (Germany, 1854–1915)

---

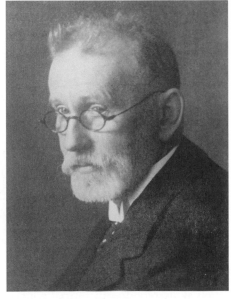

Born in Strehlen, Paul Ehrlich pursued medical studies at the universities of Breslau, Strasbourg, Freiburg, and Leipzig. He obtained his doctorate in 1882 and worked at the Charité Hospital in Berlin as an assistant medical director. Fascinated with staining tissues for microscopy since a young age, Ehrlich concentrated on histology, hematology, and color chemistry using dyes. In 1891, Robert Koch invited Ehrlich to

Paul Ehrlich. (*Wikimedia / United States Library of Congress, Prints and Photographs Division*)

---

35. https://www.nobelprize.org/nobel_prizes/medicine/laureates/1972/press.html.

join the staff at his Berlin Institute of Infectious Diseases. Five years later, Ehrlich became the founding director of its new branch, the Institute for Serum Research and Testing, which had been established for his area of specialization. In 1899, the Institute was moved to Frankfurt and expanded into the Institute of Experimental Therapy, where Ehrlich focused his research on chemotherapy and infectious disease.

In addition to selectively staining tissues for histologic examination, German chemists had developed a technique for selectively staining bacteria on a microscope slide. Ehrlich reasoned that it should also be possible to develop toxic compounds that would selectively target a disease-causing microscopic organism in the human body. This was Ehrlich's dream of the "magic bullet," which would kill only the targeted organism while not affecting normal body cells.

Ehrlich and his assistants studied hundreds of chemical substances to treat disease. In 1907, he demonstrated that an injection of the 606th drug tested was effective in clearing large syphilitic sores in rabbits and eliminating the causative spirochete from the animal's blood. Immediately, Ehrlich embarked on an unprecedentedly large clinical trial of this new drug, now known by the trade name Salvarsan ("safe" or "healing" arsenic), on tens of thousands of patients, with a pharmaceutical company supplying the drug free of charge to clinics and hospitals in Germany. The results were remarkable, with reports of dramatic cures due to this first effective medical treatment for syphilis. When complications were reported, Ehrlich developed "Neosalvarsan," which had a lower arsenic dose and twice the curative power, though repeated injections were often required. Nevertheless, the drug was an overwhelming success, decreasing the incidence of syphilis in Europe by up to 75%. This launched the age of chemotherapy, a term that Ehrlich coined.

Ehrlich is well known for his concept of the side-chain theory to explain the immune response in reaction to infection. He proposed that living cells have side-chains just like those in dyes, which are related to their coloring properties. These side chains can link with a particular toxin, in a manner similar to Emil Fischer's suggestion that enzymes must bind to their receptors "like a key in a lock." Ehrlich theorized that a cell under threat grew additional side-chains to bind the toxin, and that these additional side chains broke off to become antibodies that circulate through the body. Ehrlich described these antibodies as "magic bullets," which could search for infectious agents and then bind with and inactivate them. Ehrlich also made substantial contributions to the development of an antiserum to fight diphtheria and conceptualized a method for standardizing therapeutic serums.

Ehrlich shared (with Elie Metchnikoff) the 1908 Nobel Prize in Physiology or Medicine "in recognition of their work on immunity," the first two Jews to be so honored.

## Feldmann, Marc  (Poland, 1944–)

Michael Feldmann was born in Lvov, near the Russian border, into a Jewish family that managed to get to France immediately after World War II. He immigrated to Australia at age eight, later earning a doctoral degree in immunology at the University of Melbourne. Moving to London in the 1970s, Feldmann has worked at several research institutes and now is a professor at Oxford University.

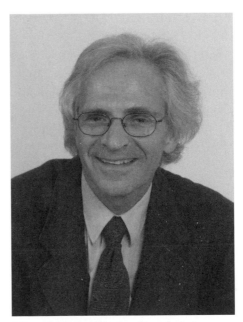

Marc Feldman. (*Lasker Foundation*)

In the 1980s, Feldmann published a new hypothesis for the mechanism of induction of autoimmune diseases, highlighting the role of cytokines. These are a large family of molecules that act as signals in cell-to-cell communication in immune responses and stimulating the movement of cells toward sites of inflammation, infection, and trauma. Examples include interleukin and interferon, which are involved in regulating the response of the immune system to inflammation and infection. In autoimmune diseases, the immune system attacks and damages the body's own tissues, leading to diseases of various organs. A major autoimmune disease is rheumatoid arthritis, a severe destructive process that attacks the joints. Feldmann and his colleagues demonstrated that diseased joints have much more pro-inflammatory cytokines than normal, and they identified one of these (Tumor Necrosis Factor Alpha; abbreviated TNFα) as the key. In laboratory experiments and clinical trials, Feldmann showed that blocking TNFα reduced the levels of other pro-inflammatory cytokines and was a successful treatment for rheumatoid arthritis. Pharmaceutical companies rushed to develop TNFα inhibitors, which have become the therapy of choice for stopping the inflammatory and tissue-destructive pathways of rheumatoid arthritis and other autoimmune diseases, such as Crohn's disease, ulcerative colitis, ankylosing spondylitis, and psoriatic arthritis.

For the discovery of anti-TNFα therapy for rheumatoid arthritis and other autoimmune diseases, Feldmann and rheumatologist Ravinder Maini received the 2003 Lasker Award for Clinical Medical Research.

## Freund, Jules                                    (Hungary, 1890–1960)

After receiving his medical degree at the Royal Hungarian University in Budapest, Jules Freund served in the Austrian Army in World War I before returning to the Department of Preventive Medicine at his alma mater. Freund moved to the United States in 1922 for a joint fellowship at Harvard University and the Massachusetts Antitoxin and Vaccine Laboratory. After positions in New York, North Carolina, and Pennsylvania, Freund became a member of the Department of Pathology at Cornell University Medical College (1932–1945) and Assistant Director of the New York City Department of Health (1938–1945). Freund was the first Chief of the Division of Applied Immunology of the Public Health Research Institute (1943–1956), and

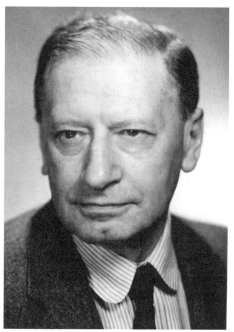

Jules Freund. (*The American Association of Immunologists Collection, Center for Biological Sciences Archive, University of Maryland, Baltimore County*)

in 1957 he was appointed chief of the Laboratory of Immunology at the National Institute of Allergy and Infectious Diseases (NIAID).

Freund received the 1959 Lasker Award for Basic Medical Research "for new findings in the field of immunology and allergy which have strengthened immunization procedures against such diseases as tuberculosis, malaria, rabies and poliomyelitis." In early investigations of poliovirus vaccines made from brain tissue, he demonstrated that brain tissue virus produced antibody responses only with the aid of an adjuvant or auxiliary agent that he developed ("Freund adjuvant"). As the Lasker Foundation noted, "Techniques of scientific study developed by him have advanced knowledge in basic immunology and have provided tools used routinely in laboratory research by immunologists throughout the world today."[36]

---

### Haffkine, Waldemar Mordechai Wolff (Russia, 1860–1930)

Born in Odessa, Waldemar Haffkine was a student at the Faculty of Natural Science at Odessa University when Tsar Alexander II was assassinated, leading to civil repression and pogroms that especially affected the Jews. As a member of the Jewish League for Self-Defense, Haffkine was defending a Jewish home from a group of military cadets when he was seriously wounded, arrested, and placed on trial. Unlike many other student activists, however, Haffkine was actively supported by his mentor, Elie Metchnikoff, who used his influence to spare Haffkine from execution or exile. Realizing that he had no future in Russia, where an unbaptized Jew was effectively

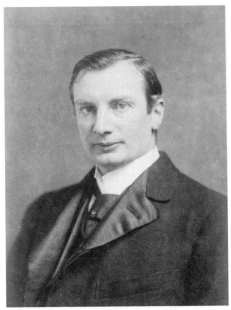

Photograph of Waldemar Haffkine by Elliot & Fry Photo Co. (*Wikimedia / National Library of Israel, Schwadron Collection*)

barred from a professorial position, Haffkine worked for a year with Moritz Schiff in Geneva before following Metchnikoff to join the Louis Pasteur Institute in Paris.

In 1893, the brother of the king of Siam visited Paris to ask Louis Pasteur, the discoverer of attenuated vaccines, to produce a vaccine for cholera, a disease that had been devastating Asia. Pasteur assigned this task to Haffkine, who had distinguished himself by observing how the rod-shaped bacteria that caused typhoid fever adapted to various conditions. A decade earlier, Robert Koch had isolated and bred a pure culture of *Vibrio cholera*, the comma-shaped bacterium responsible for causing cholera. Using a highly virulent culture of cholera bacteria, Haffkine determined that at 39° Celsius (about the temperature of the human body) the organism would continue multiplying, but in a weakened form. When injected under the

---

36. http://www.laskerfoundation.org/awards/show/freunds-adjuvent/.

skin of a human or animal host, these weakened bacteria would produce a mild infection that generally produced immunity to subsequent infection by the more virulent strain. Risking his own life, Haffkine performed the first human test on himself, injecting a dose four times stronger than was later used, recording his reactions, and determining that his vaccine was safe for human use. For the next several years, Haffkine performed field trials in India. He showed that a prophylactic inoculation of attenuated cholera bacteria could produce a 75% reduction in mortality from the disease.

When a pandemic of plague, the Black Death that killed a third of the population in medieval Europe, returned to ravage India in 1896, the government asked Haffkine to come to Bombay (where the infection was most acute) to develop a vaccine against the disease. Haffkine was among the first scientists to suspect that rat-borne fleas were the carriers of the plague bacteria. (This microorganism, known as *Yersinia pestis*, had been first isolated at the Pasteur Institute by Alexandre Yersin.) Haffkine determined that an attenuated vaccine, like the one he had developed for cholera, might not be as successful in preventing the much more virulent plague bacteria. Consequently, he killed the plague bacteria by heating them for an hour at 90° Celsius and then exposing them to carbolic acid. When inoculated in a sufficient dosage, this mixture triggered a strong immune response without the risk that those who had been injected could develop the deadly disease. After the prophylactic vaccine produced a 90% decrease in mortality rate from plague, Haffkine was knighted in Queen Victoria's Diamond Jubilee Year honors in 1897. In 1925, the Plague Research Laboratory where he had worked in Bombay was renamed the Haffkine Institute in his honor.

In his later years, Haffkine returned to Orthodox Jewish practice. In 1916, he wrote an article entitled *A Plea for Orthodoxy*, in which he advocated traditional religious observance, decrying the lack of such observance among "enlightened" Jews and stressing the importance of community life. He also created the Haffkine Foundation, which still exists, to foster religious, scientific, and vocational education in Eastern European *yeshivot*.

---

**Heidelberger, Michael**                                    (USA, 1888–1991)

---

Born in New York City, Michael Heidelberger received a doctorate in organic chemistry from Columbia University, where he spent almost his entire academic career. Heidelberger was one of the fathers of modern immunology and the founder of immunochemistry, the branch of biochemistry that examines the mammalian immune system on a molecular level. With the bacteriologist Oswald Avery, in 1923 Heidelberger made the seminal discovery that the powerful antigens of pneumococcus bacteria are polysaccharides. For the first time, this established a relationship between chemical constitution and immunological specificity of antigens, thereby putting the field of immunology on a firm biochemical footing. It also disproved the prevailing assumption among scientists that only proteins could act as antigens. This discovery led the way to a new understanding of infectious diseases, their treatment, and their prevention. Heidelberg received the 1953 Lasker Award in Clinical Medical Research.

Previously, Heidelberger had

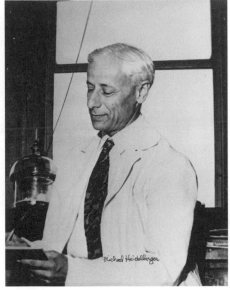

Michael Heidelberger. (*The American Association of Immunologists Collection, Center for Biological Sciences Archive, University of Maryland, Baltimore County*)

participated in the synthesizing of many chemotherapeutic drugs (aromatic arsenicals) for the treatment of infectious diseases, specifically syphilis and African sleeping sickness.

## Metchnikoff, Elie                                           (Russia, 1845–1916)

Born in Karkov, Ukraine, Elie Metchnikoff's Jewish grandfather allowed himself and his family to be baptized so as to live in St. Petersburg, which was beyond the Pale of Settlement where Jews were legally permitted to live. Nevertheless, Metchnikoff later wrote, "I ascribe my love for science to my descent from the Jewish race."[37]

Metchnikoff studied natural sciences at Karkov and began his doctoral research at the University of Giessen (Germany). Returning to Russia, Metchnikoff received his doctorate from the University of St. Petersburg and eventually joined the faculty at the University of Odessa. In 1888, Metchnikoff moved to Paris to join the Pasteur Institute, where he worked in bacteriology and immunology. Remaining at the Institute for

---

37. Frank Heynick, *Jews in Medicine: An Epic Saga* (NJ: KTAV Publishing House, 2002), p. 307.

the rest of his career, Metchnikoff became deputy director and succeeded Pasteur as director in 1904.

Metchnikoff is best known for his identification of the process of phagocytosis, in which a specific type of white blood cells (macrophages) surround, engulf, and then destroy harmful bacterial invaders. This established the concept of cell-based immunity, a fundamental part of the body's immune response. For this work, Metchnikoff shared (with Paul Ehrlich) the 1908 Nobel Prize in Physiology or Medicine – the first two Jews to be so honored.

Metchnikoff also identified an apparent link between acidophilus-type bacteria producing lactic acid and extended lifespan for humans. This led to the relatively modern discipline of probiotics, dietary supplements containing potentially beneficial bacteria and yeasts. Among his major works are *Immunity in Infectious Diseases* (1901) and *The Nature of Man* (1938).

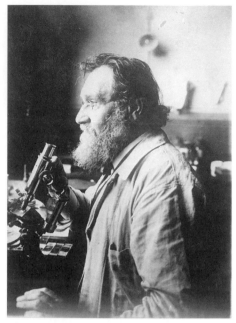

Elie Metchnikoff in his laboratory, circa 1910. (*Wikimedia / Library of Congress*)

---

## Rose, Harry Melvin                                    (USA, 1906–1986)

---

Born in Meredith, New Hampshire, Harry Rose became paraplegic from childhood polio and also contracted tuberculosis. After studying medicine at Cornell University, Rose specialized in microbiology and immunology, eventually becoming Professor of Microbiology and Immunology at Columbia University in 1952.

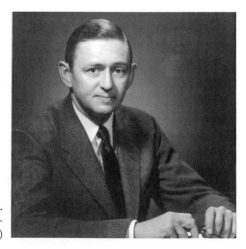

Harry Melvin Rose.
(*The American Association of Immunologists Archive / The Rose Family*)

Rose is best known for the discovery of the rheumatoid factor, made independent of the work of Erik Waaler in Norway. With colleague Charles Ragan, Rose developed an agglutination test that permitted an accurate diagnosis of rheumatic arthritis by allowing differentiation of this condition from other rheumatic diseases. For their work, Rose and Ragan were among the first recipients of the Gairdner Foundation International Award in 1959.

An editor of the Journal of Immunology, Rose also performed research in virology and the mechanism of antibiotic action and contributed to the development of influenza vaccines.

## Sela, Michael (Poland, 1924–)

Born as Mieczyslaw Solomonowicz in Tomaszów Mazowiecki, Michael Sela earned his doctorate at the Weizmann Institute of Science in Rehovot. Sela has assumed many roles at the Weizmann Institute, including Chairman of the Immunology Department, President of the Institute (1975–1985), and Deputy Chairman of the Board of Governors.

Sela is known for his research in immunology, particularly on the molecules (synthetic antigens) that trigger the immune system to attack. This has led to the discovery of genetic control of the immune response and the design of vaccines based on synthetic molecules. Sela has investigated strategies for treating autoimmune diseases and was a co-developer (with Ruth Arnon) of copaxone, a drug to combat multiple sclerosis. In 1959, Sela was awarded the Israel Prize in the Natural Sciences.

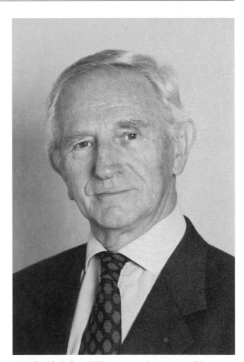

Micheal Sela. (*Weizmann Institute of Science*)

## Steinman, Ralph Marvin                    (Canada, 1943–2011)

Born in Montreal, Ralph Steinman received his degree from Harvard Medical School and was an immunologist and cell biologist at Rockefeller University. Steinman shared half (with Bruce Beutler and Jules Hoffman) of the 2011 Nobel Prize in Physiology or Medicine for "his discovery of the dendritic (antigen-processing) cell and its role in adaptive immunity."

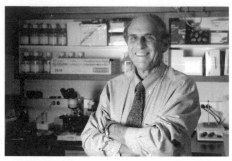

Ralph Marvin Steinman in his laboratory. (*Rockefeller University*)

His work focused on finding a vaccine to protect against cancer and other malignant tumors in humans. Ironically, the selection committee was not aware that Steinman had died three days earlier from pancreatic cancer. Although the rules stipulate that the Nobel Prize cannot be awarded posthumously, the committee determined that, since the decision to award the prize "was made in good faith," it would still be given to Steinman. Steinman had received the 2007 Lasker Award in Basic Medical Research for "dendritic cells and the immune response."

## Strominger, Jack Leonard                    (USA, 1925–)

Born in New York City. Jack Strominger studied medicine at Yale University and joined the faculty at the Washington University School of Medicine in St. Louis. In 1974, Strominger became a Professor of Biochemistry at Harvard Medical School and a staff member at the Dana-Farber Cancer Institute.

Specializing in the structure and function of human histocompatibility proteins and their role in disease, Strominger's research transformed the science of molecular immunology. He precisely defined the parameters of immune recognition by T cells, and translated cellular immunology into the language of atoms. For these achievements, Strominger received the 1995 Albert Lasker Award for Basic Medical Research.

## Yalow, Rosalyn Sussman (USA, 1921–2011)

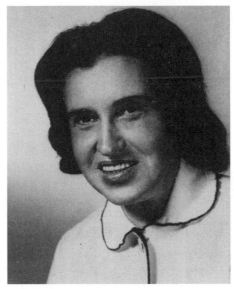

Rosalyn Sussman Yalow. (*NLM*)

Born Rosalyn Sussman in New York City, she received her doctoral degree in physics from the University of Illinois, the only woman among the 400 members of the department and the first in more than 25 years. She married Andrew Yalow, fellow student and the son of a rabbi, and they kept a kosher home. In 1977, Yalow became the second woman to ever win the Nobel Prize in Physiology or Medicine, sharing the honor with Roger Guillemin and Andrew Schally. Yalow had received the 1976 Lasker Award in Basic Medical Research for "radioimmunoassay for detecting hormones in blood."

After graduation, Yalow joined the Bronx Veterans Administration Medical Center to help set up its radioisotope service to diagnose and treat disease. There she collaborated with Solomon Berson to develop the technique of radioimmunoassay (RIA), for which she won the Nobel Prize. Radioimmunoassay refers to the use of radioistopic tracers to measure the concentration of a wide array of pharmacologic and biologic substances in the blood and other fluids of the human body, animals, and plants.

Yalow initially invented radioimmunoassay in 1959 to measure the amount of insulin in the blood of adult diabetics. Since then, this technique has subsequently been used to measure hormones, vitamins, and enzymes, which were too small to be detected previously. It also can screen blood donations for various types of hepatitis and to detect foreign substances, including some cancers. Although radioimmunoassay had great commercial potential, Yalow and Berson refused to patent their method.

In 1968, Yalow was appointed Research Professor in the Department of Medicine at Mount Sinai Hospital, and in 1976 she hosted a five-part dramatic series on the life of Madame Curie for PBS. Despite her extensive research activities, Yalow served as an inspiration to young women interested in science by showing that it was possible to combine family (two children) and a career.

## PHARMACOLOGY

Eichengrun played a major role in the synthesis of aspirin, which was performed by a student under his direction. Vane showed how aspirin produces pain relief and anti-inflammatory effects and demonstrated that it blocks the action of prostaglandins in platelets, leading to the use of aspirin for decreasing blood clots to prevent heart attacks and strokes.

Pincus showed that repeated injections of progesterone stopped ovulation. Djerassi and Colton synthesized compounds that were key components of the first oral contraceptive pills, and Colton synthesized the first anabolic steroid.

Eichengrun developed Protargol, the highly successful anti-gonorrhea agent, which remained the standard treatment for 50 years until the adoption of antibiotics. Einhorn synthesized procaine, which he patented under the name Novocaine. Reichstein synthesized vitamin C (ascorbic acid) and later collaborated with Kendall and Hench in studying hormones of the adrenal cortex, work that culminated in the isolation of cortisone and the discovery of its therapeutic value in the treatment of rheumatoid arthritis. Fried discovered synthetic fluorosteroids, leading to the development of a new class of topical steroid compounds to treat a variety of skin diseases.

Kosterlitz and Snyder explored the opiate receptors in the brain, resulting in the development of synthetic pain-killing substitutes with diminished potential for addiction. Sternbach discovered the benzodiazepines, a class of non-sedating tranquilizers first introduced as Librium and then in an improved version named Valium.

The work of Elion and her associates resulted in the first immunosuppressive drug for kidney transplants (azathioprine), a treatment for gout (allopurinol); and an antibacterial agent for meningitis, septicemia, and infections of the urinary and respiratory tracts (Septra). They also developed the important antiviral drug acyclovir, used to treat herpes virus infections. Horwitz first synthesized the chemical compound azidothymidine to interfere with the division and growth of cancer cells. Now known as AZT, it is a major drug to combat against HIV-AIDS.

Tishler led the pharmaceutical research teams that synthesized and developed the commercial processes for the mass production of ascorbic acid, riboflavin, pyridoxine, pantothenic acid, nicotinamide, methionine, threonine, and tryptophan, as well as the production of large quantities of cortisone that opened a new era in the treatment of inflammatory diseases. Goodman showed the value and safety of curare as a muscle relaxant in some surgical procedures. Brodie discovered the effectiveness of procaine amide for treating patients with severe irregularities in heart rhythm and pioneered the concept that blood drug levels must guide therapeutic dosages. Known as the father of toxicology, Lewin developed a system of classifying psychoactive drugs according to their pharmacologic actions.

Elion, Farber, and Goodman and Gilman respectively developed 6-mer-captopurine, aminopterin, and nitrogen mustard as pioneering chemo-therapeutic agents against cancer. Rosenberg demonstrated that certain compounds containing platinum inhibited cell division and cured solid tumors, leading to the development of the chemotherapeutic agent cispla-tin. A co-founder of Biogen, Weissmann was the first to clone and express human alpha-interferon genes in *E.coli*, which led to the manufacture of a family of drugs that are used today to treat hepatitis and some forms of cancer. Goodman and Gilman authored the standard pharmacology text-book used by generations of medical students.

---

## Brodie, Bernard Beryl (England, 1907–1989)

Born in Liverpool, Bernard Brodie received a doctorate in chemistry at New York University, remaining on the faculty for 15 years until joining the National Institutes of Health in 1950 as Head of the Laboratory for Clinical Pharmacology. Retiring in 1970, Brodie remained active as a senior consultant with Hoffmann-LaRoche laboratories in Nutley, New Jersey.

Widely considered the founder of modern pharmacology and the person who brought this field to prominence in the 1940s and 1950s, Brodie was a major figure in the field of drug metabolism – the study of how drugs interact in the body and how they are absorbed. According to Brodie, his most sig-

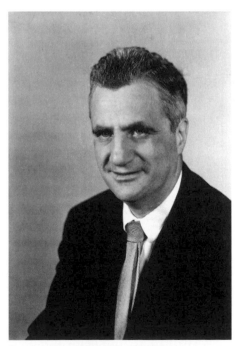

Bernard Beryl Brodie. (*NLM*)

nificant discovery was that animal and human responses to drugs do not differ significantly. He pioneered the concept that blood drug levels must guide therapeutic dosages, establishing the basis for the chemotherapy of malaria. Brodie discovered that procaine amide was effective in treating patients with severe irregularities in heart rhythm, and he developed a drug therapy for gout. Dr. Brodie was the first scientist to determine how two neurohormones, serotonin and norepinephrine, affect the functioning of the brain. This led to an understanding of how anti-psychotic drugs could be used effectively in the treatment of mental and emotional disorders.

In 1967, Brodie received the Lasker Award for Basic Research for his more than 30 years of extraordinary contributions to biochemical pharmacology. His work had a profound influence on the use of drugs in the treatment of cardiovascular diseases, mental and emotional disorders, and cancer.

## Colton, Frank Benjamin                        (Poland, 1923–2003)

Frank Colton immigrated to the United States in 1934 and received his doctorate in chemistry from the University of Chicago. Joining the G.D. Searle Company as a senior research chemist in 1952, Colton was the first to synthesize the progestin noretynodrei, which when combined with estrogen mestranol as Enovid was approved by the U.S. Food and Drug Administration in 1956 to treat menstrual disorders and then as the first oral contraceptive pill four years later. Working with Paul D. Klimstra, Colton synthesized progestine tynodiol diacetate, which combined with the estrogen mestranol as Ovulen was approved in 1965 as Searle's second oral contraceptive drug. Several years previously, Colton had synthesized norethandrolone, which under the tradename Nilevar was approved as the first oral anabolic steroid.

## Djerassi, Carl                                (Austria, 1923–2015)

Born in Vienna to physician parents, Carl Djerassi spent his first years in Sofia, Bulgaria. After his parents divorced, Carl lived with his mother in Vienna. However, when Austria refused him citizenship and after the Anschluss, his father briefly remarried his mother to allow Carl and his mother to escape the Nazi regime and flee to Sofia, where he lived with his father for a year. In 1939, Djerassi immigrated with his mother to the United States, where he eventually earned a doctorate in organic chemistry from the University of Wisconsin in Madison. His thesis examined the series of chemical reactions through which the male sex hormone testosterone could be transformed into the female sex hormone estradiol. Remaining in the pharmaceutical industry throughout this career, Djerassi served as Professor of Chemistry at Wayne State University in Detroit (1952–1959) and then at Stanford University (1960–2002).

Djerassi initially worked on developing one of the first commercial antihistamines. In 1949, Djerassi became Associate Director of Research at Syntex in Mexico City, where his team worked on a new synthesis of cortisone from a substance derived from a Mexican wild yam. At the time, it was well known that high levels of estrogen and progesterone inhibited ovulation. However, synthesizing

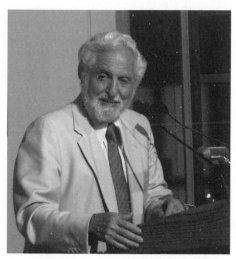

Carl Djerassi receiving the Gold Medal of the American Institute of Chemists, 2004. Photograph by Douglas A. Lockard. (*Wikimedia / Chemical Heritage Foundation*)

them from animal or plant extracts had proven expensive and ineffective for use as oral contraceptives. Djerassi and colleagues at Syntex succeeded in synthesizing norethisterone, the first highly active progestin analogue that was effective when taken by mouth and far stronger than the naturally occurring hormone. However, he was not equipped to test, produce, and distribute. First administered to animals by Gregory Goodwin Pincus and to women by John Rock, this became a key component of the first oral contraceptive (birth control pill).

In the ensuing years, Djerassi lectured widely to promote the pill. However, he faced controversies over possible side effects, including increased risks of blood clots, cancer, and excessive bleeding during menstruation. Although he dismissed such claims, the estrogen and progestin doses in the pill were later reduced to cut the risk of side effects.

## Eichengrün, Arthur (Germany, 1867–1949)

Born in Aachen, Arthur Eichengrün received a doctoral degree in chemistry at the university in his native city. In 1896, Eichengrün started working in the pharmaceutical laboratory of Bayer. Quitting twelve years later, he founded his own pharmaceutical factory, the *Cellon-Werke* in Berlin, which was taken over by the Nazis as part of their policy of "Aryanization." In 1944, Eichengrün was sent to Theresienstadt, but freed one year later when Soviet troops liberated the concentration camp.

Eichengrün developed Protargol, the highly successful anti-gonorrhea medication that remained the standard treatment for 50 years until the adoption of antibiotics. He also made pioneering contributions in plastics, co-developing (with Theodore Becker) the first safety film (cellulose diacetate), which was put into use by Eastman Kodak in 1909.

However, Eichengrün is best known as one of the two figures in the controversy over who invented aspirin. Salicylic acid, derived from

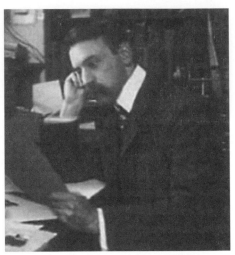

Arthur Eichengrün, circa 1900. (*Wikimedia / Aspirin and Related Drugs*, Fig. 1.7, *Google Books*)

the bark of willow trees, has long been known as having analgesic properties. However, salicylic acid is poorly tolerated by the digestive tract and therefore of limited medicinal value. Earlier attempts to reduce its toxicity by acetylation failed to produce acetylsalicylic acid sufficiently pure to be medically useful. Traditionally, the first successful synthesis of pure acetylsalicylic acid was attributed to Felix Hoffmann of Bayer in 1897. However, in 1999, Walter Sneader of the Department of Pharmaceutical Sciences at the University of Strathclyde in Glasgow re-examined the case and concluded that Eichengrün deserved credit for the invention of aspirin, since it was synthesized by a student under his direction and would not have been introduced a century earlier without his intervention.

## Einhorn, Alfred (Germany, 1856–1917)

Born in Hamburg, Alfred Einhorn, received a doctoral degree in chemistry from the University of Tübingen and spent most of his academic career at the University of Munich.

Einhorn is best known for synthesizing procaine in 1905, which he patented under the name Novocaine. Until that time, the primary local anesthetic was cocaine, which was first used for this purpose by Carl Koller in 1884. However, the toxicity and addictive quality of cocaine led scientists to search for newer anesthetics without these undesirable side effects. Although Novocaine had weaker pain-killing effects than cocaine, it was relatively safe and effective and became the standard drug for local anesthesia, especially in dentistry. However, Novocaine could trigger severe allergic reactions and was quickly replaced for non-dental purposes when Lidocaine was introduced as a local anesthetic in 1943.

---

## Elion, Gertrude Belle      (USA, 1918–1999)

Born in New York City to Lithuanian immigrant parents, Gertrude Elion graduated from Hunter College with a degree in chemistry. Even with a master's degree from New York University (she never completed a doctorate), Elion found it difficult to get a suitable position. The manpower shortage of World War II proved a boon for Elion, and after several temporary jobs she finally found a rewarding and challenging career as a research chemist at Burroughs Wellcome, a noted pharmaceutical company, where she later became as its longtime Head of Experimental Therapy.

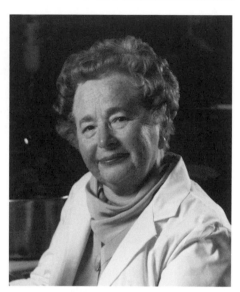

Gertrude Belle Elion. (*Wikimedia*)

In the search for new drugs that could kill or inhibit the reproduction of particular pathogens without harming the cells of the host, Elion and her associates exploited the biochemical differences between normal human cells and rapidly dividing cells such as cancer, bacteria, and viruses. She specifically used purine compounds and their derivatives to inhibit the rapid growth of pathogenic cells by blocking their synthesis of certain nucleic acids. This work resulted in the first chemotherapeutic agent for leukemia (6-mercaptopurine); the first immunosuppressive drug for kidney transplants (azathioprine), which made possible organ transplants between individuals other than identical twins; a treatment for gout (allopurinol); and an antibacterial agent for meningitis, septicemia, and infections of the urinary and respiratory tracts (Septra). Elion and colleagues also developed the important antiviral drug acyclovir, used to treat herpes virus infections. Although officially retired in 1983, Elion continued working almost full-time in her laboratory and oversaw the adaptation of AZT, which became the first drug used for the treatment of HIV-AIDS. Elion shared the 1988 Nobel Prize in Physiology or Medicine with George Hitchings (her initial supervisor at Burroughs Wellcome) and British chemist Sir James Black (discoverer of beta-blockers) "for their discoveries of important principles for drug treatment."

---

## Farber, Sidney Farber                                    (USA, 1903–1973)

---

Born in Buffalo, New York, Sidney Farber graduated from SUNY Buffalo. However, a strict quota system for Jews made it impossible for him to gain admission to an American medical school. Fluent in German, Farber was able to take his first year of medical school at the universities of Heidelberg and Freiberg. After an excellent performance in his classes, Farber was permitted to enter the second year of medical school at Harvard University. Specializing in pediatric pathology and a founder of the field, Farber became the first full-time pathologist at Children's Hospital in Boston.

Farber is often regarded as the father of modern chemotherapy for neoplastic disease. While working at Harvard Medical School on a research project funded by a grant from the American Cancer Society, Farber showed that folic acid stimulated leukemic cell growth and progression of the disease. Reasoning that folic acid antagonists would inhibit or arrest the proliferation of cancer cells, Farber carried out both the preclinical and clinical evaluation of aminopterin, a folic acid antagonist, in children with acute lymphoblastic leukemia. His studies demonstrated for the first time that it was possible to achieve clinical and hematological remission in this disease. These observations led to the development and use of other chemotherapeutic agents, such as methotrexate, which could be used singly or in combination to treat previously fatal childhood and adult malignancies. Farber also introduced actinomycin D for the treatment of localized and metastatic Wilms tumor, a pediatric cancer of the kidney. Farber received the 1966 Lasker Award in Clinical Medical Research for "therapy for childhood leukemia."

In 1947, Sidney Farber founded the Children's Cancer Research Foundation, dedicated to providing compassionate, state-of-the-art treatment for children with cancer while developing the cancer preventatives, treatments, and cures of the future. The foundation officially expanded its programs to include patients of all ages in 1969, and five years later it became known as the Sidney Farber Cancer Center. In 1983, it received its present name of the Dana-Farber Cancer Institute, acknowledging the long-term support of its activities by the Charles A. Dana Foundation.

## Fried, Josef (Poland, 1914–2001)

Born in Przemysl, Josef Fried attended universities in Leipzig and Zurich before fleeing the Nazis in 1938 and completing his doctorate in organic chemistry at Columbia University in New York. Fried worked for the Squibb Institute for Medical Research in New Brunswick, New Jersey, holding nearly 200 patents for biologically active compounds.

A pioneer in organic chemistry, Fried discovered a family of synthetic chemicals known as fluorosteroids, which led to the development of a new class of dermatological compounds used to treat everything from psoriasis to skin allergies. Prior to this time, sufferers from these dermatological conditions used coal tar, oatmeal baths, and many other unusual remedies to obtain relief. Since the advent of steroids, many afflicted with skin disease have had their symptoms dramatically reduced or even cured. Fried also suggested ways to modify the structure of steroids, resulting in topical medicines for specific diseases so that patients could avoid the side effects of oral anti-inflammatory steroid therapy. His studies of sex steroids resulted in medications used to regulate fertility, as well as some types of birth control pills and treatments to control acne in teenage girls.

After nearly 20 years at Squibb, Fried became a professor at the University of Chicago, where he worked on the synthesis of highly active hormone regulators called prostaglandins. This laid the foundation for the development of compounds used to treat pulmonary artery hypertension and clogged arteries in the legs.

## Gilman, Alfred Zack (USA, 1908–1984)

Born in Bridgeport, Connecticut, Alfred Gilman received a doctorate in Physiological Chemistry from Yale University and then joined the pharmacology faculty, where he taught courses with Louis Goodman. The two began to develop a popular textbook, first published as *The Pharmacological Basis of Therapeutics* (1941), which in multiple editions has been the standard classic for generations of medical students.

While at Yale, in 1942 Gilman and Goodman were recruited by the US Department of Defense to conduct research on possible therapeutic applications of mustard gas. This devastating chemical warfare agent had been used in World War 1, but was banned by the Geneva Protocol in 1925. Observing that mustard gas was too volatile an agent to be suitable for laboratory experiments, Gilman and Goodman exchanged a nitrogen molecule for sulfur to produce a more stable compound, nitrogen mustard (mechlorethamine). A year after the start of their research, a German air raid in Bari, Italy, led to more than 1,000 people being exposed to mustard gas bombs. Stewart Francis Alexander, an expert in chemical warfare called in by the US Army to investigate the situation, determined that the victims had severe suppression of their white blood cells. Noting that the chem-

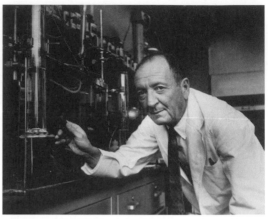

Photograph of Alfred Zack Gilman by Ted Burrows, 1963. (*Wikimedia / American Society for Pharmacology and Experimental Therapeutics*)

ical agent seemed to primarily affect rapidly growing cells, Alexander proposed that this property might suppress the division of certain types of cancerous cells. Gilman and Goodman reasoned that nitrogen mustard could be used to treat lymphoma. After a series of experiments in mice, they arranged for nitrogen mustard to be injected into a patient with radiation-resistant lymphoma and demonstrated a dramatic decrease in the tumor mass. Although this effect lasted only a few weeks, requiring that the patient return for another set of treatment, this and subsequent use of nitrogen mustard in additional patients with radiation-resistant lymphatic malignancies was the first indication that cancer could be treated by pharmacological agents. Nitrogen mustard became a model for the discovery of other classes of anticancer drugs, and chemotherapy became a standard treatment for many cancers, often in combination with surgery and radiation.

Gilman's son, Alfred, whose middle name was taken from Louis Goodman, followed his father into pharmacology and was awarded the 1994 Nobel Prize in Physiology or Medicine.

---

**Goodman, Louis Sanford**                                    (USA, 1906–2000)

---

Born in Portland, Oregon, Louis Goodman studied medicine at the University of Oregon and joined the faculty of the Yale University School of Medicine. There Goodman met Alfred Gilman, Sr., with whom he taught pharmacology courses. They also began to develop a popular textbook, first published as *The Pharmacological Basis of Therapeutics* (1941), which in multiple editions has been the standard classic for generations of medical students.

While at Yale, in 1942 Goodman and Gilman were recruited by the US Department of Defense to conduct research on possible therapeutic applications of mustard gas. This devastating chemical warfare agent had been used in World War 1, but was banned by the Geneva Protocol in 1925. Observing that mustard gas was too volatile an agent to be suitable for laboratory experiments, Goodman and Gilman exchanged a nitrogen molecule for sulfur to produce a more stable compound, nitrogen mustard (mechlorethamine). A

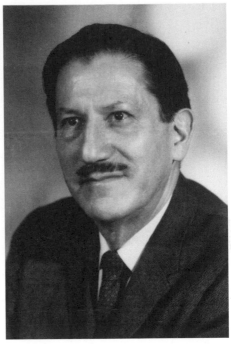

Louis Sanford Goodman. (*Wikimedia / NLM*)

year after the start of their research, a German air raid in Bari, Italy, led to more than 1,000 people being exposed to mustard gas bombs. Stewart Francis Alexander, an expert in chemical warfare called in by the US Army to investigate the situation, determined that the victims had severe suppression of their white blood cells. Noting that the chemical agent seemed to primarily affect rapidly growing cells, Alexander proposed that this property might suppress the division of certain types of cancerous cells. Goodman and Gilman reasoned that nitrogen mustard could be used to treat lymphoma. After a series of experiments in mice, they arranged for nitrogen mustard to be injected into a patient with radiation-resistant lymphoma and demonstrated a dramatic decrease in the tumor mass. Although this effect lasted only a few weeks, requiring that the patient return for another set of treatment, this and subsequent use of nitrogen mustard in additional patients with radiation-resistant lymphatic malignancies was the first indication that cancer could be treated by pharmacological agents. Nitrogen mustard became a model for the discovery of other classes of anticancer drugs, and chemotherapy became a standard treatment for many cancers, often in combination with surgery and radiation.

Goodman later became the Chair of Pharmacology and Physiology at the University of Vermont and then at the University of Utah, where he performed a daring experiment. The profound muscle relaxant property effects of curare, used by South American Indians as a poison, were well known. However, curare and similar drugs were rarely used clinically because of the fear that they would lead to permanent paralysis. Goodman and his team totally paralyzed Scott Smith, the Chair of Anesthesia, with curare and showed that that the effect was only temporary. The experiment demonstrated that curare does not alter consciousness, and that additional anesthetic agents were needed because curare does not kill pain. Curare and other muscle relaxants produce their effect with a minimal concentration of anesthetic agent. This allows patients to recover quickly and reduces the risk of postoperative pneumonia and other complications associated with surgery under general anesthesia.

## Horwitz, Jerome Phillip                                    (USA, 1919–2012)

Born in Detroit, Jerome Horwitz received a doctorate in chemistry from the University of Michigan. Horwitz joined Wayne State University as a medical researcher in 1956 and remained there for almost five decades. He also was on the staff of its affiliated institution now known as the Bar-

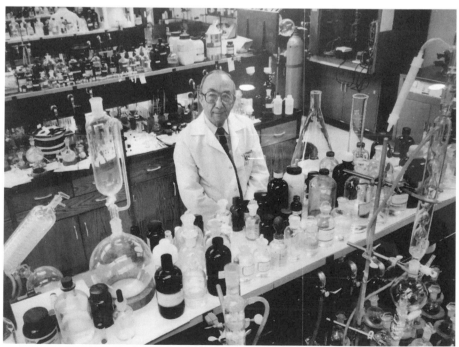

Jerome Phillip Horwitz in his laboratory. (*Courtesy of the Horwitz Family*)

bara Ann Karmanos Cancer Institute, and was later appointed Professor of Internal Medicine in the Oncology Division.

As director of chemistry at the oncology center, in 1960 Horwitz first synthesized the chemical compound azidothymidine to interfere with the division and growth of cancer cells. However, when this inhibiter of the viral enzyme reverse transcriptase failed to cure mice with leukemia, Horwitz wrote a paper on the topic, decided not to pursue a patent, and put the compound on a shelf.

Two decades later, as the AIDS epidemic claimed thousands of victims, the urgency for a cure increased. The pharmaceutical company Burroughs Wellcome began testing chemical compounds that would possibly hinder the then-untreatable human immunodeficiency virus (HIV). One of these was Horwitz's semi-forgotten anti-viral azidothymidine. After tests in animals, in 1985 the Food and Drug Administration deliberated for only one week before agreeing to allow human testing. Two years later, the FDA licensed the commercial distribution of this first AIDS treatment, now known as AZT, which significantly decreased HIV-related mortality rates. AZT later was combined with other less toxic drugs that curbed deaths even further.

Burroughs Wellcome patented and marketed AZT, earning billions of dollars because of Horwitz's work. Although the company established a chair at Wayne State in Horwitz's name, the chemist never shared a penny of the profits.

---

**Kosterlitz, Hans Walter** (Germany, 1903–1996)

---

Born in Berlin and a graduate of the medical school at the University of Berlin, Hans Kosterlitz fled to Scotland when the Nazis seized power in Germany. He joined the staff at Aberdeen University, later serving as Professor of Pharmacology and Chemistry and from 1973 the director of the university's drug addiction research unit.

Kosterlitz is best known for his pioneering work in exploring the opiate receptors in the brain, first described by Solomon Snyder. Kosterlitz proposed that the real function of these opiate receptors was not their interaction with alien alkaloids of the opium poppy, such as morphine, but with compounds having similar actions that naturally occur in the nervous system of animals and human beings. This led Kosterlitz to discover and determine the chemical structure of two enkephalins, opiate-like substances in the brain that serve as neurotransmitters of messages relating to pain and emotional behavior. Kosterlitz was awarded (with Snyder) the 1978

Lasker Award for Basic Medical Research Award for his "early and innovative contributions that have major implications for understanding the natural factors that influence pain, narcotic addiction, and the emotions . . . and which have resulted in the development of synthetic pain-killing substitutes with diminished potential for addiction."[38]

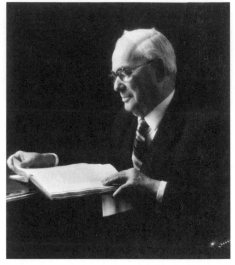

Hans Walter Kosterlitz. (*NLM / Lasker Award Archives*)

## Lewin, Louis                                                   (Germany, 1850–1929)

Born in the West Prussian town of Tuchel, Louis Lewin received his medical degree from the University of Berlin. Lewin became an assistant at the Pharmacological Institute of the university. Later, Lewin was admitted to the medical faculty as *privatdozent*, and in 1897 was appointed professor.

Lewin published the first methodical analysis of the peyote cactus (1886), a variant of which was named *Anhalonium lewinii* in his honor. He is best known as the founder of toxicology for developing a system for classifying psychoactive drugs and plants according to their pharmacologic action. His original five categories were: Inebriantia (Inebriants, such as alcohol or ether); Exitantia (Stimu-

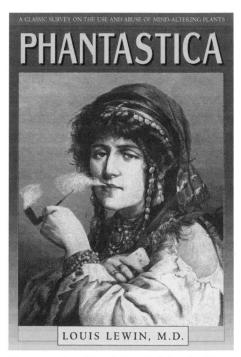

Front cover of Louis Lewin's book, *Phantastica*. (*Amazon.com*)

38. http://www.laskerfoundation.org/awards/show/opiate-receptors-and-enkephalins/.

lants, such as khat or amphetamine); Euphorica (Euphoriants or Narcotics, such as heroin); Hypnotica (tranquilizers such as kava); and Phantastica (Hallucinogens or Entheogens, such as peyote or ayahuasca).

## Pereira, Jonathan (England, 1804–1853)

Born in London and originally trained as a pharmacist, Jonathan Pereira was a physician who was appointed Professor of Materia Medica and lecturer in chemistry at the new Aldersgate Medical School. He also was a popular lecturer on pharmacology at the London Hospital.

Pereira concentrated his research on so-called "crude drugs" – naturally occurring, unrefined substances derived from organic or inorganic sources such as plant, animal, bacteria, organs, or entire organisms intended for use in the diagnosis, cure, mitigation, treatment, or prevention of disease in humans or other animals. He

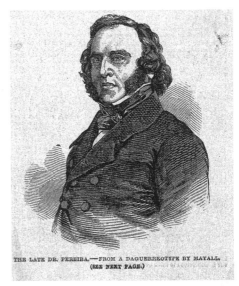

THE LATE DR. PEREIRA.—FROM A DAGUERREOTYPE BY MAYALL.
(SEE NEXT PAGE.)

Wood engraving of Jonathan Pereira from a daguerreotype by Mayall. (*Wikimedia / Wellcome Trust*)

transformed this extensive knowledge into *Materia Medica* (1842), the first great English work on pharmacology. Pereira's colleagues recognized his contribution to the scientific usage of drugs by electing him as a Fellow of the Royal Society.

## Pincus, Gregory Goodwin (USA, 1903–1967)

Born in Woodbine, New Jersey, and the son of Polish immigrants, Gregory Pincus received his doctoral degree from Harvard University. Pincus pursued postgraduate research studies at Cambridge University in England and at the Kaiser Wilhelm Institute for Biology in Berlin, where he began to investigate steroid control of reproductive cycles.

In 1934, Pincus made national headlines by achieving in-vitro fertilization of rabbits. However, this accomplishment, coming soon after the publication of Aldous Huxley's *Brave New World*, produced a vision of test-tube rabbits and brought him notoriety rather than fame, resulting in Pincus being denied tenure at Harvard. After several teaching appointments, in 1944 Pincus cofounded (with Hudson Hoagland of nearby Clark University) the Worcester Foundation for Experimental Biology in Shrewsbury, Massachusetts.

After meeting him at a dinner, Margaret Sanger (vice president of Planned Parenthood) offered Pincus a small grant to begin research on a new form of hormonal contraceptive research. He and associate Min Chueh Chang performed studies confirming earlier research showing that repeated injections of

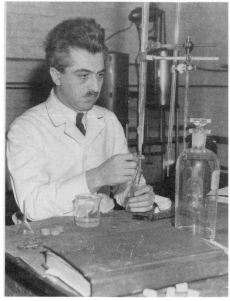

Gregory Goodwin Pincus. (*History of Medicine Collections, David M. Rubenstein Rare Book & Manuscript Library, Duke University, Durham, NC, USA*)

progesterone, which is present in increased amounts during pregnancy, stopped ovulation in animals. Fortuitously, two drug companies had recently created orally effective forms of synthetic progesterone. They allowed Pincus and fertility specialist John Rock to use them in clinical testing, initially in Puerto Rico, which showed the pill to be virtually 100% effective in preventing conception. The oral contraceptive pill was simple and safe and revolutionized family planning.

---

## Reichstein, Tadeus                          (Poland, 1897–1996)

---

Born in Włocławek, Tadeus Reichstein moved with his family to Kiev. In the wake of anti-Semitic pogroms, the family left Russia and arrived in Basel, Switzerland, when Reichstein was age 8. After receiving a degree in chemistry from E.T.H. (Swiss Federal Institute of Technology) in Zurich, Reichstein spent nine years researching the composition of the aromatic and flavoring substances in roasted coffee and chicory, which he discovered was a complex problem and resulted in a series of articles.

In 1933, Reichstein succeeded, independently of Sir Norman Haworth and his collaborators in Birmingham, UK, in synthesizing vitamin C (ascorbic acid), using what is now called the Reichstein process. He isolated and explained the constitution of aldosterone, a hormone of the adrenal cortex, and later collaborated with Edward C. Kendall and Philip. S. Hench in their work on the hormones of the adrenal cortex, which culminated in the isolation of cortisone and the discovery of its therapeutic value in the treatment of rheumatoid arthritis. For this work, Reichstein, Kendall, and Hench shared the 1950 Nobel Prize in Physiology or Medicine.

---

**Rosenberg, Barnett** (USA, 1926–2009)

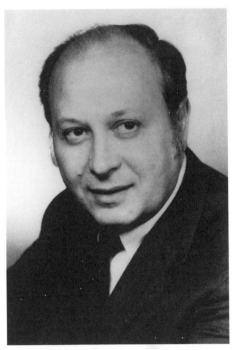

Born in New York City and receiving his doctorate in Physics from New York University, Barnett Rosenberg joined the faculty of Michigan State University in 1961 and remained on the faculty for more than 35 years. While investigating the effects of an electric field on the growth of bacteria, Rosenberg observed that bacteria ceased to divide when placed in an electric field. He eventually realized that the cause of this phenomenon was the platinum electrode he was using. Rosenberg subsequently demonstrated that certain compounds containing platinum inhibited cell division and cured solid tumors. His work eventually resulted in development of the chemotherapeutic agent cisplatin, which was approved by the FDA in 1978 and became a widely used drug to treat cancer.

Barnett Rosenberg. (*Wikimedia / National Cancer Institute*)

---

**Snyder, Solomon Halbert** (USA, 1938–)

Born in Washington, DC, Solomon Snyder received his medical degree from Georgetown University. After serving two years as a research associate at the National Institutes of Health, Snyder completed a psychiatry residency at Johns Hopkins University and remained on the faculty, rising to professorships in both pharmacology and psychiatry.

In researching addiction and its effects on the brain, Snyder discovered the opioid receptors in the mammalian nervous system, the major neurotransmitters in the brain. He mapped their regional distribution and explained the actions of psychoactive drugs, such as the blockade of dopamine receptors by antipsychotic medications. Snyder also described novel neurotransmitters such as the gases nitric oxide and carbon monoxide and the D-isomers of amino acids, notably D-serine, and identified the role of sodium in the differentiation of opiate ag-

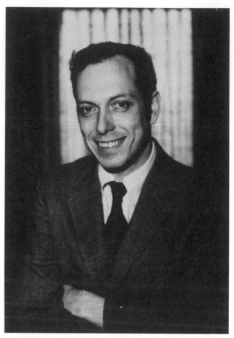

Solomon Halbert Snyder, 1979. (*NLM / Lasker Award Archives*)

onists from antagonists. For his demonstration of the nature and distribution of the opiate receptors in the brain and a series of follow-up studies that illuminated the importance of this system in human physiology, Snyder received (with Hans Kosterlitz) the 1978 Lasker Award for Basic Medical Research.

---

## Sternbach, Leo Henryk                    (Croatia, 1908–2005)

---

Born in Opatia, Leo Sternbach received his doctoral degree in organic chemistry from the Jagiellonian University in Krakow, Poland. Sternbach worked for the large pharmaceutical company Hoffmann-La Roche in Basel, Switzerland. In 1941, fearful of a possible Nazi invasion, the company arranged to transfer Sternbach and other Jewish scientists in its employ to offices in the United States. Therefore, Sternbach's discoveries took place at the Roche research laboratory in Nutley, New Jersey.

Sternbach initially discovered a way to synthesize biotin (vitamin H), which is important for strengthening nails and hair, and he also worked on anesthetics for bloodless surgery. By the mid-1950s, Roche assigned Sternbach to work on a tranquilizer that could compete with

Miltown, made by its competitor Wallace Laboratories, which was the first major anti-anxiety drug but had substantial side effects. After extensive investigations, Sternbach discovered the benzodiazepines, a class of non-sedating tranquilizers. First introduced as Librium in 1960, three years later Roche released an improved version named Valium, which from 1969–1982 was the most prescribed drug in the United States. In its peak year of 1978, some 2.3 billion doses of Valium were sold. Although having few side effects and non-toxic, Valium was later shown to be addictive.

In all, Sternbach held 241 patents, and his discoveries helped turn Roche into a pharmaceutical industry giant.

## Stokvis, Barend Joseph (Netherlands, 1834–1902)

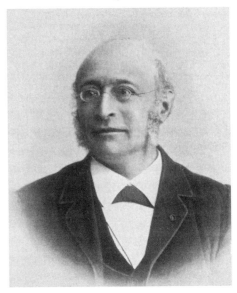

Barend Joseph Stokvis was the most prominent of Holland's major medical dynasty. After studies in medicine at the universities of Amsterdam and Utrecht, Stokvis established a medical practice in Amsterdam and became Professor of Physiology and Pharmacology at the University of Amsterdam. Stokvis made valuable contributions to the understanding of diabetes and cholera, the metabolism of glycogen and uric acid, and the toxicity of atropine and the nature of heart sounds. Recognized as an expert in tropical medicine and a renowned medical educator,

Barend Joseph Stokvis. (*NLM*)

Stokvis is best known for his description of an acute illness provoked by the newly introduced hypnotic drug sulfonmethane. Observing the patient's unusual dark red urine, he discovered that it contained porphyrins and coined the name "porphyria" for the condition. The patient was probably suffering from acute intermittent porphyria, which is now known to be provoked by various medications.

Stokvis authored a major textbook in pharmacology. Elected a member of the Royal Netherlands Academy of Arts and Sciences, Stokvis was one of the founders (in 1896) of *Janus*, an international journal for the history of medicine. Together with Samuel Siegmund Rosenstein, Professor of Medicine in Leiden, Stokvis was a supporter of Aletta Jacobs, the first woman to qualify as a doctor in the Netherlands.

In addition to his medical work, Stokvis succeeded his father as president of the charitable Jewish Poor Board of Amsterdam, was a member-founder of the Dutch Jewish Institute for the Insane, and a board member of the Jewish Institute for the Aged and the Amsterdam Jewish Hospital.

## Tishler, Max (USA, 1906–1989)

Born in Boston and earning a doctorate in inorganic chemistry from Harvard University, Max Tishler was president of Merck Sharp and Dohme Research Laboratories. He led the pharmaceutical research teams that synthesized and developed the commercial processes for the mass production of ascorbic acid, riboflavin, pyridoxine, pantothenic acid, nicotinamide, methionine, threonine, and tryptophan. The ability of Merck to provide large quantities of cortisone opened a new era in the treatment of inflammatory diseases. Tishler also developed the fermentation processes for actinomycin, vitamin $B_{12}$, streptomycin, and penicillin.

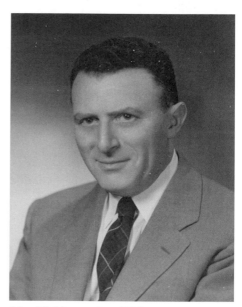

Max Tishler, 1987. (*Wikimedia / National Science and Technology Medals Foundation*)

## Vane, John Robert (England, 1927–2004)

Born in Tardebigge, Worcestershire, John Vane was the son of a Russian Jewish immigrant and a local English woman. Vane obtained his doctorate in pharmacology from Oxford University and joined the Institute of Basic Medical Sciences at the University of London, rising to Professor of Experimental Pharmacology at the Royal College of Surgeons in 1966.

Vane focused much of his research on how aspirin produces pain relief and anti-inflammatory effects. He demonstrated that aspirin blocks the action of prostaglandins, a group of physiologically active lipid compounds that have effects on circulation, inflammation, and control of muscular contractions. There are two major classes of prostaglandins affecting blood vessels and clotting. Prostacyclins are powerful locally acting vasodilators and inhibit the aggregation of blood platelets, thus preventing needless clot formation and regulating the contraction of smooth muscle tissue. In contrast, thromboxanes (produced by platelet cells) are vasoconstrictors

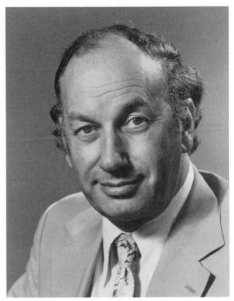

John Robert Vane. (*Wikimedia*)

and facilitate platelet aggregation and clot formation (thrombosis). Vane demonstrated that a small dose of aspirin (75 mg per day) could decrease blood clotting by blocking the prostaglandin thromboxane in platelets, leading to new treatments for heart and blood vessels disease to prevent heart attacks and strokes. This work resulted in Vane sharing (with Sune Bergström and Bengt Samuelsson) the 1982 Nobel Prize in Physiology or Medicine "for their discoveries concerning prostaglandins and related biologically active substances." Vane had shared the 1977 Lasker Award in Basic Medical Research for "prostaglandins as hormone-like regulators."

Vane also performed important research on angiotensin-converting enzyme (ACE) inhibitors, pharmaceuticals used primarily for the treatment of hypertension and congestive heart failure. These drugs relax blood vessels and decrease blood volume, thus lowering blood pressure and decreasing oxygen demand on the heart.

## Weissmann, Charles (Hungary, 1931–)

Born in Budapest, Charles Weissmann earned doctoral degrees in both medicine and organic chemistry from the University of Zurich. He then entered the new field of molecular biology, co-founding the biotech company Biogen in Geneva. Previously Director of the Institute for Molecular Biology in Zurich and President of the Roche Research Foundation,

Weissmann is currently Chairman of the Department of Infectology at the Scripps Research Institute in Florida.

Weissmann was the first to clone and express human alpha-interferon genes in *E.coli*. This discovery led to the manufacture of a family of drugs that are used today to treat hepatitis and some forms of cancer. Also an important contributor to understanding the life cycle of RNA bacterio-phages, Weissmann developed site-directed mutagenesis and reverse ge-netics. In recent years, Weissmann has made breakthroughs in the investi-gation of diseases caused by prions (small proteinaceous infectious particles that resist inactivation by procedures that modify nucleic acids), which affect both animals ("mad cow" disease) and humans (Creutzfeldt-Jacob disease).

## PHYSIOLOGY

Loewi, Katz, and Axelrod proved the existence of chemical messengers, now called neurotransmitters (the first one identified being acetylcho-line), which transmit nerve impulses linking motor neurons to muscles and stimulate contractions that regulate both the sympathetic and parasym-pathetic portions of the autonomic nervous systems. While studying how analgesics (pain killers) work, Axelrod discovered acetaminophen, which is now marketed as Tylenol. Greengard discovered how dopamine and other transmitters exert their action in the nervous system, while Kandel investigated the physiological basis of memory storage and its implications for normal and abnormal behavior. Erlanger and Gasser discovered the highly differentiated function of single nerve fibers. Traube investigated the effect of the vagus nerve on pulmonary function, while Schiff showed the effect of the vagus nerve on heart function. Van Deen proved that the dorsal columns in the spinal cord convey sensory impulses and the anterior columns motor impulses, while Stern described the blood–brain barrier.

Heidenhain demonstrated the process by which muscles self-regulate their expenditure of energy. Zuntz carried out experiments to examine human physiology in extreme environments and was the founding father of modern aerospace medicine. Evans described the unifying mechanism through which hormones control body metabolism, embryonic develop-ment, and reproduction. Levi-Montalcini discovered nerve growth fac-tor (NGF), released by tumor tissue, while her colleague Stanley Cohen discovered epidermal growth factor (EGF). Valentin demonstrated the function of the pancreas and its secretions in the digestion of food, Schiff showed the restoration to the liver of bile salts passing through the intestine, and Wald identified vitamin A in the retina of the eye and demonstrated that it is essential for retinal function. Cyon developed new methods and techniques in physiological experiments that served as a guide in many European medical centers.

## Axelrod, Julius (USA, 1912–2004)

Born in New York City to Polish immigrant parents, Julius Axelrod received a bachelor's degree in biology from City College of New York, but was rejected from every medical school to which he applied. After working briefly as a laboratory technician at New York University, Axelrod was hired by the New York City Department of Health and Mental Hygiene to test adding vitamin supplements to food. He attended night school and received a master's degree in

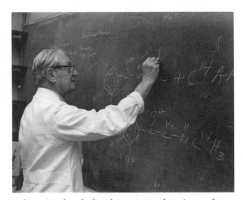

Julius Axelrod checking a student's work on the chemistry of catecholamine reactions in nerve cells. (*Wikimedia / NIH*)

science from New York University. Unfortunately, an exploding ammonia bottle in his laboratory injured his eye, forcing Axelrod to wear an eyepatch for the rest of his life.

In 1946, Axelrod began research work under Bernard Brodie at Goldwater Memorial Hospital on how analgesics (pain killers) work. Investigating cases of blood abnormalities developing in patients using non-aspirin analgesics, they discovered that the culprit was its main ingredient, acetanilide. At the same time, they found that one of the metabolites also was an analgesic (acetaminophen, given the trade name Tylenol), recommending that it be used instead.

Three years later, Axelrod began work at the National Heart Institute, focusing on the mechanisms and effects of caffeine. This led him to investigate the sympathetic nervous system and its main neurotransmitters, epinephrine and norepinephrine. During this time, Axelrod also conducted research on codeine, morphine, methamphetamine, and ephedrine, as well as performing some of the first experiments on LSD. Realizing that he could not advance his career without a doctorate, Axelrod requested a leave of absence to attend George Washington University, where he succeeded in earning a Ph.D. in one year when he was permitted to submit some of his previous research toward his degree.

Axelrod shared (with Bernard Katz and Ulf von Euler) the 1970 Nobel Prize in Physiology or Medicine "for their discoveries concerning the humoral transmitters in the nerve terminals and the mechanism for their storage, release and inactivation." Working on monoamine oxidase (MAO) inhibitors, Axelrod showed that the catecholamines in the brain (epinephrine, norepinephrine, and the later-discovered dopamine) continue to produce their effects after being released into the synapse through a process whereby they are recaptured (taken up again) by the pre-synaptic nerve ending and recycled for later transmissions. Axelrod proposed that epinephrine is held in tissues in an inactive form and released by the nervous system when needed. This research paved the way for the discovery of selective serotonin re-uptake inhibitors, such as Prozac, which block the re-uptake of another neurotransmitter, serotonin.

Axelrod also made important contributions to understanding the sleep-wake cycle and the role of the pineal gland as a biological clock. He showed that the hormone melatonin, derived like serotonin from tryptophan, enables the pineal to regulate the release of serotonin and thus control the circadian rhythm of the body.

---

**Cyon, Elias von**                                    (Russia, 1843–1912)

Born Ilya Fadeyevich Tsion in what is now Lithuania, Cyon graduated from medical school at the University of Kiev and later studied in Berlin and France. In 1870, Cyon became the first Jewish professor in Russia, when he was appointed as the Chair of Physiology at the University of St. Petersburg. Two years later, Cyon became Professor at the Medico-Surgical Academy in St. Petersburg, where he reformed the teaching of physiol-

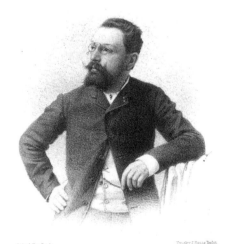

Lithograph of Elias von Cyon by Georg Engelbach, circa 1880. (*Wikimedia / Gesammelte physiologische arbeiten, 1888*)

ogy by introducing the method of illustrative experiments. The victim of political intrigues and student protests related to his political views, Cyon was forced to resign from the Academy and relocate to Paris, becoming a French citizen and working with famed physiologist Claude Bernard.

Cyon published original work on the physiology of the nervous system and the heart, the mechanism of blood pressure, the application of electrotherapy, and a monograph on the inner ear. His treatise on new methods and techniques in physiological experiments served as a guide in many European medical centers. His name is associated with "Cyon's nerve" (aortic nerve), a branch of the vagus nerve that is composed entirely of afferent fibers and terminates in the aortic arch and base of the heart.

Converting to Catholicism in 1908, Cyon later testified for the prosecution in a blood-libel case and was a supporter of anti-Semitic causes.

---

**Erlanger, Joseph** (USA, 1874–1965)

Born in San Francisco, the son of Jewish immigrants from Germany, Joseph Erlanger received his medical degree from Johns Hopkins University in Baltimore, remaining on the faculty for several years. In 1906, Erlanger moved to the University of Wisconsin in Madison, where he began collaborating in research with one of his students, Herbert Gasser. Four years later, Erlanger became the first Chair of Physiology at the Washington University in Saint Louis, where he and Gasser embarked on studies of the effect of electronics on physiological investigations.

Although much of Erlanger's early work dealt with the physiology of the circulatory system, he and Gasser began focusing their efforts on neurosciences. They modified a Western Electric cathode-ray oscilloscope to run at low voltages, which allowed them to observe small amounts of neural activity. Erlanger and Gasser observed that action potentials occurred in two phases – a spike (initial surge) followed by an after-spike (a sequence of slow changes in potential). In addition, they discovered that there were many forms of neurons (nerve cells), each with their own function and potential for excitability, and that the velocity of action potentials was directly proportional to the diameter of the nerve fiber. Erlanger and Gasser shared the 1944 Nobel Prize in Physiology or Medicine "for their discoveries relating to the highly differentiated function of single nerve fibers."

## Evans, Ronald Mark

(USA, 1949–)

Born in Los Angeles, Ronald Evans received his doctoral degree in microbiology at UCLA and joined the Salk Institute and the Department of Biology, Biomedical Sciences, and Neuroscience at UCSD. He is currently Professor in the Gene Expression Laboratory and March of Dimes Chair in Molecular and Developmental Neurobiology at the Salk Institute.

Evans is best known for discovering and isolating the first of a series of gene control switches that have widespread medical significance as a blueprint for the development of drugs for a broad spectrum of medical problems including inflammation, diabetes, heart disease, and cancer. Evans shared (with Pierre Chambon and Elwood Jensen) the 2004 Lasker Award in Basic Science Research for their combined discovery of the superfamily of nuclear hormone receptors and the unifying mechanism through which hormones control body metabolism, embryonic development, and reproduction.

## Gasser, Herbert Spencer

(USA, 1888–1963)

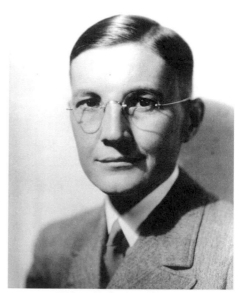

Born in Platteville, Wisconsin, Herbert Gasser received his undergraduate degree and began his medical studies at the University of Wisconsin. There he studied physiology under Joseph Erlanger, with whom he later collaborated on major projects. After finishing his clinical studies at Johns Hopkins University, Gasser eventually joined the faculty at Washington University in St. Louis (where he was reunited with Erlanger) and became Professor of Pharmacology in 1921.

After some initial work related to blood coagulation, Gasser and Erlanger began focusing their efforts on neurosciences. They modified a Western Electric cathode-ray oscilloscope to run at low voltages, which allowed them to observe small

Herbert Spencer Gasser. (*The Rockefeller University*)

amounts of neural activity. Gasser and Erlanger observed that action potentials occurred in two phases – a spike (initial surge) followed by an after-spike (a sequence of slow changes in potential). In addition, they discovered that there were many forms of neurons (nerve cells), each with their own function and potential for excitability, and that the velocity of action potentials was directly proportional to the diameter of the nerve fiber. Gasser and Erlanger shared the 1944 Nobel Prize in Physiology or Medicine "for their discoveries relating to the highly differentiated function of single nerve fibers."

In 1931, Gasser moved to New York City to become Professor of Physiology at Cornell Medical College. Four years later, Gasser was named the second Director of the Rockefeller Institute for Medical Research, succeeding the long-running tenure of founder Simon Flexner, and he remained in that position until 1953.

## Greengard, Paul (USA, 1925–)

Born in New York City, Paul Greengard received his doctoral degree from Johns Hopkins University in the field of molecular and cellular function of neurons. Greengard's major academic positions have been at Yale University and Rockefeller University.

Greengard shared (with Arvid Carlsson and Eric Kandel) the 2000 Nobel Prize for Physiology or Medicine. He was recognized for discovering how dopamine and other transmitters exert their action in the nervous system. Greengard showed that the neural transmitter initially acts on a receptor on the cell surface, which then triggers a cascade of reactions that affect a set of "key proteins," which in turn regulate specific functions within the nerve cell. These proteins undergo a change in shape and function due to the addition or removal of phosphate groups, a mechanism that enables the transmitters to carry their messages from one nerve cell to another. Disturbances in this signal transduction mechanism can result in neurological and psychiatric diseases, and an understanding of this system has the potential to permit the development of new drugs to treat them.

## Heidenhain, Rudolf Peter Heinrich (Germany, 1834–1897)

The son of a Jewish doctor who converted to Protestantism shortly before his birth, Rudolf Heidenhain studied medicine at the Universities of Halle and Berlin. In 1859, Heidenhain was appointed as the Chair of Physiology at the University of Breslau, where he remained for the rest of his career. His laboratory produced voluminous contributions by himself, his pupils, and his assistants.

Heidenhain is best known for his research on muscle and nerve physiology. In his doctoral dissertation, Heidenhain refuted the view of Moritz Schiff that the vagus nerve initiates the rhythmic contractions of the heart, showing that its real function is to regulate heart activity that he believed to originate in the ganglia of the heart. Heidenhain demonstrated the process by which muscles self-regulate their expenditure of

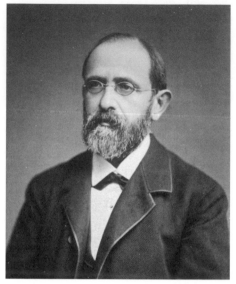

Photograph of Rudolf Heidenhain by N. Raschkow from Breslau. (*Wikimedia*)

energy. He showed that a muscle's total output of energy (heat and mechanical work) increases with an increased load (i.e., when resistance to its contraction is greater). In addition, when a muscle is fatigued, it has the ability to work more economically. In studying the production of heat during muscular activity, Heidenhain was able to detect and measure a small increase in temperature during the slightest muscular movement.

Heidenhain also investigated the secretory and absorption processes of the glands in the stomach. He demonstrated that there were two distinct types of cells in the gastric glands, one that secreted the enzyme pepsin and the other that secreted hydrochloric acid. He also embarked on systematic studies of the function of the pancreatic and mammary glands and the lymph nodes. After witnessing a public performance by a hypnotist and the power of suggestion, Heidenhain conducted scientific experiments on the physiologic mechanisms of "animal magnetism."

## Kandel, Eric Richard                                              (Austria, 1929–)

Born in Vienna, at age 9 Eric Kandel and his brother escaped the German occupation of their homeland by boat to join their uncle in Brooklyn, and they were later followed by their parents. Tutored in Judaic studies by his grandfather, Kandel graduated from the Yeshiva of Flatbush. Kandel studied medicine at New York University School and spent three years at the National Institutes of Health before taking a residency in clinical psychiatry at Harvard Medical School. After several years in a newly formed neurophysiology group at New York University, in 1972 Kandel moved to Columbia University as founding Director of its Center for Neurobiology and Behavior.

Kandel's research focused on the biological basis of memory and its implications for normal and abnormal behavior. He performed the first intracellular recordings of individual nerve cells in the portion of the brain believed to govern memory in an attempt to establish the physiological and molecular basis of this crucial function of the brain. Kandel initially focused on the relatively simple Mediter-

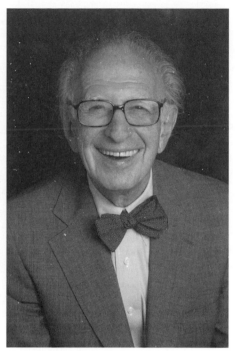

Eric Richard Kandel. (*Courtesy of Dr. Kandel*)

ranean sea snail, *Aplysia*, which has nerve cells that are especially large and well-suited to laboratory studies. He later progressed to the memory center (hippocampus) in mice, because he believed that only simple systems would give insight into understanding the incredibly complex function of consciousness in humans. In his research, Kandel ended previous speculation by clearly establishing that memory involves the connections between nerve cells and the patterns of protein synthesis within them.

Kandel shared (with Arvid Carlsson and Paul Greengard) the 2000 Nobel Prize in Physiology or Medicine for his research on the physiological basis of memory storage in neurons. He demonstrated the molecular mechanisms for modifying the efficiency of synapses, which is central for learning and memory. To generate short-term memory, Kendal showed the important role of adding phosphate groups to proteins. Development of long-term memory also requires a change in protein synthesis, which can lead to alterations in shape and function of the synapse.

## Katz, Bernard                                    (Germany, 1911–2003)

Born in Leipzig to a Jewish family originally from Russia, Bernard Katz earned a medical degree from the university in his native city. Graduating in 1934, Katz fled Germany to escape the rise of Nazism and moved to London, where he finished his doctorate in biophysics. After serving in the Pacific in World War II, Katz returned to University College London. In 1952, he became the Head of Biophysics, remaining in that position throughout the rest of his career,

Katz uncovered fundamental properties of synapses, the junctions across which nerve cells signal to each other and to other types of cells. He studied the biochemistry and action of acetylcholine, a molecule found in synapses, which links motor neurons to muscles and stimulates contractions. Katz

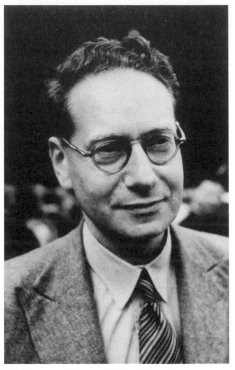

Sir Bernard Katz, FRS. (*The Physiological Society*)

discovered the "quantal" nature of neurotransmitter release. This means that at any particular synapse, the amount of neurotransmitter released is never less than a certain amount; if more, it is always an integral number times that amount. Today, it is understood that this phenomenon occurs because transmitter molecules are situated in subcellular packages (synaptic vesicles) before being released across a synapse. Moreover, in the post-war period, it was shown that organophosphates and organochlorines used as nerve agents and pesticides act by disrupting the complex enzyme cycle at the neuromuscular synapses.

Katz shared (with Julius Axelrod and Ulf von Euler) the 1970 Nobel Prize in Physiology or Medicine "for their discoveries concerning the humoral transmitters in the nerve terminals and the mechanism for their storage, release and inactivation." He was knighted by Queen Elizabeth in the same year.

## Levi-Montalcini, Rita (Italy, 1909–2012)

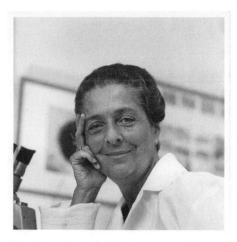

Rita Levi-Montalcini, circa 1975. (*Bernard Becker Medical Library, Washington University School of Medicine, St. Louis, MO*)

Born in Turin to a wealthy Sephardic family, Rita Levi-Montalcini received her medical degree from the University of Turin. She remained at the university until the 1938 laws barring Jews from academic and professional careers. Inspired by neurohistologist Giuseppe Levi's passion for the developing nervous system, Levi-Montalcini spent much of World War II in a home laboratory studying the growth of nerve fibers in chick embryos. Since she was a member of the "Jewish race," the results of her experiments could not be published in Italy, but they did appear in Belgium and established her scientific reputation. In 1946, Montalcini-Levi accepted the offer of a one-semester research fellowship in the laboratory of Victor Hamburger at Washington University in St. Louis. This turned into a research associate position that lasted for 30 years as she ascended the academic ladder. From 1961 onward, Levi-Montalcini established a second laboratory in Rome, where she spent part of her time each year.

As a communication from the Lasker Foundation noted when she received their Award for Basic Medical Research in 1986, Levi-Montalcini focused her research on the biochemical communications network that enables specific groups of cells to respond to the needs of the organism as a whole. She initially observed that tumor tissue, implanted in chick embryos, caused sympathetic and sensory nerve fibers to grow and branch into the tumor tissue. After a series of further studies, Levi-Montalcini concluded that this effect was produced by a soluble substance, nerve growth factor (NGF), which was released by the tumor tissue. Implanting the same tumor tissue in the membrane of a fertilized egg, even without direct contact with the embryo, caused nerve cells to grow into inappropriate organs and tissues. Levi-Montalcini later found the same substance in snake venom and mouse salivary glands, and she devised a simple in vitro assay for it that is still in use in laboratories around the world.

For her discovery and isolation of NGF, Levi-Montalcini shared the

1986 Nobel Prize in Physiology or Medicine with Stanley Cohen, her colleague at Washington University who discovered epidermal growth factor (EGF). As the Nobel Committee noted, these two discoveries led to improved understanding of many disease states, such as developmental malformations, degenerative changes in senile dementia and Alzheimer's disease, delayed wound healing, and tumors, paving the way for new therapeutic agents and treatments for these and other clinical diseases.

---

**Loewi, Otto**                                                (Germany, 1873–1961)

Born in Frankfurt, Otto Loewi studied medicine at the University of Strasbourg, which then was a part of Germany. After graduation, Loewi worked in a hospital, but was frustrated by the high mortality in many cases of far-advanced tuberculosis and pneumonia for which there was no effective treatment. Consequently, Loewi left clinical medicine and devoted his career to research in basic medical science, especially pharmacology.

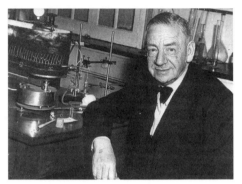

Otto Loewi in his laboratory, 1950s. (*Wikimedia / Institute of Pharmacology at University of Graz, Austria*)

Loewi moved to the University of Marburg, where he became an assistant of Hans Horst Meyer, a renowned pharmacologist. He initially worked in the field of metabolism, where he showed that animals are able to rebuild proteins from their degradation products, the amino acids – an essential discovery with regard to nutrition. Loewi later accepted a professorship at the University of Graz in Austria, where he remained until being imprisoned for two months, deprived of all his possessions, and expelled by the invading Nazis in 1938. Immigrating to the United State, Loewi became a research professor at the New York University College of Medicine.

Almost a century previously, Robert Remak had discovered a component of the nervous system that controlled the movement of involuntary muscles and glandular secretions. In the 1920s, Loewi pondered how this system could act upon structures throughout the body, such as the heart, digestive tract, and kidneys. He postulated that this process had to involve the nerves releasing tiny quantities of chemicals that affect the muscles. To prove this supposition, Loewi develop a "cross-heart perfusion experiment," in which he electrically stimulated the vagus nerve of one frog and then transfused its blood to a second frog to see whether it could slow down the second heart without directly stimulating the vagus nerve that supplied it. In a similar experiment, Loewi was able to speed up the heart of the second frog after stimulating the appropriate nerve of the first frog and transfusing its blood. In these experiments, Loewi proved the existence of chemical messengers, now called neurotransmitters (the first one he identified being acetylcholine), which transmit nerve impulses that regulate both the sympathetic and parasympathetic portions of the autonomic nervous system. For this discovery, Loewi shared the 1936 Nobel Prize for Physiology or Medicine with his longtime friend, Sir Henry Hallett Dale.

---

**Rosbash, Michael Morris** (USA, 1944– )

Born in Kansas City, Missouri to Jewish refugees who left Nazi Germany in 1938 (his father was a cantor), Michael Rosbash moved to Boston at age two. A graduate of the California Institute of Technology, Rosbash received a doctoral degree in biophysics in 1970 from the Massachusetts Institute of Technology. After three years in a postdoctoral fellowship in genetics at the University of Edinburgh, Rosbash joined the faculty at Brandeis University in 1974, where he now serves as Director of the Brandeis National Center for Behavioral Genomics.

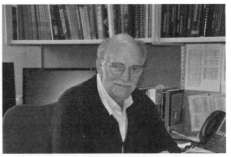

Michael Morris Rosbash, 2012. (*Gairdner Foundation*)

In 2017, Rosbash shared (with Jeffrey C. Hall and Michael W. Young) the Nobel Prize for Physiology or Medicine "for their discoveries of molecular mechanisms controlling the circadian rhythm." As the Nobel Committee noted, living organisms, including humans, have an internal, biological clock that enables them to adapt their biological rhythm so that it is synchronized with the revolutions of the earth. Using fruit flies (*Drosophila*) as a model organism, they isolated a gene that controls the normal daily biological rhythm, demonstrating that it encodes a protein that accumulates in the cell during the night and is then degraded during the day. Subsequently, they identified additional protein components of this machinery that produce a self-sustaining internal biological clock inside the cell that regulates many of our genes. This carefully calibrated circadian rhythm adapts our physiology to the different phases of the day, precisely regulating such critical functions as behavior, hormone levels, sleep, body temperature, and metabolism. Any temporary mismatch between the external environment and this internal biological clock can result in so-called "jet lag," as when humans rapidly travel across several time zones. Chronic misalignment between our lifestyle and the rhythm dictated by our internal biological clock can be associated with an increased risk for various diseases. As the Nobel Committee concluded, the discoveries by Rosbash and colleagues have led to "a vast and highly dynamic research field, with implications for our health and wellbeing."

## Schiff, Moritz                                      (Germany, 1823–1896)

Born in Frankfurt, Moritz Schiff studied medicine at the University of Göttingen. After graduation, Schiff moved to Paris to pursue postdoctoral studies in brain physiology under French physiologist François Magendie. At the same time, he worked on animal specimens at the Jardin des Plantes. Upon returning to his native Frankfurt in 1846, Schiff became director of the ornithology collection of the city's *Zoological Museum*, cataloging rare bird specimens. When the insurrection of 1848 broke out, Schiff served as a military surgeon in the revolutionary army of Baden. Captured and condemned to death, Schiff escaped and spent the next several

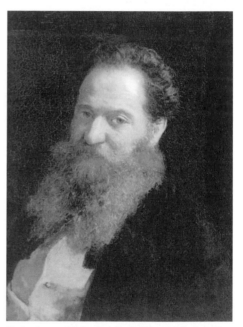

Painting of Moritz Schiff by Nikolai Ge, 1876. (*Wikimedia*)

years immersed in his work, writing multiple articles on the neurology of the spinal column, heart, lungs, bones, and gastrointestinal tract. Schiff was the first to note the influence of the cerebral cortex on blood circulation, the role of the vagus nerve in heart function, and the restoration to the liver of bile salts passing through the intestine. Schiff demonstrated that removing the thyroid glands from dogs was fatal, but later demonstrated that thyroid grafts or injection of thyroid extracts could prevent death. This eventually led to the development of successful treatments for a variety of thyroid abnormalities in humans.

Although qualified for a high academic post, Moritz was denied a position in Germany because of his participation in the failed revolution and the fear that he would adversely affect the impressionable young minds of his students. Therefore, he moved to Switzerland to become the first Professor of Microscopic Anatomy and Pathology at the University of Bern. Moritz later held professorial positions at the medical schools in Florence and Geneva. Although attacked by the Anti-Vivisection Society for alleged cruelty to animals, Schiff consistently anesthetized his experimental animals, a practice that was not standard at that time. His major literary work was a four-volume *Collected Contributions to Physiology*, written in 1894–96.

Although not religious, Schiff was proud of his own Jewish origins and helped the many young Russian Jews who came to Swiss universities because they were denied educational opportunities in their homeland. Among these was Waldemar Haffkine, who later developed vaccines for cholera and plague.

---

**Stern, Lina Solomonovna** (Russia, 1878–1968)

Born in Libau (today in Latvia), Lina Stern was educated at the University of Geneva and pursued an academic career in biochemistry and neurosciences. In 1918, Stern became the first woman to be awarded a professorial rank at the University of Geneva. Because of ideological convictions, in 1925 Stern returned to the Soviet Union and served for more than 20 years as Professor of the 2nd Medical Institute. In 1929, Stern became the first woman to be admitted as a full member of the USSR Academy of Sciences, where she founded its Institute of Physiology, which she directed until it was discontinued in 1948. Stern also was a recipient of the Stalin Prize in 1943.

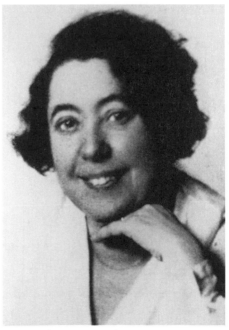

Lina Solomonovna Stern, 1910s. (*Wikimedia*)

Stern is best known for her pioneering work on the blood–brain barrier, which she described in 1921. This highly selective permeability barrier separates circulating blood from the extracellular fluid in the brain and central nervous system (CNS). The blood–brain barrier is formed by brain endothelial cells, which are connected by tight junctions. It permits the passage of water, some gases, and lipid-soluble molecules by passive diffusion, as well as the selective transport of molecules (glucose and amino acids) that are necessary for neural function. However, the blood–brain barrier prevents the entry of potential neurotoxins. The results of Stern's work were later implemented in clinical practice, saving thousands of lives at the fronts in World War II.

When World War II broke out, Stern was selected as a member of the Jewish Anti-Fascist Committee (JAC). During the 1948–1949 purges in the Soviet Union, she was accused of "rootless cosmopolitanism." Of the 15 convicted, Stern was the only one whose death sentence was commuted to a prison term followed by a period of exile. After the death of Stalin in 1953, Stern was allowed to return to Moscow and establish a laboratory to continue her research work. Until her death, Stern headed the Department of Physiology at the Biophysics Institute.

## Traube, Ludwig                                    (Germany, 1818–1876)

Born in Ratibor in Silesia (now Poland), Ludwig Traube studied medicine in Breslau, Berlin, and Vienna, receiving his doctorate for a study of pulmonary emphysema. An expert on the techniques of auscultation and percussion, Traube acceded to the requests of some young physicians and began giving courses on these subjects that made him well known. Traube became the Head Physician of the Department of Internal Medicine at the Charité Hospital, while developing intensive clinical and research work. Despite his Jewish ancestry. Traube eventually was appointed a professor at the University of Berlin.

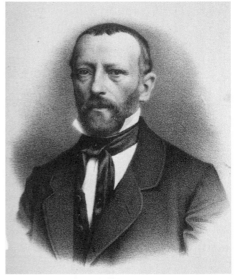

Ludwig Traube. (*Wikimedia / NLM*)

Traube was a pioneer of pathophysiologic research in Germany, investigating the effect of the vagus nerve on pulmonary function, the regulation of body temperature, and the scientific basis for digitalis therapy. He introduced the measurement of temperature as a routine clinical examination and produced the first graphic presentation of the course of a fever, with simultaneous recording of the pulse and respiratory rates. Among the many eponyms associated with him are Traube's bruit, corpuscles, dyspnea, and pulse.

---

## Valentin, Gabriel Gustav                    (Germany, 1810–1883)

Born in Breslau and receiving a solid Jewish education, Gabriel Valentin studied medicine at the university of Breslau, where his most influential teacher was the famed physiologist, Jan Purkinje. In additon to practicing medicine in his native city, in 1835 Valentin was awarded the Grand Prix des Sciences Physiques from the Institute of France for his *Handbook of the History of Man*, a comparative study on the evolution of mammals and birds. His rapid rise in academic circles led to Valentin receiving offers of full professorships from several univeristies at age 25. The only requirement was that he renounce his Jewish faith and become baptized, which Valentin adamantly refused to do. When Valentin received an offer to become a Professor of Physiology and Animal Anatomy at the University of Bern, he asked about the

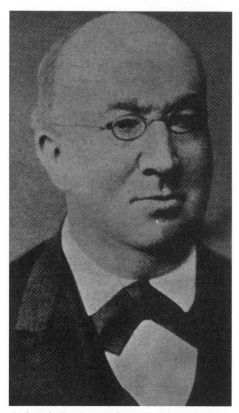

Gabriel Gustav Valentin. (*Wikimedia / NLM*)

baptismal requirement. Valentin was assured that "religion would be no obstacle in the mind of any enlightened personality,"[39] but since some at

---

39. Frank Heynick, *Jews in Medicine: An Epic Saga* (NJ: KTAV Publishing House, 2002), p. 253.

the university were apparently not that enlightened, it would be best if he were baptized before accepting the post. Disturbed by this, Valentin replied that "such a step, if connected with the attainment of any worldly goal, becomes despicable and discreditable. It means yielding to old prejudices, abandoning one's own people because one desires to join the group of better human beings."[40] Strongly wanting to recruit this talented researcher, the university and the Bern government agreed to waive this requirement, and in 1836 Valentin became the first unbaptized Jewish full professor at a German-speaking university, a position he held for 45 years. When later naturalized as a "burger" of Bern, Valentin may have became the first unbaptized citizen with full civil rights in Switzerland!

Valentin published two textbooks on human physiology, performed extensive studies integrating physics (especially mathematics) into medicine, researched the two nervous systems regulating the heart, and discovered the function of the pancreas and its secretions in the digestion of food.

---

## Van Deen, Izaak                                    (Germany, 1805–1869)

Born in Germany and moving with his family to Denmark at a young age, Izaak Van Deen attended medical school at the University of Copenhagen. Subsequently the family moved to Groningen, where his father became Chief Rabbi. This Danish background explains his name, with Van Deen meaning "from Denmark."

To obtain a medical license in The Netherlands, Van Deen earned a doctorate in Leiden with a thesis on the nervous system, which remained the focus of his research. Van Deen studied transmission of nervous impulses and reflexes in animals after partial

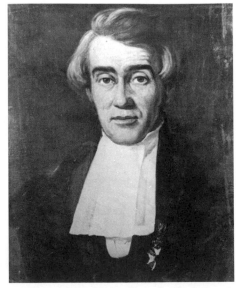

Painting of Izaak Van Deen by Onbekend, circa 1870. (*Wikimedia*)

transection of their spinal cords. In this way, he showed that the dorsal columns convey sensory impulses and the anterior columns motor impulses.

---

40. Ibid.

His data was explicitly cited by Brown-Sequard in his later well-known studies in humans. The Van Deen test (also known as the Almen test for blood) entails adding glacial acetic acid, gum guaiac solution, and hydrogen peroxide to an aqueous suspension of a suspected stain. If occult blood or blood pigment is present, it develops a blue color. In 1851, Van Deen was appointed Professor and Chair of the Department of Physiology at Groningen, the first Jew to be given a university chair in The Netherlands.

## Wald, George (USA, 1906–1997)

Born in New York City to immigrant parents from Eastern Europe, George Wald was a member of the first graduating class at Brooklyn Technical High School. Wald received a doctorate in zoology from Columbia University and was awarded a travel grant to study with Nobel laureate Otto Warburg in Germany. With the rise of the Nazis, Wald returned to the Unites States and in 1934 joined the faculty at Harvard University.

While researching the biochemistry of vision, Wald identified the presence of vitamin A in the retina of the eye and showed that it was essential for retinal function. He then made major discoveries in the molecular makeup and chemi-

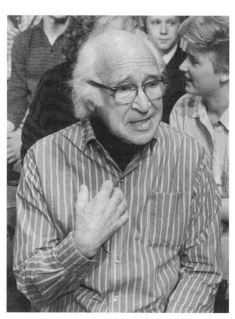

Photograph of George Wald by Bart Molendijk, 1987. (*Wikimedia / Dutch National Archives*)

cal interactions within the eyes of all species. For this work, Wald shared (with Haldan Keffer Hartline and Ragnar Granit) the 1967 Nobel Prize in Physiology or Medicine "for their discoveries concerning the primary physiological and chemical visual processes in the eye." Wald had received the 1953 Lasker Award in Basic Medical Research for "chemistry of the visual cycle."

## Zuntz, Nathan                                    (Germany, 1847–1920)

Born in Bonn, Nathan Zuntz studied medicine at the University of
Bonn. After an initial academic
position in Bonn, in 1881 Zuntz became Professor of Animal
Physiology at the Royal Agricultural College in Berlin, where he
remained for almost four decades
until his retirement. During this
period, Zuntz carried out experiments examining human physiology in extreme environments. He
developed the treadmill, later add-

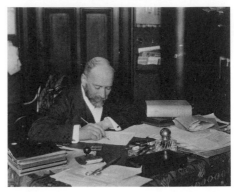

Nathan Zuntz on Tenerife, 1910. (*Wikimedia*)

ing an x-ray apparatus to observe changes in heart volume during exercise,
as well as a portable gas clock to provide real-time measurements of metabolism. He also opened the first sports medicine laboratory in Germany.

At the research station of Mount Rosa in Switzerland (14,000 feet eleva-
tion), Zuntz performed studies in high-altitude physiology, which resulted
in his classic *High Altitude Climate and Mountaineering and their Effect on
Humans* (1906). This work was expanded during hot air balloon trips (up
to 27,000 feet) and later in airplanes. In *The Physiology and Hygiene Involving Aviation* (1912), Zuntz established himself as the founder of modern
aerospace medicine.

# THE AGE OF SPECIALIZATION
~: Clinical Medicine :~

---

## CARDIOLOGY, CARDIAC SURGERY

Kantrowitz developed the plastic heart valve; electronic heart-lung machine; intra-aortic balloon pump (IABP) which alternately expands and contracts within the aorta to reduce strain on the heart; and left ventricular assist device (LVAD), which allows a patient with severe chronic heart failure to pump blood more effectively and leave the hospital with a permanent implant. Master and Dack were instrumental in developing and implementing the first cardiac stress test. Zoll made important improvements to the pace makers of his day, while Mower and Mirowski developed the automatic implantable cardiac defibrillator (AICD). Bing pioneered the use of nitric oxide to measure cardiac blood flow and collaborated in developing the use of radioactive tracers to measure cardiac blood flow and produce images of the heart, which laid the foundation for modern PET (positron emission tomography) scanning. Kantrowitz led the surgical team that performed the first human heart transplant in the United States, while Vineberg developed the technique for implanting the left mammary artery directly into the wall of the left ventricle of the heart to relieve myocardial ischemia. Taussig proposed the idea for an operation to treat children with Tetralogy of Fallot, the most common cause of anoxemia or "blue bay" syndrome. Corday was a pioneer in invasive cardiology and contributed to the development of coronary intensive care units.

## Bamberger, Heinrich von                                    (Austria, 1822–1888)

Born near Prague, Heinrich von Bamberger studied medicine at the University of Prague. After a clinical assistantship in Vienna, in 1854 Bamberger became Professor of Therapeutic Pathology at the University of Würzburg, returning to the University of Vienna in 1872 as Professor of Special Pathology and Therapy.

A specialist in respiratory and circulatory pathology, Bamberger is best known for his research on diseases of the pericardium, heart, and great vessels. The eponymous "Bamberger's disease" is characterized by spasms of the leg muscles.

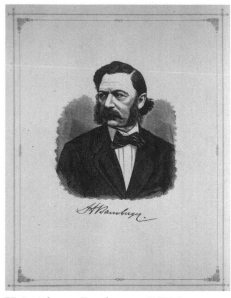

Heinrich von Bamberger. (*NLM*)

In 1857, Bamberger published his *Handbook of Diseases of the Heart*, one of the first textbooks dedicated to cardiac pathology.

## Bing, Richard John                                    (Germany, 1909–2010)

Born in Nuremburg, Richard Bing studied music at the local conservatory while also interested in medicine. After an indifferent reception from Richard Strauss, Bing earned a medical degree at the University of Munich. His Jewish family fled Nazi Germany shortly after Bing graduated, but he continued his studies at the University of Bern, where he was awarded another

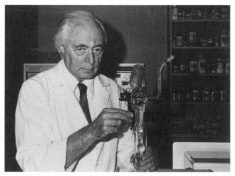

Richard John Bing (*NLM*)

medical degree. Bing then received a fellowship to Columbia University, enabling him to come to the United States.

After serving in the military, Bing joined the faculty of the Johns Hopkins

University School of Medicine. There he focused his research on cardiac metabolism, especially cardiac blood flow and the pumping mechanism of the heart. With cardiac surgeon Alfred Blalock and the cardiologist Helen B. Taussig, Bing founded the first catheterization laboratory dedicated to the diagnosis of congenital cardiac anomalies and measurement of mechanical efficiency in the heart. After moving to the Huntington Medical Research Institutes in California, Bing studied the chemistry of heart attacks, developing techniques for high-speed photography of the coronary vessels that facilitated the diagnosis and treatment of congenital cardiac malformations. He also pioneered the use of nitric oxide to measure cardiac blood flow and collaborated in developing the use of radioactive tracers to measure cardiac blood flow and produce images of the heart, which laid the foundation for modern PET (positron emission tomography) scanning. As Life President of the International Society for Heart Research, a group that he helped found, Bing established the *Journal of Molecular & Cellular Cardiology*, the official publication of the society.

Bing's interest in music continued throughout his life, and he composed more than 300 scores for chamber ensemble, orchestra, and chorus, some of which have been performed around the world.

## Corday, Eliot (Canada, 1913–1999)

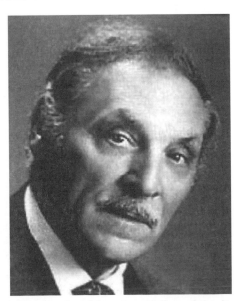

Born in Prince Rupert, British Columbia, Eliot Corday received his medical degree from the University of Alberta. After serving in the Royal Canadian Air Force during World War II, Corday came to the United States to specialize in cardiology. He then moved to Los Angeles, where he became a Clinical Professor of Medicine at UCLA and Chief of Cardiology at Cedars of Lebanon Hospital, which merged with Mount Sinai to form Cedars-Sinai.

Corday played a major role in conveying American cardiovascular expertise to other countries. To help achieve this goal, Corday

Eliot Corday. (*American College of Cardiology*)

founded the international education program of the American College of Cardiology, which supported groups of cardiologists traveling to underdeveloped countries to give instruction in cardiovascular diagnosis and treatment, thus greatly improving patient care. Corday was a leading force in initiating Federal support of cardiovascular research.

Clinically, Corday contributed to fundamental practices of cardiology. He helped pioneer invasive cardiology and collaborated on research that led to modern stress testing and nuclear cardiology. His interests in sudden cardiac death and ischemic ("silent") heart disease contributed to the development of coronary intensive care units. Invited by President Ronald Reagan to head the United States Information Agency's Medical Science Advisory Committee, Corday arranged live televised communication sessions between American cardiologists and cardiologists in the Middle East, India, Hungary, and Russia. From 1967 to 1977, Corday was national consultant in cardiology to the Surgeon General of the Air Force, rising to the rank of major general.

---

**Dack, Simon**                                        (USA, 1908–1994)

---

Born in New York, Simon Dack received his degree from New York Medical College. While an intern at Mount Sinai Hospital, Dack worked with Arthur M. Master to develop the first cardiac stress test, a precursor of the treadmill stress test, in which patients climbed steps to increase their heart rate. Dack remained at Mount Sinai for most of his career, joining the faculty when its School of Medicine was established in 1966.

Dack focused his efforts in teaching, lecturing, and trying to raise the level of knowledge in clinical cardiology. To this end, Dack was among the founding Fellows of the American College of Cardiology (1949) and Editor-in-Chief of *The Journal of American Cardiology* for 30 years from its inception in 1958.

---

**Kantrowitz, Adrian**                                 (USA, 1918–2008)

---

Born in New York City, Adrian Kantrowitz received his degree from the Long Island College of Medicine (now SUNY Downstate Medical Center) and specialized in cardiovascular surgery. Kantrowitz became Director of Surgical Services at Maimonides Medical Center in Brooklyn and later served as Professor of Surgery at New York University and Chairman of the Department of Surgery at Sinai Hospital in Detroit.

Kantrowitz was a pioneer in bioengineering related to the heart and cardiovascular surgery. He is best known as leading the surgical team that performed the first human heart transplant in the United States in 1967, just three days after the first heart transplant performed by Christiaan Barnard in South Africa. Although Kantrowitz's patient lived for less than seven hours, this operation was a crucial step in the development of heart transplantation, which has almost become routine today.

Kantrowitz designed numerous devices used to treat individuals with severe cardiac disease. In addition to a plastic heart valve

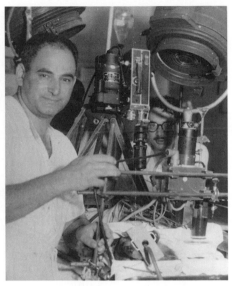

Dr. Adrian Kantrowitz (left) with assistants in the laboratory making an image of the mitral valve in situ, 1951. (*NLM*)

and electronic heart-lung machine, Kantrowitz invented the intra-aortic balloon pump (IABP), which alternately expands and contracts within the aorta to reduce strain on the heart. This can be inserted without a surgical procedure and save the lives of the 15% of heart attack patients who go into severe shock. Kantrowitz invented the left ventricular assist device (LVAD), which allows a patient with severe chronic heart failure to pump blood more effectively and leave the hospital with a permanent implant. He also invented an early version of the implantable pacemaker and a technique for taking movies inside the living heart that could show the sequential opening and closing of the mitral valve. Inspired by the way that heart muscles were stimulated, Kantrowitz was the first physician to enable paraplegic patients to move their limbs by stimulating their muscles electronically.

---

## Katz, Louis Nelson (Poland, 1897–1973)

---

Born in Pinsk, at age 3 Louis Katz immigrated with his family to the United States, settling in Cleveland. After studying medicine at Western Reserve University, Katz specialized in cardiology. He decided to combine clinical medicine with research in physiology, joining the faculty as an instructor in physiology but retaining his clinical interests as a consulting cardiologist at St. Luke's Hospital in Cleveland.

Katz pursued research studies in a broad spectrum of cardiovascular diseases, including hemodynamics, electrocardiography, hypertension, experimental atherosclerosis, the coronary circulation, myocardial metabolism, and the psychosomatic and epidemiological aspects of heart disease. In 1930, Katz moved to Chicago to become Director of the Cardiovascular Department of the newly established Michael Reese Institute and Assistant Professor of Physiology at the University of Chicago. His reasons for going to a private community hospital in a non-university medical environ-

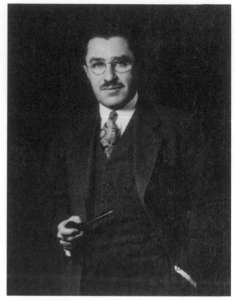

Louis N. Katz. (*NLM*)

ment included the freedom to build his own department and take responsibility for raising private funds to support his research, as well the opportunity to work at a place that attracted bright young Jewish physicians who at that time were not welcomed by many university departments. Katz also accepted into his laboratory scientists fleeing from the Nazi takeover of most of Europe.

A prolific writer, Katz published hundreds of articles on electrocardiography, physiology, and clinical cardiology, and he was the author of an electrocardiography textbook (1946) that became a standard reference in the field. Katz received the 1956 Lasker Award for Clinical Medical Research for "modeling atherosclerosis."

---

## Master, Arthur M.                                    (USA, 1895–1973)

---

Born in New York City, Arthur Master graduated from Cornell University Medical College and specialized in cardiology. Most of his career was spent at the Mount Sinai Medical Center, where he became Chief of the Cardiac Clinics and of the Electrocardiography Department. Although primarily a practicing physician, rather than a researcher, Master published many scientific articles, as well as five books on the cause and detection of heart disease.

Master's name is virtually synonymous with the two-step exercise test. Formulating a protocol taking into consideration the age, gender, weight, and height of the patient, it provided a standard workload to evaluate the heart rate and blood pressure responses as measures of cardiac function. Working with British physiologist E.T. Oppenheimer, they showed that cardiac efficiency declined with age and detected the effect of obesity on cardiac function, demonstrating that weight reduction improved the exercise tolerance of the patient.

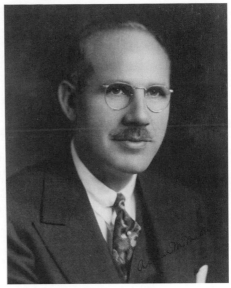

Arthur Master, 1940. (*NLM*)

Convinced of the importance of detecting "silent" coronary disease, Master stressed that even patients with severe coronary artery disease could have a normal resting electrocardiogram (ECG). Therefore, he advocated a two-step ECG for everyone over age 35. Master was one of the first cardiologists to write that victims of certain types of heart attacks could make a complete recovery without being bedridden for the rest of their lives. One of his studies showed that more than half of a sampling of 1,620 heart attacks occurred during sleep or rest, disputing the widely held theory that most heart attacks were brought on by heavy exercise.

## Mirowski, Michel (Poland, 1924–1990)

Born Mordechai Frydman in Warsaw, when Germany invaded Poland in the fall of 1939, his father renamed his son Mieczysław Mirowski in an attempt to protect him from rampant anti-Semitism. Later, his French wife called him Michel, by which he became known. To escape the Nazis, Mirowski fled to Ukraine, surviving under terrible conditions. After the war, he registered as a medical student in Gdansk, but his Zionist leanings led him to immigrate to the Land of Israel. However, there were no medical schools in the Land of Israel during the early post-war years, so Mirowski returned to Europe and in 1954 eventually earned his medical degree in Lyon. He returned to Israel to become first assistant to the chief

of medicine at Tel Hashomer Hospital in Tel Aviv and then the sole cardiologist at the nearby Asaf Harofeh Hospital in Hadera.

When his close friend and colleague died suddenly due to ventricular
tachycardia (a dangerous rapid heart rhythm), Mirowski conceived the idea
of implanting a defibrillator in the body that would detect ventricular fibrillation and other arrhythmias when they occurred and automatically deliver
a high-energy shock to convert the heart to a normal rhythm. Mirowski
met substantial resistance from Israeli cardiologists, who informed him
that the defibrillators (weighing 30–40 pounds at the time) could not be
miniaturized to the size of a cigarette box. Therefore, Mirowski moved
his family from Israel to Baltimore, where he collaborated with Morton
Mower at Sinai Hospital to develop the first automatic implantable cardiac defibrillator (AICD) as a substitute for portable defibrillators in patients with chronic cardiac problems. They worked on this project for 12
years until they were able to implant the first defibrillator into a patient
at Johns Hopkins Hospital in 1980. Since that time, the device Mirowski
and Mower invented has been much improved and further miniaturized,
and millions of patients have received them.

---

## Mower, Morton M.                                  (USA, 1933–)

Born in Baltimore, Morton Mower received his medical degree from the
University of Maryland and joined the Department of Cardiology at Sinai
Hospital in his native city. There Mower collaborated with Israeli cardiologist Michel Mirowski to develop the automatic implantable cardiac
defibrillator (AICD) as a substitute to portable defibrillators for patients
with chronic cardiac problems.

Normally, the natural pacemaker in the heart regulates the contraction
of the ventricles. When there are irregularities in the electrical signals from
the pacemaker, ventricular fibrillation and ventricular tachycardia occur,
causing the ventricles to contract abnormally and preventing blood from
circulating throughout the body. If not treated immediately, ventricular
fibrillation and tachycardia can lead to sudden cardiac death. An AICD
is a device implanted under the skin through an incision in the shoulder,
with leads passing through a vein into the heart. The leads are attached
to electrodes that monitor the electrical activity in the heart. When it de-
tects irregular electrical activity, the defibrillator delivers a shock to restore
normal electrical activity.

Many cardiology experts doubted the potential of the AICD for clinical
success. In 1972 Bernard Lown, the inventor of the external defibrillator,

wrote in the journal *Circulation*: "The very rare patient who has frequent bouts of ventricular fibrillation is best treated in a coronary care unit and is better served by an effective antiarrhythmic program or surgical correction of inadequate coronary blood flow or ventricular malfunction. In fact, the implanted defibrillator system represents an imperfect solution in search of a plausible and practical application."[41] Eight years later, Mower and Mirowski implanted the first defibrillator into a patient at Johns Hopkins Hospital. Since that time, the device they invented has been much improved and further miniaturized (the size of a deck of cards and weighing nine ounces), and millions of patients have received them.

Mower has played an important role in numerous Jewish organizations in the Baltimore area and serves on the Board of Directors of the Jewish National Fund.

---

**Taussig, Helen Brooke**                                    (USA, 1898–1986)

---

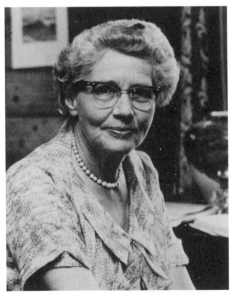

Born in Cambridge, Massachusetts, Helen Taussig suffered from severe dyslexia during her early school years but received her bachelor's degree from the University of California, Berkeley. Taussig later studied histology, bacteriology, and anatomy at both Harvard Medical School and Boston University, though neither school allowed her to earn a degree. Eventually, Taussig was accepted at Johns Hopkins University, where she completed her medical degree. By the time she graduated, Taussig had lost her hearing and relied on lip-reading and hearing aids for the rest of her career, compensating for this deficit through the use of her hands for palpating the chests of her patients.

Photograph of Helen Brooke Taussig taken for the cover of *Modern Medicine*, 1963. (*NLM / Modern Medicine*)

Working in Baltimore and Boston, Taussig founded the field of pediatric cardiology. For years, Taussig specialized in anoxemia or "blue baby"

---

41. Implanted standby defibrillators. Circulation 1972; 46:637-639.

syndrome, the congenital heart condition caused by a defect that prevents the heart from receiving enough oxygen. Taussig used fluoroscopy, a new x-ray technique, to establish that babies suffering from anoxemia had a leaking septum (the wall that separates the ventricles of the heart) and an underdeveloped pulmonary artery leading from the heart to the lungs. In 1941, Taussig proposed an idea for an operation that might help children with Tetralogy of Fallot, the most common cause of "blue baby" syndrome, and suggested it to her colleagues at Johns Hopkins – surgeon Alfred Blalock and surgical technician Vivien Thomas. After extensive experimentation, three years later they performed the first new operation on a child with anoxemia and reported this and two other successful cases in the *Journal of the American Medical Association*. The technique, named the Blalock-Taussig operation, was soon used worldwide. Taussig continued her research on cardiac birth defects, and her 1947 publication of *Congenital Malformations of the Heart* is often considered the beginning of pediatric cardiology as an independent field.

After a trip to Germany, where she worked with infants suffering from severe limb deformities (phocomelia), Taussig played a major role in banning the drug thalidomide, which when given to pregnant women caused catastrophic effects on their newborns. Her testimony before Congress in 1967 led to thalidomide being banned in the United States and Europe.

In 1954, Taussig received the Lasker Award for Clinical Medical Research for the "first successful 'blue baby' operation."

---

**Vineberg, Arthur Martin**                              (Canada, 1903–1988)

Born in Montreal, Arthur Vineberg studied medicine at McGill University. From 1933 until his death, Vineberg served as a cardiac surgeon on the staff of the Royal Victoria Hospital, the original teaching facility of the institution.

Vineberg is best known for the surgical procedure that bears his name. Introduced in 1950, it involves implantation of the left mammary artery directly into the wall of the left ventricle of the heart to relieve myocardial ischemia. The Vineberg procedure provides the heart with an alternate flow of blood, circumventing the dangerous blockages resulting from atherosclerosis in gravely ill heart patients. Variations of the procedure were removing the outer lining of the heart to permit other vessels to supply blood to the organ, or even surrounding the heart with tissue rich in blood vessels and taken from the patient's abdominal cavity. Thousands of patients benefitted from the Vineberg procedure before it was replaced by direct aorto-coronary artery bypass grafting as a more efficient means of revascularizing the myocardium.

Vineberg was the author of *How to Live with your Heart; the Family Guide to Heart Health* (1975); and *Myocardial Revascularization by Arterial/Ventricular Implants* (1982). His third book, *The Complete Guide to Heart Health*, was being prepared for publication at the time of his death.

## Zoll, Paul Maurice (USA, 1911–1999)

Born in Boston, Paul Zoll studied medicine at Harvard University and became a member of the cardiology department at the Beth Israel Hospital in his native city.

Having observed numerous open-heart surgeries during his military service in World War II, and noting how the heart responded reflexively to the slightest touch, Zoll became involved in attempts to regulate the heartbeat and treat myocardial infarctions. At the time, emergency resuscitation for cardiac arrest was crude – a doctor would cut open the patient's chest and squeeze the heart with his hand to pump blood through

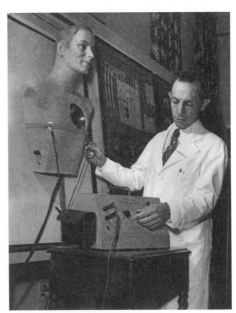

Paul Maurice Zoll. (*NLM*)

the body. Zoll experimented with closed-chest electrical cardiac stimulation to resuscitate two patients whose hearts had stopped, one of whom survived for 11 months after 52 hours of electrical stimulation. Zoll then focused his efforts on developing external pacemakers to restore normal rhythms in patients whose hearts were beating erratically and dangerously. However, this research was met with much opposition by physicians who questioned whether such "artificial" methods were unethical or even blasphemous. Zoll concentrated on improving the cardiac pacemakers of his day, which were massive, inefficient external machines that often caused burns, involuntary muscle contractions, and even intolerable pain to their users. Zoll's new designs were the forerunners of the miniaturized permanent pacemakers that are currently implanted in hundreds of thousands of patients each year. Zoll also worked to improve electrocardiographic monitoring devices and founded a company to develop and market new defibrillator designs.

Despite his numerous contributions to medical technology, Zoll received only limited recognition until 1973, when he won the Lasker Award for Clinical Medical Research for "cardiac pacemakers and defibrillators."

## DERMATOLOGY

A specialty that was generally disdained by Gentile physicians, dermatology became popular among Jewish physicians. Auspitz, Hebra, Kaposi, and Unna played important roles in describing a host of skin disorders, such as lupus, eczema, impetigo, erythema multiforme, exfoliative dermatitis, seborrheic dermatitis, mycosis fungoides, and the skin manifestations of syphilis. Bloch and Jadassohn instrumental in introducing the patch test for contact dermatitis and allergic conditions. Jadassohn used immunological techniques to study skin diseases, especially tuberculosis and trichophytosis, while Klein introduced topical steroids and other medications to treat skin irritations and superficial cancers. Kligman discovered the active ingredient of a medication to improve acne and reduce facial wrinkles, Neumann demonstrated that prematurely aged skin was caused by over-exposure to extreme weather conditions, and Sulzberger made valuable contributions to the understanding and treatment of the dermatoses caused by poison gases, burns, and tropical skin diseases during World War II. Kaposi's name was given to what at the time was a rare, slow-growing malignancy, which in recent decades became a major diagnostic marker of AIDS. As in other specialties, Jewish dermatologists became heads of leading academics departments (especially Hebra, who founded the New Vienna School of Dermatology) and edited major textbooks in the field.

---

**Auspitz, Heinrich**                              (Moravia, 1835–1886)

Son of a Jewish surgeon, Heinrich Auspitz studied medicine at the University of Vienna, specializing in dermatology and syphilis. Part of the so-called Vienna School of Dermatology, Auspitz worked as a *privatdozent* (private lecturer) and then Professor of Dermatology and Syphilis at the University of Vienna, and in 1872 was named director of the general polyclinic.

A pioneer in tissue pathology, Auspitz described the pinpoint bleeding following removal of a psoriasis scale that bears his name (Auspitz's sign).

He also published a seminal article on mycosis fungoides, the most common form of cutaneous T-cell lymphoma that produces a characteristic rash and itchy skin.

Auspitz co-founded the first German-language dermatology journal, and since 2005 the Hcinrich Auspitz Prize has been awarded to promote scientific research in the field of dermatology.

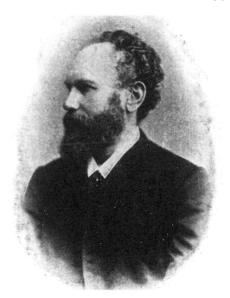

Heinrich Auspitz. (*Wikimedia / Pagel: Biographisches Lexikon hervorragender Ärzte des neunzehnten Jahrhunderts. Berlin, Wien 1901, Sp. 61–62*)

## Bloch, Bruno                          (Switzerland, 1878–1933)

After completing medical school at the University of Basel, Bruno Bloch pursued further training in dermatology in Basel, Vienna, Berlin, Paris, and Bern, where he worked under Josef Jadassohn. In 1908, Bloch was appointed Head of Dermatology at the University of Basel. He eventually became the head of the newly established Chair of Dermatology at the University of Zurich, where he remained until his death.

Bloch was influenced by Jadassohn in applying laboratory techniques to the study of skin disorders. He expanded his mentor's clinical and experimental work in patch testing, which is often cited as the Jadassohn-Bloch technique,

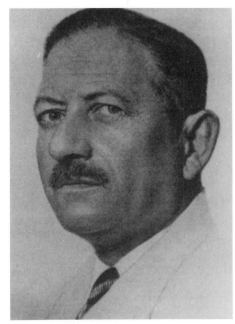

Bruno Bloch. (*Alumni Medizinische Fakultät Basel*)

and played a major role in developing a standard series of allergens. Bloch made important contributions in the field of allergy and was an expert on disorders of pigmentation. He discovered and developed the Dopa reaction in staining, specifically those mammalian cells that have the capacity to form melanin pigment.

## Hebra, Ferdinand Ritter von                     (Austria, 1816–1880)

Born in Brno, Ferdinand von Hebra graduated from medical school at the University of Vienna. Known as the founder of the New Vienna School of Dermatology, an illustrious group of physicians who established the foundations of modern dermatology, Hebra collaborated with Carl Rokintansky and Josef Skoda in transforming the Vienna medical faculty to among the best in the world.

Focusing his attention on microscopic investigation of multiple skin rashes, Hebra authored one of the most influential books on dermatology, the *Atlas der Hautkrankeiten* (Atlas of Skin Diseases). Hebra stressed that diseases of the skin were related to local irritation,

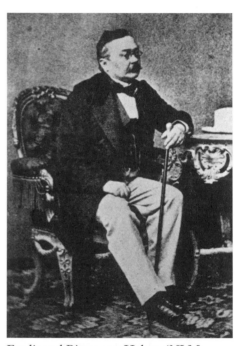

Ferdinand Ritter von Hebra. (*NLM*)

disproving the humoral doctrine that they reflected a general metabolic disruption due to blood poisoning. As an example, he demonstrated that scabies, a highly contagious itchy disease, was caused by infestation by a mite. Haber described numerous skin disorders, such as lupus, eczema, impetigo, erythema multiforme, exfoliative dermatitis, and the skin manifestations related to syphilis.

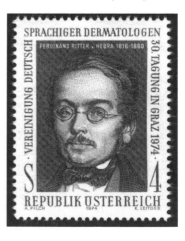

Ferdinand Ritter von Hebra depicted on Austrian stamp, 1974. (*Author's private collection*)

Hebra became Professor of Dermatology at the University of Vienna in 1869, attracting students from all over the world, and was elevated to the nobility by Emperor Franz Joseph I.

---

**Jadassohn, Josef** (Germany, 1863–1936)

Born in Liegnitz in Silesia (now Poland), Josef Jadassohn studied medicine in Göttingen, Heidelberg, and Leipzig before receiving his doctorate in Breslau. After serving as an assistant to Albert Neisser at the Allerheiligen Hospital in Breslau, in 1896 Jadassohn became Professor and Director of the Dermatological Clinic at the University of Bern. From 1917, he was Professor of Dermatology at the University of Breslau.

An excellent clinician and teacher, Jadassohn devoted much of his time to research. He was among the first to utilize immunological techniques in the study of dermatological disorders, especially tuberculosis and trichophytosis, and is credited with introducing the patch test for the

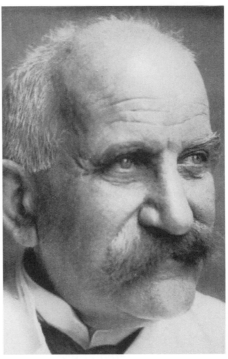

Josef Jadassohn. (*Wikimedia / British Journal of Dermatology, Vol. 48, 1937*)

diagnosis of contact dermatitis. He was the first to identify maculopapular erythematosa, a scaling condition of the skin that is known as "Jadassohn's disease." His name is also associated with the Jadassohn-Bloch skin test for allergic conditions. A prolific writer, Jadassohn was the co-editor of the *Archiv fuer Dermatologie und Syphilis* (Archives of Dermatology and Syphilis).

---

**Kaposi, Moritz** (Hungary, 1837–1902)

Born Moritz Kohn to a poor Jewish family in Kaposvar, he changed his surname to Kaposi (a play on Kaposvar, the town of his birth) when he converted to Catholicism (1871). Kaposi studied medicine at the University of Vienna and immediately was appointed assistant to Ferdinand Ritter von Hebra, the noted Austrian dermatologist, whose daughter he married. Kaposi became a professor at the University of Vienna, a member of the board of the Vienna General Hospital, and director of its clinic of skin diseases, as well as the Chairman of the Vienna School of Dermatology after his mentor's death.

Together with Ferdinand von Hebra, Kaposi authored *Textbook of Skin Diseases* (1878). However, Kaposi's major work was *Pathology and Therapy of the Skin Diseases in Lectures for Practical Physicians and Students*, which was published two years later and is considered one

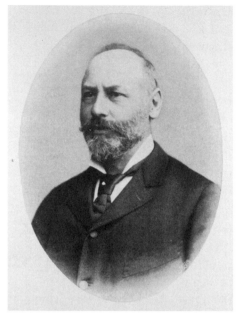

Moritz Kaposi, circa 1890. (*Wikimedia / J.F. Lehmann, Munich, 1902; NLM*)

of the most significant books in the history of dermatology. Throughout his career, Kaposi emphasized the use of pathologic examination in the diagnosis of dermatologic diseases.

Kaposi wrote some of the early descriptions of lupus erythematosus of the skin, terming the classic appearance a "butterfly" rash. However, he is most famous for being the first (1872) to describe a type of skin cancer that he encountered in five elderly male patients, which he termed "idiopathic multiple pigmented sarcoma." Renamed Kaposi's sarcoma, for years it was considered a rare, slow-growing malignancy. However, more than a century later, an HIV-associated Kaposi's sarcoma became a major diagnostic marker of AIDS, as well as the most common neoplastic complication of that disease. It also has become the most commonly reported cancer in parts of sub-Saharan Africa.

---

**Klein, Edmund**                                              (Austria, 1922–1999)

Born in Vienna, Edmund Klein and his family moved to Canada when the Nazis rose to power. A graduate of the medical school at the University of Toronto, Klein was long a Research Professor of Medical Dermatology and Experimental Pathology at the School of Medicine at the State

University of New York at Buffalo and Head of Dermatology at the Roswell Park Memorial Institute.

Klein realized that an aging population would result in more people suffering from skin cancer due to long exposure to sunlight. Because this would increase the need to develop nonsurgical treatment for skin cancer, Klein devoted his research efforts toward identifying drugs that could be applied directly to skin cancers and precancerous lesions. He developed a topical treatment for skin cancer with 5-fluorouracil and one of the first effective treatments for Kaposi's sarcoma. In 1972, Klein

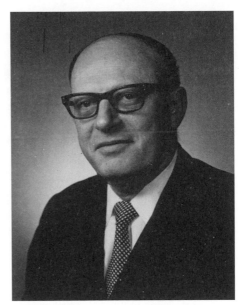

Edmund Klein, 1972. (*NLM*)

received one of the first Lasker Awards for Clinical Medical Research for developing the means of treating superficial cancers with a topical ointment containing potent anticancer chemicals – a form of therapy that is still used today, especially for premalignant growths.

Klein also focused his efforts on the use of immunotherapy, which enables the body's own defenses to ward off tumors. Application of agents to stimulate the immune system led to the use of interferon and interleukins in modern cancer therapy. Klein also developed a technique to separate whole human blood into its component parts of plasma, platelets, white blood cells, and red blood cells. This greatly increased the efficiency of the blood transfusions, making it possible for three people to benefit from a single donor instead of one. Red blood cells could be used for treating a person with anemia, platelets as therapy for those with bleeding disorders, and plasma for individuals with decreased blood volume. For this work, Klein received the first prize for originality of research from the International Society for Hematology in 1956.

---

## Kligman, Albert Montgomery (USA, 1916–2010)

---

Born in Philadelphia to immigrant parents, Albert Kligman received a doctorate in botany and then a medical degree from the University of Pennsylvania. Kligman specialized in dermatology and joined the faculty at the Hospital of the University of Pennsylvania.

Kligman is best known for his discovery that tretinoin, the active ingredient in Retin-A, could improve acne and reduce facial wrinkles. This generated substantial royalties, which Kligman used to donate millions of dollars to the Dermatology Department at Penn. He was credited with coining the terms "photoaging," to describe the wrinkles and discoloration that result from a lifetime of overexposure to the sun, and "cosmeceuticals," to describe skin care products that are part cosmetic and part drug. By feeding chocolate bars to teenagers with acne in a controlled study, Kligman was able to debunk the myth that chocolate makes acne worse.

Despite his significant scientific contributions, Kligman gained notoriety for the human experiments he performed on inmates at Holmesburg Prison in Philadelphia and the scandal it generated years later. At a time when prisoners were routinely paid for volunteering as subjects for drug testing, Kligman performed dozens of such experiments financially supported by pharmaceutical companies and government agencies. From 1965–1966, Kligman exposed about 75 prisoners at Holmesburg to high doses of dioxin to test the toxicity of the chemical warfare agent, which was later determined to be responsible for the toxicity of Agent Orange. In 2000, soon after the publication of a book on the Holmesburg experiments was published, nearly 300 former prisoners sued Kligman and other defendants, alleging that their exposure 35 years previously had caused debilitating health problems. These suits were dismissed by the courts, which ruled that the statute of limitations had expired. However, public reaction to the testing program contributed to the enactment of federal regulations restricting medical studies in prisons.

---

**Lassar, Oskar**                                              (Germany, 1849–1907)

---

Born in Hamburg and earning a medical degree, Oskar Lassar worked briefly as a hospital assistant at the Berlin Charité Hospital before establishing a private hospital for dermatology and syphilis in Berlin. Technologically advanced, Lassar's clinic was the first to have a Finsen ultraviolet light therapy device and X-ray machine. In 1902, Lassar became a Professor of Dermatology at the University of Berlin.

At a time when the poor in Germany and Austria had no access to private baths, Lassar spearheaded the creation of public bath houses for these low-income individuals to provide public hygiene. One slogan for these bathhouses (Volksbaden, in German) was "a weekly bath for every German."[42]

Lassar developed a topical zinc oxide paste with salicylic acid for treatment of skin irritations. This material forms a barrier on the skin to protect it from irritants and moisture and is still known as "Lassar's paste." In 1893, Lassar founded the German dermatology journal, *Dermatologische Zeitschrift*, which he edited until his death. One hundred years later, this major publication was renamed *Dermatology*.

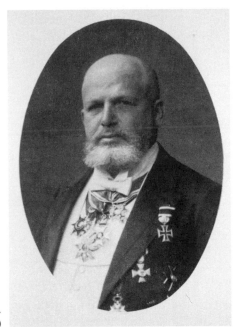

Oskar Lassar with medals, 1908. (*Wikimedia*)

## Neumann, Isidor (Moravia, 1832–1906)

Born in Miroslav, Isidor Neumann studied medicine at the University of Vienna. A student at the so-called Vienna School of Dermatology under Ferdinand Ritter von Hebra, Neumann eventually was appointed Professor of Dermatology and director of the clinic for syphilis. During the occupation of Bosnia-Herzogovina, the Austrian government sent Neumann to manage the public health problems of syphilis and leprosy.[43]

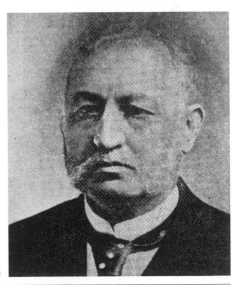

Isidor Neumann. (*NLM*)

42. Albrecht Scholz, et al., *Geschichte der deutschsprachigen Dermatologie (History of German language dermatology)* (Wiley-Blackwell, 2009). Also cited in Wikipedia, https://en.wikipedia.org/wiki/Oskar _Lassar.

43. L. Whaley, *Women and the Practice of Medical Care in Early Modern Europe, 1400–1800* (New York: Palgrave MacMillan, 2011).

In an 1886 publication, he described a type of the skin disease pemphigus vulgaris, which later became known as "Neumann disease," Neumann also was the first to publish a detailed study of prematurely aged skin caused by over-exposure to extreme weather conditions, which later was called "sailors' skin."

---

## Sulzberger, Marion Baldur                                    (USA, 1895–1983)

Born to a wealthy family in New York City, Marion Sulzberger served as an aviator in World War I before beginning his medical studies in Switzerland, first in Geneva and then at the University of Zurich, where he specialized in dermatology under Bruno Bloch. Returning to the United States, Sulzberger entered private practice. During World War II, Sulzberger served with the Naval Reserve as a lieutenant commander and was decorated by the United States and France for his outstanding contributions to the understanding and treatment of the dermatoses caused by poison

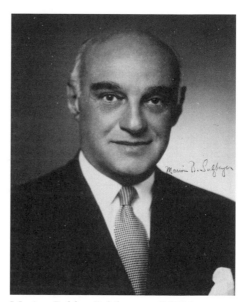

Marion Baldur Sulzberger. (*NLM*)

gases, burns, and tropical skin diseases. Becoming Professor of Dermatology and Syphilology of the New York University-Bellevue Medical Center in 1949, Sulzberger retired for several years before accepting an appointment as Professor of Clinical Dermatology at the University of California in San Francisco, where he founded a dermatological research unit that later became the Letterman Army Institute of Research.

Sulzberger was a major figure in establishing the modern specialty of dermatology in the United States. His most famous paper on Compound F (later named cortisone) introduced the use of topical corticosteroids applied directly to the skin as a treatment for various dermatologic diseases. Sulzberger was known for his work in dermatologic obstetrics and described a phenomenon now called specific immunologic tolerance, which plays an important role in modern immunologic research. He also was a leader in the study of contact allergies, such as those due to poison ivy.

Cited as "Mr. Dermatology" and "Dermatology's Man of the Century" in obituaries in the *Journal of the American Medical Association*, Sulzberger was the founder of the *Journal of Investigative Dermatology* in 1937 and served for a decade as its first editor.

## Unna, Paul Gerson (Germany, 1850–1929)

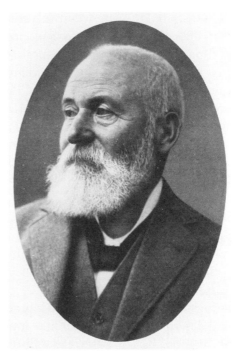

Paul Gerson Unna (*Wikimedia / NLM*)

The son of a prominent Jewish physician from Hamburg, Paul Unna initially studied medicine at the University of Heidelberg, but this was interrupted when he enlisted to fight in the Franco-Prussian war and was seriously injured. Unna eventually completed his medical education in Strasbourg, with a dissertation on the histology and developmental history of the epidermis. Seeking further intensive training in dermatology, Unna traveled to Vienna to study at its famous Dermatology Institute. Unna returned to Hamburg, where he worked in his father's clinical practice before branching out to establish a private skin clinic and then a dermatology institute, which attracted many students from Germany and abroad. In 1919, Unna became a professor at the University of Hamburg and its first Chair for Dermatology.

Unna's first book, *Histopathology of Skin Diseases* (1884), summarized the entire scope of knowledge in the field. His description of all known skin diseases and proposal of new therapies made Unna one of the most prominent dermatologists of his time. Unna also conducted research on the biochemical processes of the skin, described the plasma cell, and identified seborrheic dermatitis, a common inflammatory disease of the skin characterized by scaly lesions usually on the scalp, hairline, and face that became known as "Unna's disease."

## ENDOCRINOLOGY

Minkowski demonstrated that removal of the pancreas could induce symptoms of diabetes in dogs, concluding that the pancreas secretes an anti-diabetic substance that controls blood sugar, later shown to be the hormone insulin. Levine showed that insulin lowers blood sugar by stimulating the movement of glucose from the blood into fat and muscle cells. Barron demonstrated the important relationship of the islet cells in the pancreas with diabetes. Lunenfeld was a pioneering human reproduction, extracting and purifying human menopausal gonadotropin (hgMG) and being the first to introduce it for clinical use in non-ovulatory women and hypopituitary-hypogonadotropic men. Conn described primary aldosteronism, due to an adrenal tumor that secretes a hormone that produces hypertension that can be cured by surgically removing the tumor.

**Barron, Moses**                                            (Russia, 1884–1974)

Brought to the United States by his parents at age 5, Moses Barron grew up in Minnesota and studied medicine at the University of Minnesota. After serving as a medical officer in France during World War 1, Barron returned to his alma mater and later became a Clinical Professor of Medicine.

Barron is best known for his 1920 article indicating the important relationship of the islet cells of Langerhans in the pancreas with diabetes and describing the experimental approach he had used to investigate this association. Barron described a fibrotic pancreas, in which the acinar enzyme-secreting cells had disappeared but the islet cells were intact, and referred to previous experiments in animals where almost identical pathologic changes developed after ligation of the pancreatic duct.

Barron was instrumental in the creation of Mount Sinai Hospital in Minneapolis. Prior to the hospital construction in 1949, Jewish doctors were denied admitting privileges to local hospitals. Determined to address this discrimination, the Jewish community raised the capital to build Mount Sinai Hospital in South Minneapolis. Initially, Barron pushed for a Jewish-sponsored hospital to provide opportunities for Jewish physicians returning from the war, but with Barron as the first Chief of Staff, Mount Sinai soon became the first private non-sectarian hospital in the state to accept members of minority races on its medical staff.

After winning the 1923 Nobel Prize in Physiology or Medicine (with Charles Best) for the discovery of insulin as a treatment for diabetes, Frederick Banting noted that Barron's article was the inspiration for their own successful experiments. Fittingly, Barron received the Banting Award from the American Diabetes Association in 1964.

---

## Conn, Jerome W. (USA, 1907–1994)

Born in New York City, Jerome Conn received a medical degree from the University of Michigan, where he spent virtually all his career, serving as Head of the Division of Endocrinology and Metabolism from 1943 to 1973. Conn initially worked at the Division of Clinical Investigation under Louis H. Newburgh on the relationship between obesity and non-insulin-dependent diabetes mellitus. Conn proved that normal carbohydrate tolerance could be achieved in almost all subjects when they reached normal weight.

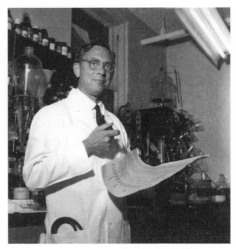

Jerome W. Conn. (*Faculty History Project, Bentley Historical Library, University of Michigan*)

Conn in best known for his 1954 description of a serious kidney disease associated with potassium loss. Now known as Conn syndrome, he termed it primary aldosteronism after determining that it stemmed from an adrenal tumor that produces excessive amounts of aldosterone, a hormone that affects the kidneys and causes the retention of salt and the excretion of potassium. Unlike many serious hypertensive diseases, primary aldosteronism can be cured completely, if recognized early enough, by surgically removing the adrenal tumor.

Conn also developed a treatment for Addison's disease, an adrenal hormonal disorder that affects the balance of substances like salt, potassium, water, glucose, and protein. He found that the administration of cortisone could restore the balance, but that it was necessary for the patient to take the medication for life.

## Levine, Rachmiel                                    (Poland, 1910–1998)

Born in eastern Poland, now part
of the Ukraine, Rachmiel Levine
was 16 years old when his father
was killed in an anti-Jewish pogrom. Unsuccessful in joining his
grandparents in the United States,
Levine was able to immigrate to
Canada, where he was adopted by
a family friend who was a physician. Levine received his medical
degree from McGill University in
Montreal. After completing an internal medicine residency at Michael Reese Hospital in Chicago,
Levine continued on the staff and
rose to become director of the department. Levine later was Chief
Physician of Internal Medicine at
the New York Medical College and

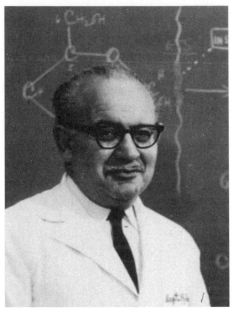

Rachmiel Levine. (*Gairdner Foundation*)

the Managing Medical Director of the City of Hope National Medical
Center, establishing it as a leading institution for diabetes research.

Levine made numerous contributions to the study of diabetes. At the
time, insulin was an established treatment, but how it regulated the use
of blood sugars was unknown. Without insulin, glucose accumulates in
the blood and cannot enter muscle and fat cells. This can cause a diabetic
coma, which can be fatal. Levine was skeptical of explanations that required
insulin to enter the cell to turn on enzymes within it. Instead, he reasoned
that insulin worked on the outside of the cell to stimulate the transport of
glucose and other sugars.

In his experiments, conducted with Maurice Goldstein and Samuel
Soskin, Levine gave dogs a form of sugar called galactose and then calcu-
lated its level of dilution. He found that the galactose was concentrated
only in the small amount of water outside the cells. After injecting insulin,
the sugar's dilution level showed that the galactose had reached the inside
of the cells. Levine concluded that insulin acted like a key that unlocked
the cell membrane, allowing the sugars to get inside.

This discovery that insulin lowers blood sugar by stimulating the movement of glucose from the blood into fat and muscle cells is known as the

Levine effect. This standard explanation of how the transport mechanism works also was shown to apply to other hormones, introducing a new era of research into how hormones modify cell functions.

## Luft, Rolf (Sweden, 1914–2007)

Born in Stockholm, Rolf Luft was a physician and medical researcher working at the Karolinska Hospital in Solna Municipality and as Professor of Endocrinology at the Karolinska Institute. Internationally known as a researcher on diabetes, the Rolf Luft Center for Diabetes Research at the Karolinska Institute is named for him, as is its annual award that recognizes a scientist who "made groundbreaking discoveries that can be of great importance for the development of new drugs for the treatment of diabetes." He also described Luft disease, the first disorder that could be linked to impaired mitochondrial function. In 1977, Luft served as President of the Nobel Committee for Physiology or Medicine.

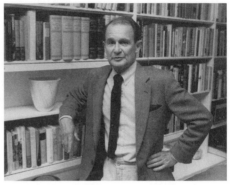

Rolf Luft. (*Courtesy of Dr. Luft's family*)

## Lunenfeld, Bruno (Austria, 1927–)

Born in Vienna, Bruno Lunenfeld was educated in Austria, the United Kingdom, and Israel before attending medical school at the University of Geneva. After receiving his medical degree, Lunenfeld returned to Israel to become a Senior Scientist at the Weizmann Institute in Rehovot. In 1969, he was appointed head of the Institute of Endocrinology at the Sheba Medical Center. In 1992, Lunenfeld was named Professor Emeritus of the Faculty of Life Sciences at Bar-Ilan University, and Medical Director of the International Fertility Institute in Ra'anana.

Lunenfeld is best known for his pioneering work in human reproduction. He extracted and purified human menopausal gonadotropin (hgMG) and was the first to introduce it for clinical use in non-ovulatory women and hypopituitary-hypogonadotropic men. Lunenfeld was instrumental in the creation of an international standard for gonadotropins, the classification of infertile patients, and description of the hyperstimulation syndrome. He also has made significant contributions to the understanding of follicular recruitment, rescue, selection, growth and development, the ovulatory cycle, and the mechanism of action of gonadotropins in ovaries and testes, as well as molecular mechanisms of cell proliferation and cell death in hormone-dependent tumors and aging.

---

### Minkowski, Oskar                                   (Russia, 1858–1931)

---

Oskar Minkowski was born in Kovno, now in Lithuania, the son of a merchant who subsidized the construction of the Choral Synagogue in that city. After receiving his medical degree at Königsberg, Minkowski held multiple academic positions in internal medicine, including professorships at Strasbourg and Breslau.

In a landmark 1889 study in collaboration with Josef von Mering, which demonstrated that removal of the pancreas could induce symptoms of diabetes in dogs, Minkowski concluded that the pancreas secretes an anti-diabetic substance that controls blood sugar. Later this was shown to be the hormone insulin, which could be provided to patients to treat the disease. Minkowski also proved that diabetic coma is accompanied by a decrease in the amount of carbon dioxide dissolved in the blood and introduced alkali therapy to counteract it.

---

### GASTROENTEROLOGY

---

Jewish gastroenterologists developed innovations for visualizing the digestive tract and collecting samples from it. Einhorn invented a tube for duodenal intubation, which made it possible to obtain specimens of bile and pancreatic secretions for examinations, as well as an ingenious means of locating the site of upper gastrointestinal bleeding by observing stains on a swallowed, weighted string. Hirschowitz developed an improved optical fiber that allowed the creation of a fully flexible fiberoptic endoscope, which provided an unobstructed view inside such hollow organs as the esophagus, stomach, and colon and the means for minimally invasive surgical procedures. Clinically, Crohn demonstrated the distinct pathologist entity, originally called regional ileitis, which now bears his name. He also was among the first to maintain that many gastric and intestinal ailments were the result of anxiety, stress, or neuroses rather than actual organic disorders. Kirsner demonstrated that stomach acid was necessary for the development of ulcers, while Lewisohn showed an increased risk of colon cancer in patients with ulcerative colitis and suggested the possibility of an infectious factor in the etiology of peptic ulcer disease. Potter is considered the father of modern hepatology, establishing diagnostic guidelines for major liver diseases and making important observations in understanding hepatitis viruses. Schiff was one of the first physicians to use the procedures of gastroscopy and percutaneous liver biopsy and was the author of the leading textbook on hepatic diseases.

---

## Crohn, Burrill B. (USA, 1884–1983)

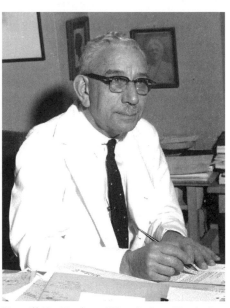

Born in New York City, Burrill Crohn studied medicine at Columbia University and spend most of his career associated with Mount Sinai Hospital. Specializing in gastroenterology, Crohn is best known for describing regional ileitis, the disease that now bears his name.

Working with Leon Ginzburg and Gordon Oppenheimer, Crohn identified 14 patients who had similar symptoms and intestinal abnormalities discovered at surgery that did not fit any previously known disease. In their classic 1932 article, "Regional Ileitis: A Pathologic and Clinical Entity," Crohn and colleagues showed that this was a distinct inflammatory

Burrill B. Crohn. (*The Arthur H. Aufses, Jr. MD Archives, Icahn School of Medicine at Mount Sinai*)

disease of the gastrointestinal tract, rather than the mistaken belief that it was a form of tuberculosis. Crohn always preferred the medically descriptive terms "regional ileitis" and "regional enteritis," but was unable to prevent the disorder from being generally known as "Crohn's disease." Crohn built a large and thriving practice treating patients with regional enteritis and served as Chief of Gastroenterology at Mount Sinai Hospital.

Crohn was among the first physicians to maintain that many gastric and intestinal ailments were the result of anxiety, stress, or neuroses rather than actual organic disorders. Elected president of the American Gastroenter-ological Association in 1932, Crohn was asked to consult on high-profile patients with ileitis from all over the world, including President Dwight D. Eisenhower in 1956. Crohn authored three books: *Affections of the Stomach* (1927), *Understand Your Ulcer* (1943), and *Regional Ileitis* (1947).

---

## Einhorn, Max                                      (Poland, 1862–1953)

One of the first clinicians to de-velop gastroenterology as a med-ical specialty, Max Einhorn was born in Grodno and attended medical school at the Univer-sity of Berlin. Immigrating to the United States in 1888, Einhorn was appointed the first Professor of Gastroenterology at the New York Postgraduate Medical School. He established a private practice at German Hospital, now the Lenox Hill Hospital.

A prolific innovator, Einhorn invented many devices to exam-ine the gastrointestinal tract. He developed a tube for duodenal in-tubation, which made it possible to obtain specimens of bile and pan-

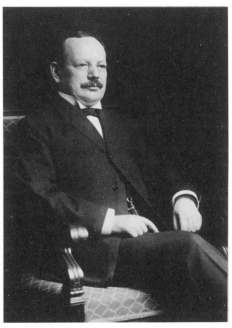

Max Einhorn. (*NLM*)

creatic secretions for examinations. Before the advent of radiography or en-doscopy, Einhorn developed an ingenious means of locating the site of up-per gastrointestinal bleeding by observing stains on a swallowed, weighted string. Other inventions included gastrodiaphany to map the stomach by introducing an electrical light into the stomach so that it became trans-parent through the anterior abdominal wall, a new esophagoscope, and an intestinal tube, as well as a stomach bucket and gastrograph, stomach spray and power blower, and duodenal bucket. Einhorn also invented the fermentation saccharometer, which was used to diagnose diabetes by es-timating the amount of sugar in the urine.

The author of several books in his specialty, Einhorn was a founding member of the American Gastrointestinal Association and served as its third president.

## Hirschowitz, Basil Isaac

(South Africa, 1925–2013)

Born in Bethal, the son of Jewish immigrants fleeing pogroms in Lithuania, Basil Hirschowitz received his medical degree from the University of the Witwatersrand in Johannesburg. Moving to the United States in 1953, Hirschowitz completed a fellowship in gastroenterology at the University of Michigan before joining the faculty. In 1959, Hirschowitz was among the elite faculty recruited to the University of Alabama School of Medicine in Birmingham. Hirschowitz founded the department of gastroenterology and remained as its director for 29 years. After Hirschowitz's retirement, an endowed chair in gastroenterology was established in his honor.

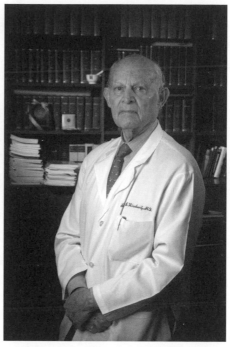

Basil Isaac Hirschowitz. (*UAB/Steve Wood*)

In 1954 while a fellow, Hirschowitz read an article by Hopkins and Kapany describing recent advances in fiberoptics. After visiting the authors in Britain to discuss the application of fiberoptics to endoscopy, Hirschowitz and associates Larry Curtis and C. Wilbur Peters developed a technique for coating and bundling hair-thin glass fibers to allow viewing over long distances and around bends. This gave an illuminated and unobstructed view inside hollow organs such as the esophagus, stomach, and colon, even providing the means for minimally invasive surgery. In 1957, Hirschowitz tested the first prototype instrument by passing it down his own throat; shortly afterward, he repeated the procedure in a patient. In collaboration with American Cystoscope Manufacturing, within three years Hirschowitz received the first production model of a fully flexible fiberoptic endoscope. This invention not only revolutionized the practice of gastroenterology, but also provided the basis for optical fiber communication in multiple industries, such as modern telecommunications.

## Janowitz, Henry D.                                    (USA, 1915– 2008)

Born in Paterson, New Jersey, Henry Janowitz studied medicine at Columbia University and specialized in gastroenterology. A pioneer in establishing this field, Janowitz served as Chief of the Gastrointestinal Clinic at the Mount Sinai Hospital from 1956–1961, afterwards remaining as Professor of Clinical Medicine. The Gastroenterology Department at Mount Sinai was named in his honor.

An internationally renowned leader in gastroenterology, Janowitz's main research interest was the pathology, natural history, and management of inflammatory

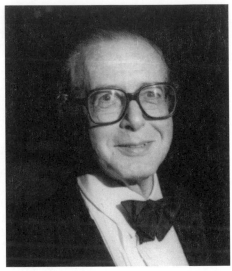

Henry D. Janowitz. (*The Arthur H. Aufses, Jr. MD Archives, Icahn School of Medicine at Mount Sinai*)

bowel diseases, and he played a major role in founding the Crohn's and Colitis Foundation of America. Janowitz emphasized meticulous history taking and involvement of the patient and family in the pursuit of diagnosis and cure. A distinguished teacher with a great interest in lay education, Janowitz authored the popular book *Good Food for Bad Stomachs* (1997), and he was an authority on medical allusions in Shakespeare.

## Kirsner, Joseph Barrett                              (USA, 1909–2012)

The son of Ukrainian Jewish immigrants, Joseph Kirsner was born in Boston and attended medical school at Tufts University. Kirsner joined the faculty at the University of Chicago in 1935, remaining there for his entire professional career. Kirsner was a major force in transforming the field of gastroenterology from an art (which he termed "speculative, impressionistic, anecdotal, almost mystical at times")[44] into a science.

Kirsner's early research involved the study of peptic ulcers and the ef-

44. https://news.uchicago.edu/article/2012/07/09/joseph-b-kirsner-pioneer-gastroenterology-1909-2012

fects of antacids on stomach-acid secretion and body chemistry. He was among the first to demonstrate that stomach acid was necessary for the development of ulcers. Kirsner later was a pioneer in the understanding and treatment of inflammatory bowel disease. He drew attention to the complex relationships between bacteria in the gut and the immune system in the development of inflammatory bowel disease and was one of the first to show an increased risk of colon cancer in patients with ulcerative colitis. Noting that patients with even mild cases of inflammatory bowel disease lost high levels of protein, Kirsner emphasized the importance of nutrition in these

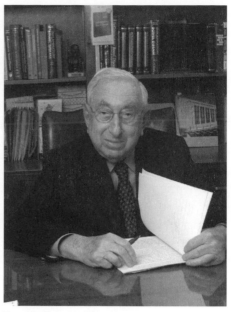

Joseph Barrett Kirsner. (*University of Chicago Medicine*)

individuals. Never forgetting the personal aspects of medicine, he always emphasized to students and young physicians the importance of combining competence with compassion when treating patients.

The author of more than 750 papers and an authoritative textbook, *Inflammatory Bowel Disease* (1975), Kirsner was among the founders of the American Gastroenterological Association.

## Lewisohn, Richard (Germany, 1875–1961)

Born in Hamburg, Richard Lewisohn received his medical degree from the University of Freiburg. Lewisohn immigrated to the United States in 1906, where he joined the staff at Mount Sinai Hospital in New York as a gastroenterologist and surgeon and later was Chief of General Surgery (1928–1936). After witnessing a subtotal gastrectomy for gastric ulcer in Europe, Lewisohn convinced Albert Berg to perform the procedure at Mount Sinai. He reported that subtotal gastrectomy resulted in a loss of acidity, whereas a simple gastrojejunostomy alone had no effect on acid production, which resulted in the subsequent development of gastrojejunal ulcers at the anastomotic site. In the same article, Lewisohn suggested the possibility of an infectious factor in the etiology of peptic ulcer disease, many years before the critical role of *Heliobacter pylori* in ulcer disease was discovered. Lewisohn also was the first to demonstrate the importance of folic acid in the biology of cancer and among the first to use folic acid antagonists in clinical treatment.

Lewisohn is best known for introducing the use of sodium citrate as an anticoagulant. In combination with the use of refrigeration, this permitted the effective storage of blood and the subsequent development of the first blood banks. Although its anticoagulant properties were known, Lewisohn proved that sodium citrate was non-toxic when used in the proper concentration (0.2%). This replaced the previous method of direct blood transfusion between donor and recipient.

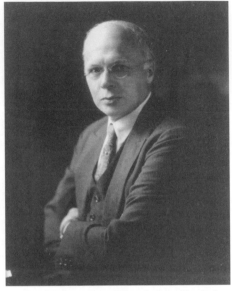

Richard Lewisohn. (*The Arthur H. Aufses, Jr. MD Archives, Icahn School of Medicine at Mount Sinai*)

---

### Popper, Hans

(Austria, 1903–1988)

Born in Vienna and the son of a prominent physician, Hans Popper followed in his father's footsteps and received his medical degree from the University of Vienna. After graduation, Popper specialized in anatomical pathology and established a biochemical laboratory, where he developed the creatinine clearance test to assess renal function. After the Nazis occupied Austria, Popper narrowly escaped

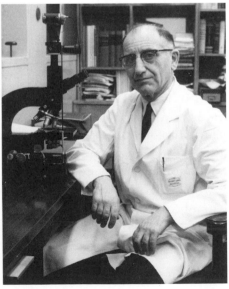

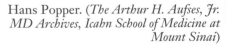

Hans Popper. (*The Arthur H. Aufses, Jr. MD Archives, Icahn School of Medicine at Mount Sinai*)

and moved to Cook County Hospital in Chicago, earning a doctorate in pathology and physiology at the University of Illinois. A leading figure in the founding of the Mount Sinai School of Medicine in New York, Popper served as Pathologist-in-Chief and the first Dean of Academic Affairs when it was established in 1963.

Popper was an international authority on liver disease and known as the founding father of modern hepatology. He demonstrated that the liver is the only organ in the body that does not deteriorate with age, research that had major ramifications in the field of liver transplantation. The author of 800 papers and 28 books, Popper established diagnostic guidelines for several major liver diseases and was instrumental in furthering the understanding of hepatitis viruses.

---

## Schiff, Leon (Latvia, 1901–1994)

Born in Riga, Leon Schiff immigrated with his family to the United States at age 5. Schiff earned his medical degree and doctorate at the University of Cincinnati. Specializing in gastroenterology, Schiff remained at his alma mater and founded the Gastric Laboratory. A distinguished clinician, teacher, and researcher, Schiff was one of the first physicians to use the diagnostic procedures of gastroscopy and percutaneous liver biopsy, both of which are standard

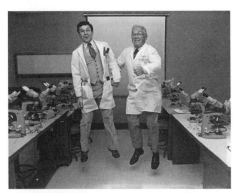

Leon Schiff (right) and his son Eugene Schiff (left) in a laboratory at the Schiff Center for Liver Disease at the University of Miami. (*Courtesy of Dr. Schiff*)

techniques today. He was the author of *Schiff's Diseases of the Liver*, recognized as the world's foremost textbook on hepatic diseases and now in its eleventh edition. Schiff also was a founding member and the first president of the American Association for the Study of Liver Diseases. In 1970, Schiff joined the faculty of the University of Miami School of Medicine, establishing the Center for Liver Diseases 20 years later.

His son, Eugene Schiff, has followed in his father's footsteps, serving as Chief of the Hepatology Section at the Miami VA Medical Center, working alongside his father at the Center for Liver Diseases, and editing later editions of *Schiff's Diseases of the Liver*.

## HEMATOLOGY

Jewish physicians were leading pioneers in the development of modern hematology. Wintrobe and Hayem developed techniques for performing accurate counts of red blood cells and platelets, respectively. Wintrobe classified anemia morphologically as microcytic, normocytic, or macrocytic, a system still used today. Beutler and Wintrobe intensively studied iron metabolism, pernicious anemia, and the hemolytic anemias related to sickle cell disease and G-6-PD deficiency. Beutler pioneered bone marrow transplantation for acute leukemia and chemotherapy for chronic lymphoma and leukemia, while Dameshek developed steroid therapy for immune thrombocytopenia and antimetabolite therapy for autoimmune diseases. Landsteiner and Hirszfeld improved the safety of blood transfusions by initially discovering the existence of three distinct antigenic groups (A, B, and O) and then showing that a blood transfusion between persons with the same blood group did not lead to the destruction of blood cells, whereas this occurred between persons of different blood groups. Landsteiner, Wiener, and Levine discovered the Rhesus (Rh) factor and introduced into clinical practice a method of preventing maternal-fetal incompatibility (erythroblastosis fetalis).

Shapiro was a pioneer in anticoagulant therapy, discovering Dicoumarol and conceiving the use of sodium warfarin as an even more effective and safer anticoagulant agent. Cohn developed a process of blood fractionation, a technique that separated the different proteins in blood plasma, allowing transfusion with purified albumin on the battlefield that saved the lives of thousands of soldiers suffering from shock.

---

**Beutler, Ernest**                                                     (Germany, 1928–2008)

---

Born in Berlin to a pair of Jewish physicians who ironically were living on a square renamed "Adolf Hitler Platz," Ernest Beutler and his family moved to the United States in 1935 to escape Nazi persecution. Raised in Milwaukee and receiving his undergraduate, medical school and residency education at the University of Chicago, Buetler specialized in hematology. After several years on the faculty, in 1959 Beutler became Chairman of the Department of Medicine of the City of Hope National Medical Center in Duarte, California. Twenty years later, Beutler assumed the Chairmanship of the Department of Clinical Research at the Scripps Clinic and Research Foundation in La Jolla, remaining there until his death.

Beutler performed research on many aspects related to red blood cells and bone marrow transplantation. He made important discoveries about the causes of the anemia due to G-6-PD deficiency and other hemolytic anemias, Gaucher's disease, disorders of iron metabolism, and Tay-Sachs disease. He also was among the first scientists to identify X-chromosome inactivation as the genetic basis of tissue mosaicism in female mammals. Beutler pioneered various medical treatments, including bone marrow transplantation for acute leukemia and chemotherapy for chronic lymphoma and leukemia.

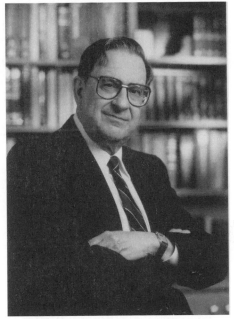

Ernest Beutler. (*American Society of Hematology*)

## Cohn, Edwin (USA, 1892–1953)

Born in New York City, Edwin Cohn received a doctorate in biochemistry at the University of Chicago. Cohn spent most of his research career at Harvard University, focusing on amino acids and peptides, the building blocks of proteins.

Cohn is best known for developing a process of blood fractionation during World War II, a technique that separated the different proteins in blood plasma. One major component is serum albumin, which is essential for maintaining the osmotic pressure in blood vessels and preventing their collapse. Transfusion with purified albumin

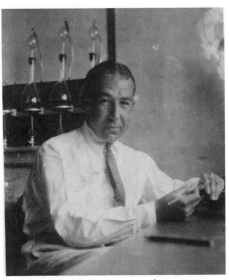

Edwin Cohn. (*Smithsonian Institution Archives. Image #SIA2008-1041*)

on the battlefield saved the lives of thousands of soldiers suffering from shock. With serum albumin in high demand as the war dragged on, Cohn oversaw the efforts to produce large quantities of this plasma fraction at high-quality standards. Gamma globulin fractions, which contain antibodies, were used to treat measles during the war, and later they were the main weapon for fighting polio until a vaccine was developed to prevent this disease.

Earlier in his career, Cohn developed a method for significantly concentrating the vital factor in liver extract, which had been shown by Minot and Murphy to be the only known specific treatment for pernicious anemia. For the next 20 years, Cohn's technique allowed for a practical treatment of this previously incurable and fatal condition.

---

## Dameshek, William                                    (Russia, 1900–1969)

---

Born Ze'ev Dameshek in Voronezh, he was brought to the United States at age 3 and renamed William. Dameshek graduated from Harvard Medical School and specialized in hematology, becoming the pre-eminent clinical hematologist of his time. After serving as Professor of Medicine at Tufts in Boston, Dameshek moved to New York to become a Professor of Medicine and attending hematologist at Mount Sinai.

In 1946, Dameshek was the founder and chief editor of *Blood*, the major clinical journal in hema-

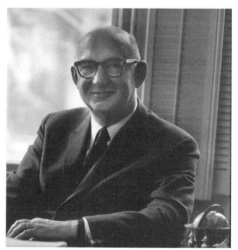

William Dameshek. (*American Society of Hematology*)

tology. He was a lead investigator in the first multi-institutional trial of chemotherapy for malignant disease, which employed nitrogen mustard to treat Hodgkin's lymphoma. Dameshek pioneered the treatment of immune thrombocytopenia with corticosteroids, introduced antimetabolite therapy for autoimmune diseases, and developed the concepts of the myeloproliferative and lymphoproliferative disorders. He also described chronic lymphocytic leukemia (CLL), a common form of leukemia in adults, proposing that the disease resulted from a gradual accumulation of lymphocytes.

Dameshek served as president of the American Society of Hematology, which established a prize in his honor to be awarded to an individual who has made an outstanding contribution in hematology. Among his major books are *Leukopenia and Agranulocytosis* (1944), *Hemolytic Syndromes* (1949), *The Hemorrhagic Disorders* (1955), and *Leukemia* (1958).

## Hayem, Georges                                         (France, 1841–1933)

Born in Paris and earning a medical degree at the University of Paris, Georges Hayem practiced in several locations in the city before becoming the Chair of Clinical Medicine at Hôpital St. Antoine.

A pioneer of modern hematology, Hayem performed seminal studies on the formation of leukocytes and erythrocytes (white and red blood cells). He developed a solution of mercury bichloride, sodium chloride, and sodium sulfate for diluting blood prior to counting erythrocytes with the hemocytometer he invented. Hayem microscopically studied the characteristics of red blood cells, describing their normal and pathological morphology and relationship with hemoglobin, as well as reporting

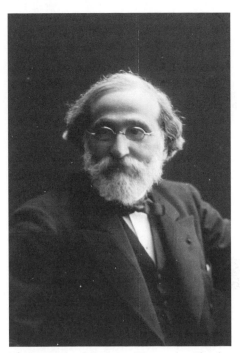

Photograph of Georges Hayem by Charles Gerschel. (*Wikimedia / NLM*)

numerous clinical studies of blood diseases and hemorrhagic diatheses. He provided classic descriptions of chronic interstitial hepatitis and acquired hemolytic jaundice (once known as the Hayem-Widal syndrome) and performed the first accurate count of blood platelets. During a cholera epidemic, Hayem introduced the intravenous administration of an isotonic solution of saline for treatment to combat the dehydration resulting from the disease, succeeding in saving 30% of his patients.

In 1872, Hayem founded the *Revue des sciences médicales en France et à l'étrang*. Hayem authored many published articles, and his 1900 textbook on hematology, *Clinical Lessons on Blood Disorders*, was widely read.

## Hirszfeld, Ludwik                                    (Poland, 1884–1954)

Born in Warsaw into the family of a rich Jewish industrialist, but later a convert to Catholicism, Ludwik Hirszfeld was unable to obtain a spot in a Polish medical school because of his faith. Therefore, Hirszfeld went to Germany to study medicine, first in Wurzburg and then in Berlin. The topic of his doctoral thesis was the agglutination of blood. After several years at the Heidelberg Institute for Experimental Cancer, Hirszfeld accepted an assistantship at the Hygiene Institute of the University of Zurich. During World War I, Hirszfeld joined the Serbian army as a serological and bacteriology adviser to a country devastated by epidemics of typhus and bacillary

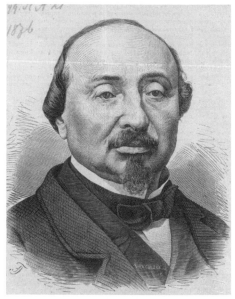

Photograph of Ludwik Hirszfeld by Aleksander Tadeusz Regulski, 1876. (*Wikimedia*)

dysentery. At the hospital for contagious diseases in Thessaloniki, Hirszfeld discovered the bacillus *Salmonella paratyphi C*, which now bears his name.

After the war, Hirszfeld returned to Warsaw to establish a serum institute modeled after the Ehrlich Institute for Experimental Therapy in Frankfurt. He became the scientific head of the State Hygiene Institute in Warsaw and a professor at the University of Warsaw, serving on many international boards. After the German army occupied Poland, Hirszfeld was dismissed as a "non-Aryan" from the Hygiene Institute, and in 1941 was forced to move into the Warsaw ghetto with his wife and daughter. There he organized anti-epidemic measures and vaccination campaigns against typhus and typhoid, as well as conducting secret medical courses. Two years later, a day before being sent to an extermination camp, Hirszfeld and his wife fled the ghetto and survived underground by using false names and continually changing their hiding place, When a part of Poland was liberated in 1944, Hirszfeld immediately participated in establishing the University of Lublin and then became Director of the Institute for Medical Microbiology at Wrocław and Dean of the Medical Faculty.

Although Gregor Mendel had discovered the laws of heredity in 1866, his work was published in an obscure journal and largely ignored. Independently rediscovered at the turn of the 20th century, it was postulated that blood types were inherited by Mendelian principles. Hirszfeld and Emil von Dungern succeeded in establishing the pattern of blood heredity via three distinct groups, A, B, and O. They showed that a child of type B and a mother of type A could never have a father who was type A or O. Similarly, it was impossible for a child of type O to have a type AB father, regardless of the blood type of the mother.

Given the heredity of blood types, Hirszfeld wondered whether there might be a pattern of their geographical distribution based on such factors as race, nationality, or ethnic origin. During World War I, Hirszfeld was fortuitously thrust into a situation in which he had access to blood samples of soldiers from throughout Europe, the Middle East, and Asia. After analyzing large numbers of samples, Hirszfeld documented a definite geographic distribution of blood type. About half of Northern Europeans were type A, and this percentage dropped as one moved eastward. In contrast, a similar percentage of Indians had type B blood, which decreased as one moved westward. He concluded that blood types originated in two parts of the world – type A in Northern Europe and type B in Asia. Population migration and interbreeding resulted in the spectrum of people with various blood types that existed in his day. Hirszfeld speculated that the type O blood group must have developed much later in human evolution.

Hirszfeld was the first to foresee the serological conflict between mother and child, which was confirmed by the discovery of the Rhesus (Rh) factor, and introduced into clinical practice a method of preventing maternal-fetal incompatibility (erythroblastosis fetalis).

In 1946, Hirszfeld published his autobiography, *The Story of One Life*, which included his memories from the Warsaw Ghetto, and Poland issued a commemorative stamp in his honor in 2009.

## Landsteiner, Karl (Austria, 1868–1943)

Born in Vienna, Karl Landsteiner was the son of a prominent Jewish journalist and editor of *Die Presse*, but he converted to Catholicism as a young adult. Landsteiner earned his medical and doctoral degrees at the University of Vienna before becoming a Professor of Pathology at that institution and a co-discoverer of the polio virus (1910). In 1922, Landsteiner joined the Rockefeller Institute for Medical Research in New York, where he remained for the rest of his career.

Landsteiner is best known for developing the modern system of classification of the main blood groups (A, B, O), based on the presence of agglutinins in the blood. During residency, Landsteiner had witnessed patients dying of hemorrhage after an accident or during surgery because physicians refused to consider replacement blood transfusion. The often violent and fatal reactions after blood transfusions were considered at the time to be secondary to some unusual hematological disease of either the donor or the recipient. To test this theory, Landsteiner had blood drawn from six healthy people, including himself, and in individual test tubes mixed the red blood cells of one person with cell-free sera from each of the others. Under the microscope, Landsteiner observed that the red blood cells of two sub-

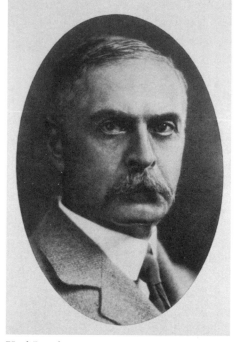

Karl Landsteiner, 1920s. (*Wikimedia / Biographical Memoirs of the National Academy of Sciences, vol. 40*)

jects were agglutinated (attacked) by the serum of the other four, but not by each other's. Another pair of subjects showed similar results. Landsteiner and the last person were immune from attack by anyone else's serum, or from the serum of each other.

Based on these experiments, Landsteiner established the existence of the three major blood groups. (Subsequent studies on a much larger group also revealed a rarer fourth blood type, AB, whose cells were agglutinated by the sera of all of the other three types.) Landsteiner demonstrated that

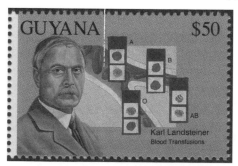

Karl Landsteiner depicted on Guyana stamp, 1993. (*Author's private collection*)

a blood transfusion between persons with the same blood group did not lead to the destruction of blood cells, whereas this occurred between persons of different blood groups. For this work, Landsteiner was awarded the 1930 Nobel Prize in Physiology or Medicine.

Recognized as the father of transfusion medicine, in 1937 Landsteiner collaborated with Alexander Wiener in identifying the Rh (Rhesus) factor, an inherited protein found on the surface of red blood cells. Individuals with this protein are termed Rh positive, while those whose blood lacks the protein are Rh negative. A person who is Rh positive can receive a blood transfusion of Rh positive or Rh negative blood. However, a person with Rh-negative blood should only get Rh-negative red blood cells, except in an extreme emergency. The reason is that an Rh-positive blood transfusion can cause a person with Rh negative blood to make antibodies against the Rh factor. The presence of these antibodies could harm any Rh-positive fetus she may have in the future, attacking its Rh positive blood cells and causing a severe and potentially fatal hemolytic anemia of the newborn. Rh incompatibility also can arise from pregnancy. The blood of the mother and fetus usually do not mix, but a small amount of fetal and maternal blood could come in contact during delivery or related to a miscarriage. If the mother is Rh negative and the fetus is Rh positive, the mother might produce Rh antibodies after exposure to the red blood cells of the fetus. This has no effect on the current pregnancy, but could prove devastating to a subsequent one. If a later fetus is Rh positive, the mother will produce Rh antibodies that can cross the placenta and damage the baby's red blood cells, leading to a miscarriage or to hemolytic anemia and jaundice or severe mental complications in the newborn. Understanding the cause eventually led to the effective treatment of this condition by replacing the blood supply of an affected infant through transfusions, usually right after birth. For this work, Landsteiner shared (with Wiener and Philip Levine) the 1946 Lasker Award for Clinical Medical Research for "Rh factor as a cause of hemolytic anemia in newborns."

## Levine, Philip (Russia, 1900–1987)

Born in Kletsk, now in Belarus, Philip Levine was brought to the United States at age 8. Levine studied medicine at Cornell University and became assistant to Karl Landsteiner at the Rockefeller Institute in New York. There he isolated three additional inherited factors in human blood (M, N, and P), which proved to be of special value in forensic medicine. After moving to the University of Wisconsin, Levine co-sponsored a model state law authorizing courts to carry out blood tests to determine paternity.

In a 1939 report about a family with a stillborn baby who had died of hemolytic disease of the newborn, Levine suggested that a mother could make blood group antibodies because of immune sensitization to the red blood cells of her fetus. Although the rhesus (Rh) factor responsible for this phenomenon was later isolated by Landsteiner and Alexander Wiener, Levine demonstrated its importance in obstetrics. He showed that the unborn child of an Rh-negative mother may inherit this factor from an Rh-positive father, which could pass through the placental circulation and sensitize the immune system of the mother to form antibodies against the blood of her own baby. Depending on the ability of other natural mechanisms to mitigate this effect, this Rh-incompatibility could result in a miscarriage or hemolytic anemia and jaundice or severe mental complications in the newborn. Understanding the cause

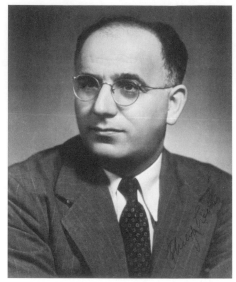

Philip Levine, 1944. (*NLM*)

eventually led to the effective treatment of this condition by replacing the blood supply of an affected infant through transfusions, usually right after birth.

Levine shared (with Landsteiner and Alexander Wiener) the 1946 Lasker Award for Clinical Medical Research for "Rh factor as a cause of hemolytic anemia in newborns."

## Shapiro, Shepard                                                          (USA, 1896–1966)

Born in Bayonne, New Jersey, Shepard Shapiro studied medicine at New York University and Bellevue Hospital Medical College. A pioneer in the concept and practice of anticoagulant therapy, Shapiro collaborated with Karl Paul Link of the University of Wisconsin, who discovered methylene dicoumarin. In 1940, they demonstrated the value of Dicoumarol as an anticoagulant in the treatment and prevention of thrombotic disease. Soon afterward, Shapiro showed that high doses of vitamin K could overcome the prothrombinopenia induced by Dicumarol (and salicylates). Shapiro conceived of using sodium warfarin as an even more effective and safer anticoagulant agent than Dicoumarol, introducing it for clinical use in 1953. With Paul Unger, Shapiro developed the vitamin K tolerance test, which made it easier to control anticoagulant therapy.

Shapiro also described the pathogenesis of sickle cell crisis and the ineffectiveness of anticoagulant therapy in that condition. With Victor Ross, Shapiro demonstrated the *in vivo* inhibition of blood coagulation by the hyperglobulinemia of multiple myeloma.

## Wiener, Alexander Solomon (USA, 1907–1976)

Born in Brooklyn, Alexander Wiener received a degree from the Long Island College of Medicine. Collaborating with Nobel Prize-winner Karl Landsteiner shortly after beginning his work at Brooklyn Jewish Hospital, where Wiener remained for the rest of his academic life, they discovered that the M Factor actually represented five distinct blood factors. In 1937, Wiener and Landsteiner discovered the Rh factor, named after the Rhesus monkeys used as test subjects, which is associated with complications in blood transfusions. Their work led subsequently to the development of

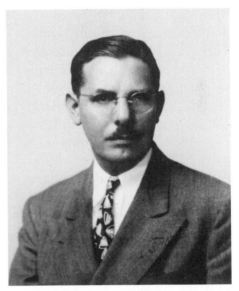

Alexander Solomon Wiener. (*NYU Health Sciences Library / NLM*)

methods of exchange transfusion, which saved the lives of countless infants with hemolytic anemia of the newborn. Wiener shared (with Landsteiner and Philip Levine) the 1946 Lasker Award for Clinical Medical Research for "Rh factor as a cause of hemolytic anemia in newborns."

All blood factors are inherited in predictable fashion and combine in a highly specific way in individuals. Therefore, Wiener pioneered the creation of a blood "fingerprint," a unique blood profile that could be used in a variety of both civil and criminal legal proceedings. Blood factor analysis became important in establishing paternity, as well as in identifying the victims and perpetrators of crimes. This technique also was used in physical anthropology, in which tribal movements can sometimes be traced by analysis of the proportions of various blood factors in different groups of people. Wiener and his father, attorney George Wiener, assisted in drafting a number of laws concerning blood testing that became part of the New York State domestic relations, civil, and criminal codes. In recognition of his contributions to forensic medicine, Wiener was made an honorary member of the Mystery Writers of America.

## Wintrobe, Maxwell Myer                           (Austria, 1901–1986)

Born Max Weintraub, at age 5 his family fled religious persecution in his native land and joined Canadian relatives living in Halifax, Nova Scotia. Wintrobe attended medical school at the University of Manitoba before moving to New Orleans, where he obtained his doctoral degree from Tulane University with a dissertation entitled "The Erythrocyte in Man." After serving on the faculty at Johns Hopkins Hospital, in 1943 Wintrobe was appointed Professor of Internal Medicine at the University of Utah, also serving as the first Chairman of the Department

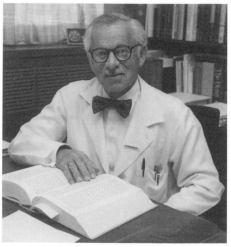

Maxwell Myer Wintrobe as President of the American Society of Hematology, 1972. (*American Society of Hematology*)

of Medicine and Physician-in-Chief for the Salt Lake County General Hospital. Wintrobe established one of the country's earliest hematology training programs, from which more than 80% of its fellows pursued careers in medical schools and research institutes around the world.

As a leading authority in hematology, in 1942 Wintrobe wrote *Clinical Hematology*, the first dedicated work in hematology that remains a definitive textbook in the field. He was the sole author of the first six editions, with multiple subsequent editions edited by others but retaining his name. Wintrobe also was one of the editors of the first edition of *Harrison's Principles of Internal Medicine* (1950).

To quantitatively assess the population of red cells in the blood, he developed the Wintrobe Hematocrit Tube. Realizing that there were no published and reliable normal blood values that physicians could use in clinical practice, Wintrobe was the first to document statistically normal values in adults and children, defining what are now known as Wintrobe indices – mean cell volume, hemoglobin, and hemoglobin concentration. Wintrobe also classified anemia morphologically as microcytic, normocytic, or macrocytic, a system still used today.

Wintrobe defined the important roles of iron and copper in the development of red blood cells and published research papers dealing with pernicious anemia, sickle-cell disease, and other anemias, as well as describing the abnormal copper metabolism in Wilson's disease. Wintrobe participated in the team that pioneered the use of chemotherapy in treating cancer, and he was one of the first to recognize the potential of chloramphenicol to produce aplastic anemia.

## INTERNAL MEDICINE

Using observations acquired during the Civil War, Da Costa described an anxiety disorder known as "soldier's heart," which combines effort fatigue, dyspnea, a sighing respiration, palpitation, and sweating. Rosenbach discovered an eponymous sign in which fine, rapid tremors when the eyelids are closed is an indication of hyperthyroidism. Goldblatt revealed that narrowing of the renal arteries causes the kidney to release renin, which in turn causes the production of angiotensin 1 and leads to the development of hypertension. Widal developed a test for diagnosing typhoid fever and prepared a vaccine that substantially reduced the contagion of this disease among allied armies. Widal recognized that excess salt could lead to nephritis (inflammation of the kidney) and cardiac edema (heart disease resulting from accumulation of excessive fluid in tissues. Feinstein challenged the belief that proper treatment after an early diagnosis of rheumatic fever kept patients from developing severe heart disease later in life, arguing that the disease had different forms, including one which causes joint pain and seldom progresses to heart disease. Metz was a strong supporter of homeopathy, a movement founded by Samuel Hahnemann that championed the use of tiny doses of substances that, if administered at full strength to a person, would produce symptoms identical to those manifest by the disease to be treated. One of the first women to keep her maiden name after marrying, Jacobs operated perhaps the first birth control clinic in the world.

**Da Costa, Jacob Mendes**                    (St. Thomas, 1833–1900)

Born into a wealthy Sephardic Jewish family on the Caribbean island of St. Thomas, then a Danish colony, Da Costa left at age four with his parents for Europe, where he received an excellent private education. Twelve years later, Da Costa decided to attend medical school in Philadelphia, where his mother was living. After graduating from Jefferson Medical College (now Thomas Jefferson University), Da Costa pursued postgraduate work in Europe.

During the Civil War, Da Costa served as a physician at the Military Hospital and Turner's Lane Hospital in Philadelphia. In 1871, using observations acquired during the war, he described an anxiety disorder known as Da Costa's syndrome or "soldier's heart," which combines effort fatigue, dyspnea, a sighing respiration, palpitation, and sweating.

Da Costa became a Professor of Clinical Medicine at Jefferson and was a popular teacher for his

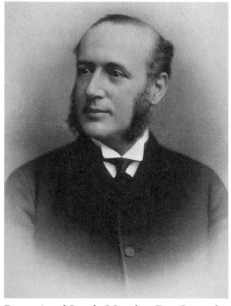

Portrait of Jacob Mendes De Costa by Thomas Eakins. (*Wikimedia / Thomas Eakins: Volume II, by Lloyd Goodrich. Harvard University Press, 1982*)

classes in physical diagnosis. His book *Medical Diagnosis* made Da Costa well known, both in the United States and Europe. In a talk he gave to a graduating class at Jefferson, Da Costa asserted that becoming a truly gifted physician required a knowledge of art and the humanities, not merely scientific learning.

## Feinstein, Alvan R.                                      (USA, 1925–2001)

Born in Philadelphia, Alvan Feinstein received his medical degree from the University of Chicago and completed residency training in Internal Medicine at the Rockefeller Institute. As Medical Director of Irvington House Institute, an affiliate of New York University, Feinstein studied a large population of patients with rheumatic fever and challenged the belief that proper treatment after an early diagnosis kept those patients from developing severe heart disease later in life. Instead, Feinstein demonstrated that the disease had different forms, including one which causes joint pain and seldom progresses to heart disease. The other, which does result in heart disease, has no symptoms to permit early detection. Consequently, Feinstein concluded that diagnosis of rheumatic fever at an early stage leads to a favorable outcome not because of early treatment, but because those patients tend to have a less-virulent form. Similarly, Feinstein showed that breast cancers grew at differing rates, so that aggressive treatments were not necessarily appropriate for cancers detected at an early stage by mammograms. Those detected early are often slow-growing and relatively benign.

In 1962, Feinstein joined the faculty of the Yale University School of Medicine, and he became the founding director of the Robert Wood Johnson Clinical Scholars Program in 1974. As the prestigious Sterling Professor of Medicine and Epidemiology at

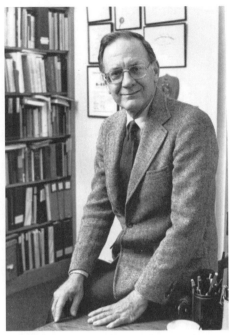

Alvan R. Feinstein. (*Gairdner Foundation*)

Yale, Feinstein utilized his undergraduate studies in mathematics to develop what he called "clinimetrics." Now used widely today, Feinstein stressed the importance of maintaining consistency among assessments made by doctors through clinical indexes and rating scales for evaluating conditions like pain, distress, and disability. Feinstein focused much of his research on basic issues in the design and analysis of clinical investigation. The author of several of the most widely referenced books in epidemiology, Feinstein was the founder of the Journal of Clinical Epidemiology. Unfortunately, this journal under his editorship published numerous articles and opinion pieces by Feinstein and his colleagues minimizing the deleterious effects of smoking, effectively supporting the false claims of the tobacco industry.

## Goldblatt, Harry (USA, 1891–1977)

The son of Jewish immigrants from Lithuania who arrived in the United States five years before his birth, Harry Goldblatt studied medicine at McGill University in Montreal. He specialized in pathology and joined the faculty at Case Western Reserve University in Cleveland, eventually becoming Professor of Experimental Pathology (1935–1946). Goldblatt then headed the Institute for Medical Research at Cedars of Lebanon Hospital

in Los Angeles, later returning to
Cleveland to head the research laboratories at Mount Sinai Hospital.

Goldblatt is best known for his
experimental research in hypertension. Having noted a characteristic narrowing of the renal blood
vessels in patients who had died of
hypertension, Goldblatt reasoned
that decreased blood flow, and an
associated lowering of the oxygen supply to the kidneys, might
somehow trigger hypertension. To
test this theory, Goldblatt partially
constricted the major renal arteries
of dogs using a self-styled adjust-
able silver clamp. In his 1934 article, Goldblatt reported that partial

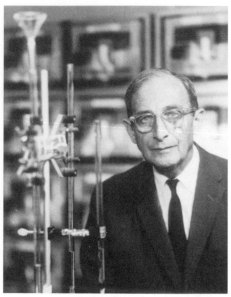

Harry Goldblatt. (*NLM*)

constriction of both renal arteries resulted in a reproducible and persistent
rise in blood pressure, even if there was no evidence of renal failure. Clamp-
ing other large arteries (splenic, femoral) produced no similar effect. Subsequent experiments by Goldblatt and others revealed that constriction of
the renal arteries triggers a chemical chain reaction leading to hypertension.
Narrowing of the renal arteries causes the kidney to release renin, which
in turn causes the production of angiotensin 1. This substance is benign
until it reacts with the angiotensin converting enzyme (ACE) to become
angiotensin 2, a major cause of hypertension. Goldblatt summarized this
pathway for the relatively rare cases of secondary hypertension in his 1943
monograph, "The Origin of Renal Hypertension."

## Gutman, Alexander                                              (1902–1973)

Born in New York City and the son of a successful practicing physician,
Alexander Gutman received a doctorate in experimental biology at Cornell
University and then went to Vienna for his medical degree. Gutman joined
the research staff at Columbia University, and from 1951 to 1968 served as
Physician-in-Chief and Director of the Department of Medicine at Mount
Sinai Hospital during its transition into an academic medical center.

Gutman performed pioneering work on serum proteins and phospha-
tases. In 1961, he received the Gairdner International Award "in recog-

nition of his contributions to the knowledge of rheumatology and biochemistry, and especially for his achievements in elucidating the metabolic defects present in gout, and in demonstrating the action of certain drugs which increase the excretion of uric acid, thus leading to the present situation in which it is possible to exercise almost perfect control over attacks of acute gouty arthritis."

Gutman was the founding editor of the American Journal of Medicine, popularly known as the "Green Journal," and served in this capacity for 25 years, during which it became recognized as one of the

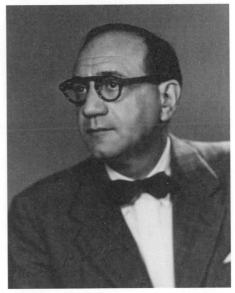

Alexander Gutman, 1950. (*Gairdner Foundation*)

best and most prestigious publications in internal medicine.

---

## Jacobs, Aletta Henriette (Netherlands, 1854–1929)

Daughter of a provincial Jewish doctor, at age 17 Aletta Henriette Jacobs was admitted to the University of Groningen and became the first female student to study medicine in the Netherlands, obtaining her degree in 1879. One of the first women to keep her maiden name after marrying, Jacobs operated perhaps the first birth control clinic in the world. This earned the wrath of Holland's male medical establishment, which attacked her for everything from promoting adultery to threatening the economic future of the country.

Although Jacobs had her own medical practice, she became in-

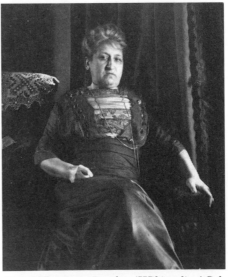

Aletta Henriette Jacobs. (*Wikimedia / Collectie Spaarnestad Photo/Het Leven/Fotograaf onbekend via Nationaal Archief*)

creasingly active in a variety of social causes. Her fight for equal rights for women led to her assuming an active role in the women's movement. In 1903, Jacobs became the head of the Association for Women's Suffrage, devoting herself to revising the Dutch constitution in order to give women the right to vote and to be elected. Her years of intense struggle finally succeeded in 1919, when Queen Wilhelmina signed the Jacobs Act giving Dutch women the full right to vote.

## Jacoby, Johann                                                    (1805–1877)

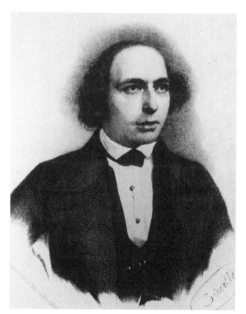

Born in Königsberg, Johann Jacoby studied medicine at the Albertina University of Königsberg and began practicing in his native city. However, he soon became involved in liberal political activities.

Jacoby's first published brochures called for Emancipation of the Jews, not as a special favor but because of their natural right as human beings. In later writings, Jacoby called for reform of the medical services in Prussia and attacked what he deemed an oppressive judicial system and state censor. Although prosecuted for his writings, Jacoby was eventually acquitted. During the revolu-

Johann Jacoby. (*NLM*)

tionary upheaval in 1848–1849, Jacoby was a radical delegate in both the Prussian National assembly and the All-German Frankfurt Parliament. When the latter was dissolved, Jacoby fled to Stuttgart and set up a rump parliament with the goal of proclaiming a German republic.

An outspoken opponent of Otto von Bismarck, Jacoby remained adamantly against the policies of the "Iron Chancellor," even after Bismarck's success in achieving the unification of Germany. After the creation of the new German Second Reich, Jacoby joined the Social Democratic Party. He was elected to the Reichstag in 1874, but refused to take his seat as an act of political protest.

## Katznelson, Judah Leib (Russia, 1846–1917)

Also known by his pen name, Buki Ben Yogli, Judah Katznelson was born in the Ukraine and attended the rabbinical seminary in Zhitomir before beginning his medical studies at the University of St. Petersburg. After graduating, Katznelson served as a military physician in the Ottoman–Russian War before returning to St. Petersburg, where he practiced medicine until his death.

Katznelson worked for Hebrew-language newspapers, acting as an editor and contributing articles on scientific matters. He devoted much of his time to writing articles showing the relevance of the Talmud to modern medicine, eventually assembling these works in his book, *The Wisdom of the Talmud and Medicine.* Analyzing the parallels between vitiligo and the biblical skin disease of *tzara'at*, Katznelson concluded that they were identical. A supporter of the *Haskalah* (Enlightenment), Katznelson was a lecturer at the Institute of Jewish Studies in St. Petersburg and later its head.

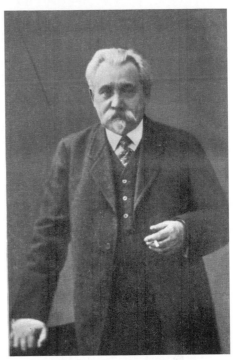

Judah Leib Katznelson. (*Wikipedia*)

Although Katznelson did not identify as a Zionist at the beginning of his public career, he eagerly promoted Jewish-owned agricultural advances, especially in southern Russia and the Jewish colonies in Argentina. In 1909, Katznelson visited the Land of Israel and toured Jewish settlements, leading to his support of practical Zionism.

## Metz, Carl August (Germany, 1798–1848)

Born Sekkin Amschel, Carl August Metz was a Jewish physician, educated at Marburg, who wrote several books on homeopathy for physicians and laymen. This movement was founded by Samuel Hahnemann, a physician who rebelled against the use of powerful drugs and poisons that traditional medicine prescribed for treating illness. Instead, Hahnemann championed the use of tiny doses of substances that, if administered at full strength to a person, would produce symptoms identical to those manifest by the disease to be treated. Although Hahnemann was not Jewish, the concept of homeopathy had some correlates in ancient and medieval Jewish remedies. For example, there is a midrash in which an herb that would blind a sighted individual could restore the sight of one who was blind.

## Rosenbach, Ottomar Ernst Felix                        (Germany, 1851–1907)

The son of a physician practicing in Krappitz in Silesia, Ottomar Rosenbach studied medicine at the universities of Berlin and Breslau, interrupted by a year as a volunteer in the siege of Paris during the Franco-Prussian war. After several years of assistantship in Jena, Rosenbach joined All Saints' Hospital in Breslau, where he subsequently became Physician-in-Chief of the Department of Medicine. Rosenbach later moved to Berlin, where he practiced medicine until his death.

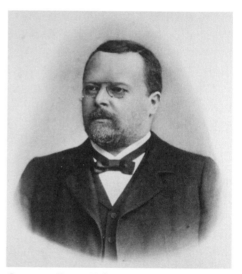

Ottomar Ernst Felix Rosenbach. (*NLM*)

Rosenbach is best known for the discovery of fine, rapid tremors when the eyelids are closed (Rosenbach's sign), which is an indication of hyperthyroidism. He was skeptical of the laboratory based methods favored by pathologists and bacteriologists of his era, preferring instead to focus on energetic conditions that he termed "functional" diagnostics. Rosenbach engendered controversy by rejecting the bacterial theory, instead emphasizing psychosomatic causes and features of disease and championing the value of psychotherapy and the power of suggestion.

## Widal, Georges-Fernand Isidor                         (Algeria, 1862–1929)

Born in Dellys and the son of an army surgeon, Georges-Fernand Widal studied medicine in Paris, remaining there for his entire professional life. As a medical intern, Widal worked at a frantic pace, performing morning rounds on an astounding 80 patients, spending long afternoons in the laboratory, and devoting his evening hours to seeing patients and writing up his research. His doctoral thesis demonstrated that *Streptococcus* was the causative bacterial agent in puerperal fever, endocarditis, and erysipelas, and Widal emerged as one of a small group of scientists with the novel idea that many different diseases could be caused by a single organism. From 1911 until his death, Widal served as a Professor of Pathology and Internal Medicine at the University of Paris.

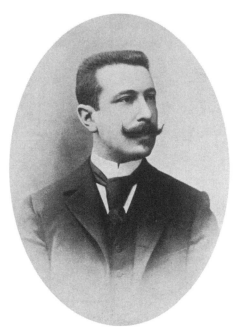

Georges-Fernand Isidor Widal. (*Wikimedia / NLM*)

Widal developed a test for diagnosing typhoid fever, based on the observation that antibodies in the blood of an infected individual cause the bacteria to bind together into clumps (Widal reaction). During World War I, he prepared a vaccine against typhoid fever that substantially reduced the contagion of this disease among allied armies. Widal also recognized that the body's retention of sodium chloride is a feature of nephritis (inflammation of the kidney) and that cardiac edema (accumulation of excessive fluid in tissues) is a result of heart disease, recommending salt deprivation in the treatment of both diseases. He demonstrated the increased fragility of red blood cells in cases of hemolytic jaundice and, with the French physician Georges Hayem, described the acquired form of hemolytic anemia (once called Hayem-Widal syndrome).

A prolific writer of medical journal articles, Widal was co-editor of 22 volumes of a medical textbook. His emphasis on relating laboratory observations to clinical patient care was a forerunner of the modern concept of translational medicine.

## MEDICAL IMAGING AND RADIATION ONCOLOGY

Bucky designed a metallic grid used to decrease scatter radiation obscuring x-ray images. Felson coined a dozen important signs in radiology and authored a major early textbook in chest radiology. Jacobson was a pioneer in correlating the radiographic appearance of diseases with their gross and microscopic appearance and co-edited a major textbook in musculoskeletal radiology. Rigler described the classic eponymous sign indicating the presence of free intraperitoneal air on a supine radiograph of the abdomen. Salomon was a surgeon and the first person to use the x-ray to study breast cancer, correlating 3,000 mastectomy specimens with radiographic images. Decades later, Gershon-Cohen, a strong advocate of screening mammography, tirelessly attempted to convince physicians and the public of the vital importance of early detection of breast cancer to increase survival. Swick developed the first relatively non-toxic intravenous contrast material that was excreted by the kidney and provided distinct images on radiographs, ushering in the new era in urologic diagnosis that allowed physicians to image stones, cysts, and tumors. Bloch and Rabi studied the magnetic properties of atomic nuclei with great precision using resonance principles, the first step in the development of the sophisticated imaging technique of magnetic resonance imaging (MRI). Sokoloff used a radioactive analogue to glucose to measure brain blood flow and metabolism and to develop images of brain activity using a positron emission tomography (PET) scanner.

Freund was the first physician known to have used ionizing radiation for therapeutic purposes. Kaplan revolutionized the practice of radiation oncology, installing the first medical linear accelerator in the Western hemisphere that enabled radiotherapy to be used as a curative, rather than merely a palliative, treatment for cancer. Friedell's research on the effects of radiation on biological systems has led to better protection from radiation exposure.

---

**Bloch, Felix**                                            (Switzerland, 1905–1983)

---

Born in Zurich, Felix Bloch received his doctorate in physics at the University of Leipzig and remained in German academia for postgraduate studies. After the Nazis came to power in 1933, Bloch immediately left Germany and moved to the United States. Bloch initially worked at Stanford University, but then relocated to the University of California, Berke-

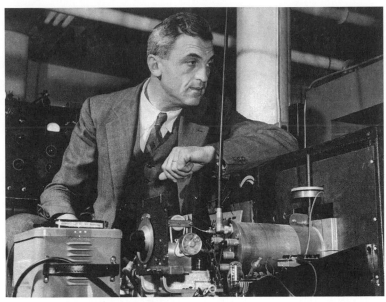

Felix Bloch in his laboratory, 1950s. (*Wikimedia / Mondadori Publishers*)

ley, where he could use its cyclotron to determine the magnetic moment of the neutron. In 1938, Bloch returned to Stanford to become its first Professor of Theoretical Physics.

During World War II, Bloch was involved in the early stages of the work on atomic energy at the Los Alamos National Laboratory and then joined the Harvard University project on counter measures against radar. This latter experience, in conjunction with his earlier work on the magnetic moment of the neutron, provided Bloch with a new approach toward the investigation of nuclear moments. Returning to Stanford after the war, Bloch developed (with W.W. Hansen and M.E. Packard) a new method of nuclear induction, a purely electromagnetic procedure for the study of nuclear moments in solids, liquids, and gases. A few weeks after the first successful experiments, Bloch received the news that the same discovery had been made independently and simultaneously by Edward Mills Purcell and his collaborators at Harvard. For their efforts, Bloch and Purcell shared the 1952 Nobel Prize in Physics for "their development of new methods for nuclear magnetic precision measurements." As the Nobel Committee noted, protons and neutrons in nuclei act as small rotating, spinning magnets. Therefore, atoms and molecules align in a magnetic field. When returning to the original spin position, electromagnetic radiation is emitted with a frequency characteristic of the particular atom or molecule.

Since that time, nuclear magnetic resonance has become an important tool in nuclear physics and chemistry. It also led to the subsequent development of magnetic resonance imaging (MRI), an important diagnostic modality in modern medicine.

In 1954, Bloch took a leave of absence to serve for one year in Geneva as the first Director General of CERN – the European Organization for Nuclear Research, which now operates the largest particle physics laboratory in the world.

## Bucky, Gustav Peter                                    (Germany, 1880–1963)

Born in Leipzig, Gustav Bucky studied medicine at the universities of Geneva and Leipzig, specializing in the new field of radiology. In those early days, scatter radiation (secondary rays) from the x-ray tube greatly obscured the radiographic image. In 1913, Bucky reported the use of a stationary honeycombed, metallic grid-diaphragm between the patient and the x-ray plate, in which the grid was composed of an x-ray absorbing material such as lead and the intervening cells (composed of an x-ray transparent material) were oriented to permit the primary rays emerging directly from the focal spot of the tube to pass

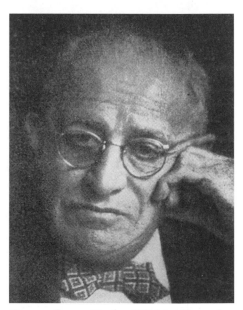

Gustav Peter Bucky (*NLM / Jerusalem Academy of Medicine*)

through. However, secondary rays emitted at other angles by atoms in the body of the patient were blocked by being absorbed in the metal strips.

Unfortunately, Bucky's original grid had a major deficit. To perform its function, the material composing the grid had to be of high atomic weight and therefore cast a marked shadow of criss-cross configuration on the x-ray plate. Thus, the price of eliminating the blurring was to superimpose an objectionable grid pattern that obscured most of the findings. In 1920, Hollis Potter reported that the grid lines could be eliminated by moving the grid at right angles to the grid lines during the exposure. If the range and speed of motion is sufficient and continues throughout the exposure, the grid lines are blurred out. This led to the development of the Bucky-Potter movable grid.

With the rise of Nazism in Germany, Bucky moved to the United States.

## Felson, Benjamin (USA, 1913–1988)

Born in Newport, Kentucky, Benjamin Felson attended medical school at the University of Cincinnati and completed a residency in radiology, specializing in diseases of the chest. After serving in Europe during World War II as Chief of Radiology at an Army hospital, Felson returned to his alma mater and rose rapidly in academic rank. Felson was promoted to Professor of Radiology in 1948 and named Department Chair three years later, continuing in that position for more than two decades.

A brilliant and humorous lecturer, Felson's *Principles of Chest Roentgenology* (1965) has remained a popular text among residents in the specialty. He coined a dozen important signs in radiology (e.g., silhouette and hilum overlay signs) and popularized the term "Aunt Minnie" as radiological shorthand referring to a lesion/finding with such a characteristic appearance that it realistically can represent only one diagnosis.

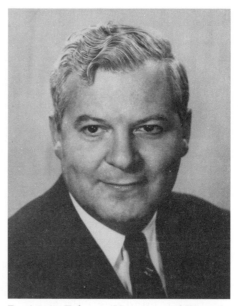

Benjamin Felson. (*University of Kentucky Archives*)

## Fleischner, Felix (Austria, 1893–1969)

Born in Vienna, Felix Fleischner received his medical degree from the University of Vienna. Specializing in radiology, Fleischner served as Professor and Head of Radiology of the Second Medical Clinic at his alma mater. After Germany annexed Austria in 1938, Fleischner moved to Boston, spending two years at the Massachusetts General Hospital and two years in private practice. In 1942, Fleischner became the first full-time radiologist at the Beth Israel Hospital. Three years later, he was appointed chair of its radiology department, a position he held until his retirement in 1960. A prolific author of scientific articles, Fleischner described many important chest imaging signs that are still used by radiologists today. In 1969, a group of radiologists specializing in thoracic imaging formed a new organization to study thoracic disease, primarily through chest radiology, which became known as the Fleischner Society.

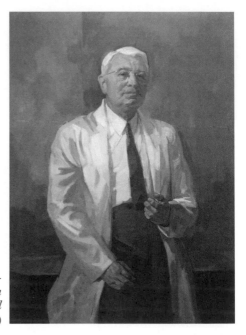

Painting of Felix Fleischner by Nathaniel Jacobson. (*Ruth and David Freiman Archives at Beth Israel Deaconess Medical Center*)

## Freund, Leopold                                                (Austria, 1868–1943)

Born in Central Bohemia, then part of the Austro-Hungarian Empire, Leopold Freund was a Professor of Radiology at the Medical University of Vienna and is considered the founder of radiotherapy. Freund was the first physician known to have used ionizing radiation for therapeutic purposes. In 1896, a year after the discovery of X-rays by Wilhelm Roentgen and the same year that Antoine Henri Becquerel discovered radioactivity, Freund successfully treated a five-year-old patient in Vienna suffering from hairy moles covering her whole back. In 1903, he published the first textbook on radiation therapy.

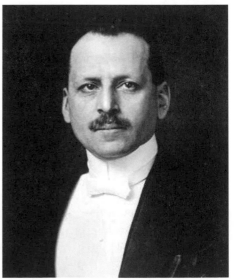

Leopold Freund. (*Picture collection Josephinum, Medical University of Vienna, MUW-FO-IR-001678-0005*)

Freund also published fundamental work on the treatment of occupational diseases with light and the use of X-rays for testing construction materials. Following the annexation of Austria by Nazi Germany in 1938, the Jewish physician moved to Belgium.

## Friedell, Hymer Louis (Russia, 1911–2002)

Born in St. Petersburg, as a young child Hymer Friedell and his family moved to Minnesota, where he later received both his medical degree and PhD in radiology from the University of Minnesota. Prior to World War II, Friedell held positions as a National Cancer Institute Fellow at Memorial Hospital in New York and at the University of California Hospital in San Francisco. In 1943, Friedell was transferred to the Oak Ridge National Laboratory in Tennessee, where he became the Executive Officer of the Manhattan Engineer District Medical Division and assisted in directing experiments to determine dose tolerances for the new radioactive isotopes.

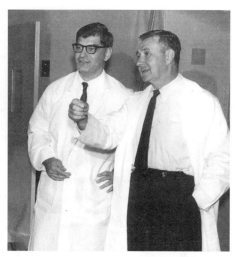

Hymer L. Friedell, Director of Radiology (right), with radiologist Benjamin Kaufman, 1967. Photograph by Dan Rothenberg. (*Stanley A. Ferguson Archives of University Hospitals Cleveland Medical Center*)

This led to his being appointed as a member on the Atomic Energy Commission and subcommittees dealing with isotope distribution and allocation of isotopes for human use.

After the war, Friedell resumed his academic and research career at Western Reserve University, where he served as Chair of Radiology, and later at the University of California, making important contributions to radiation biology. His research on the effects of radiation on biological systems has led to better protection from radiation exposure for both members of the military and civilians alike.

## Gershon-Cohen, Jacob (USA, 1899–1971)

Born in Philadelphia of immigrant parents, Jacob Gershon-Cohen attended the College and Medical School of the University of Pennsylvania. Specializing in radiology, for 18 years Gershon-Cohen was Director of Radiology at the Albert Einstein Medical Center in his native city.

In the 1950s, Gershon-Cohen was virtually the only major advocate of mammography in the United States. As early as 1938, he published an article on the radiographic examination of the normal breast, in which he stated that a precise knowledge of the normal breast at all ages and stages of activity was a prerequisite to recognizing pathologic conditions that

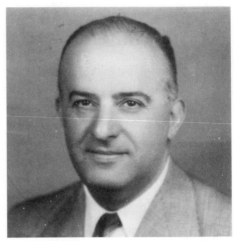

Jacob Gershon-Cohen. (*Wikimedia / NIH*)

might arise. In collaboration with renowned pathologist Helen Ingleby, Gershon-Cohen stressed the need for close correlation of radiographically detected breast lesions with the gross and microscopic specimens. This eventually permitted recognition on the films of shadows that had previously appeared unimportant.

For the next 30 years of his career, Gershon-Cohen focused on the importance of early detection of breast cancer to survival. He was the author of two textbooks: *Comparative Anatomy, Pathology and Roentgenology of the Breast* (with Helen Ingleby; 1960) and *Atlas of Mammography* (1970).

Gershon-Cohn pioneered the development of thermography in 1962, as soon as infrared-sensing devices were declassified by the military. Advocating the importance of such equipment to medicine, especially for early cancer detection, Gershon-Cohen was considered the foremost proponent of this discipline in the country and was elected the first president of the American Thermographic Society (1967–1968).

An accomplished violinist, Gershon-Cohen eventually acquired a Stradivarius, which he delighted playing in chamber music sessions with members of the Philadelphia Orchestra and students at the Curtis Institute of Music.

---

**Hertz, Saul**                                                    (USA, 1905–1950)

---

Born in Cleveland to Orthodox Jewish immigrants from Europe, Saul Hertz graduated from Harvard Medical School and specialized in endocrinology. Serving as Chief of the Thyroid Clinic at the Massachusetts General Hospital from 1931–1943, Hertz asked Karl Compton, the renowned physicist and president of the Massachusetts Institute of Technology, whether iodine could be made radioactive artificially. Learning that this was possible, Hertz collaborated with physicist Arthur Roberts at MIT on experiments in rabbits that demonstrated that the normal thyroid gland concentrated radioactive iodine and that a hyperplastic thyroid gland took up even more iodine. In 1941, Hertz was the first to administer a therapeutic dose of cyclotron-produced radioactive iodine to patients with hyperthyroidism, documenting the success and safety of this treatment. Follow-up studies led to radioactive iodine becoming the standard treatment for hyperthyroidism.

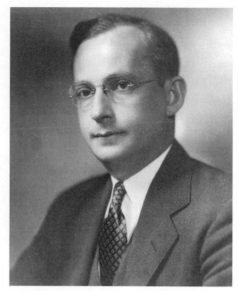

Portrait of Saul Hertz, 1940. (*Wikimedia, Courtesy Dr. Hertz's family*)

After serving during World War II as part of the Manhattan Project for Biology and Medicine for furthering medical uses of atomic energy, Hertz established the Radioactive Isotope Research Institute in Boston to apply fission products to the treatment of thyroid cancer, goiter, and a variety of malignant tumors. He also studied the application of radioactive phosphorus and the influences of hormones on cancer as displayed by isotope studies.

## Jacobson, Harold (USA, 1912–2001)

Born in Cincinnati, Harold Jacobson received his medical degree from the University of Cincinnati and completed a residency in radiology, specializing in bone disease. Although having a medical disability that disqualified him from service in World War II, Jacobson's strong obligation to serve his country led to his successfully appealing his classification and joining the Army Medical Corps. Returning to civilian life, Jacobson successively served as Chief of Radiology at the Bronx VA Hospital, Hospital for Special Surgery, and Montefiore Medical Center, before heading the Department of Radiology at Albert Einstein College of Medicine for more than 20 years.

Jacobson was a pioneer in correlating the radiographic appearance of diseases with their gross and microscopic appearance. He emphasized that this correlation enabled radiologists to better understand the imaging findings so as to arrive at a definitive diagnosis. With Ronald O. Murray, Jacobson edited the classic *Radiology of Skeletal Disorders: Exercises in Diagnosis* (1971).

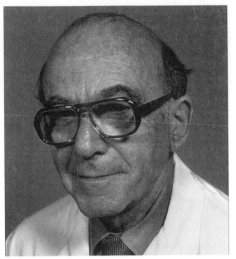

Harold Jacobson. (*"In Memoriam" by Seymour Sprayregen, MD; Radiology 223:588, 2002*)

## Kaplan, Henry Seymour                    (USA, 1918–1984)

Born in Chicago, the grandson of immigrants from the Ukraine, Henry Kaplan received a degree from Rush Medical College in his native city. After a residency in radiology at the University of Minnesota, Kaplan joined the faculty at Yale University, treating patients and setting up a laboratory to study radiation-induced leukemias and lymphomas in mice. In 1948, Kaplan was recruited by the Stanford School of Medicine to become Chair of Radiology, which at the time was a non-academic department consisting only of three primitive diagnostic x-ray machines.

During his long tenure at Stanford, Kaplan revolutionized the practice of radiation oncology. He installed the first medical linear accelerator in the Western hemi-

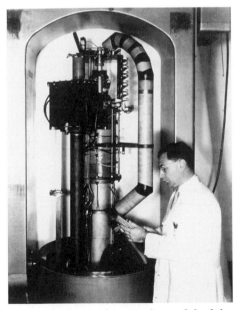

Henry Kaplan with an early model of the Linear Accelerator developed to treat cancer, 1950s. For this picture, the protective hood has been removed, revealing the electronic insides of the six-million volt machine, used for radiation treatment. (*Wikimedia / National Cancer Institute*)

sphere, a six million volt machine that enabled radiotherapy to be used as a curative, rather than merely a palliative, treatment for cancer. Kaplan's major focus was Hodgkin's disease, a malignant lymphoma that was uniformly fatal before the advent of radiation therapy but soon had a cure rate of about 75%. Kaplan and Saul Rosenberg were the first to apply chemotherapy as an adjunct to radiation therapy in Hodgkin's disease, achieving a cure rate of almost 100% for early stages of the disease.

Kaplan also was responsible for the clinical trials that established the utility of the histopathologic classification of non-Hodgkin's lymphomas proposed by Henry Rappaport. Although not widely accepted at the time, a modified version of the Rappaport classification is now the most widely used for staging and treatment of the disease.

For his pioneering work in radiation oncology, in 1969 Kaplan became the only biomedical scientist to be awarded the prestigious Atoms for Peace Award. Three years later, Kaplan was the first radiologist elected to the National Academy of Sciences.

## Rabi, Isidor Isaac (Austria, 1898–1988)

Born in Raymanov and brought to the United States as a baby, Isidor Rabi was raised in New York City and received his doctorate in physics from Columbia University with a dissertation on the magnetic susceptibility of certain crystals. In 1929, after two years of postdoctoral study in Europe, Rabi was appointed Lecturer in Theoretical Physics at his alma mater and rose through the academic ranks to be promoted to professor eight years later. During World War II, Rabi was granted leave from Columbia to work as Associate Director of the Radiation Laboratory at the Massachusetts Institute of Technology on the development of radar and the atomic bomb.

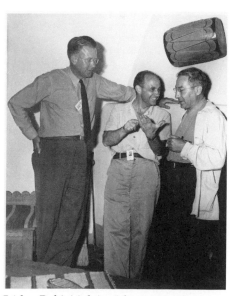

Isidor Rabi (right) with atomic physicists Ernest O. Lawrence and Enrico Fermi. (*Wikimedia / National Archives and Records Administration*)

In the 1930s, Rabi began studying the magnetic properties of atomic nuclei with great precision. By an ingenious application of the resonance principle, Rabi succeeded in detecting and measuring single states of rotation of atoms and molecules, as well as developing techniques for using nuclear magnetic resonance to determine the magnetic moment and nuclear spin of atoms. This work led to his being awarded the 1944 Nobel Prize for Physics "for his resonance method for recording the magnetic properties of atomic nuclei." As the Nobel Committee noted, protons and neutrons in nuclei act as small rotating, spinning magnets. Therefore, atoms and molecules align in a magnetic field. In his experiments, Rabi sent a beam of molecules through a magnetic field. When the beam was exposed to radio waves, the spin direction could be changed, but only in certain steps according to quantum mechanics. When returning to the original spin position, electromagnetic radiation was emitted with a frequency characteristic of the particular atom or molecule.

Since that time, nuclear magnetic resonance became an important tool for nuclear physics and chemistry and led to the subsequent development of magnetic resonance imaging (MRI), an important diagnostic modality in modern medicine.

Rabi also was involved in the development of the cavity magnetron, which is used in microwave radar and microwave ovens.

---

**Rigler, Leo George**                                     (USA, 1896–1979)

Born in Minneapolis, Leo Rigler earned his undergraduate and medical degrees from the University of Minnesota, where he spent much of his academic career. He became the first full-time Chairman of Radiology in 1933, serving in this capacity for almost a quarter century. As a full professor, Rigler was certified by the American Board of Radiology in 1934, the 68th candidate to receive this recognition in the year it was established. In 1957, Rigler moved to Los Angeles to become Executive Director of Cedars of Lebanon and Sinai Hospitals. He later be-

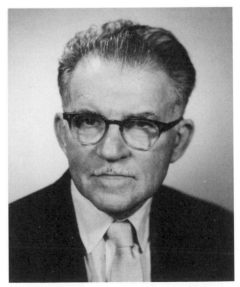

Leo George Rigler. (*NLM*)

came Professor of Radiology at the University of California, Los Angeles, and director of its postgraduate training program. In 1970, he founded the radiology research facility at UCLA, which was named the Leo G. Rigler Center for Radiological Sciences.

A leader in the development of academic radiology, Rigler played a prominent role in developing American diagnostic radiology into a clinically oriented consultative specialty and unique academic discipline. He transformed the radiology department at Minnesota into a model for radiologic education.

Among radiologists, Rigler is best known for his 1941 description of a new sign indicating the presence of free air in the peritoneal cavity. Now universally known as the Rigler sign, it allowed pneumoperitoneum to be detected on supine radiographs of the abdomen – suggesting the occurrence of a perforated viscus or other catastrophic event even before clinical signs were evident and indicating the need for early surgical intervention. Rigler authored two books, *Outline of Roentgen Diagnosis* (1938) and *The Chest* (1946).

Rigler was the first Jew to be president of the Radiological Society of North America. He also served as Chairman of the Jewish Family Welfare Association in Minneapolis and national vice president of the American Friends of Hebrew University.

---

## Salomon, Albert (Germany, 1883–1976)

---

Albert Salomon was a surgeon at the Royal Surgical University Clinic in Berlin and the first person to use the x-ray to study breast cancer. Salomon evaluated 3,000 mastectomy specimens in an attempt to correlate the radiographic appearance with the gross and microscopic anatomy of breast tumors. His primary concern was to study the extent and mode of spread of breast cancer, so that a more adequate biopsy specimen could be removed at the time of surgery.

Salomon's most important observation was the recognition that an x-ray film gave a true picture of the margins and extent of a tumor. He described the radiographic appearance of the most common forms of breast cancer, clearly differentiating the scirrhous or infiltrating type from the circumscribed or nodular forms. Salomon identified the punctate microcalcifications characteristic of ductal carcinoma, and he reported the first "clinically occult" breast cancer found by radiographic examination.

The scientific community was impressed and intrigued by his work, but Salomon never used the diagnostic technique in his own practice. Although he published his findings in 1913, mammography did not become a common life-saving practice until decades later.

With the rise of Nazism in 1933, Salomon was discharged from the University of Berlin. He was interned in a concentration camp until 1939, when he managed to go into hiding in The Netherlands. After World War II, Salomon moved to Amsterdam, where he spent his remaining years as an emeritus professor.

## Sokoloff, Louis                                          (USA, 1921–2015)

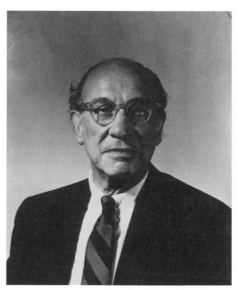

Born in Philadelphia, the son of Jewish immigrants who had fled pogroms in Ukraine and Russia, Louis Sokoloff studied medicine at the University of Pennsylvania and specialized in neurosciences. Recruited to the National Institute of Mental Health by his mentor, Seymour Kety, a major figure in the biological study of schizophrenia and other mental illnesses, Sokoloff headed the Laboratory for Cerebral Metabolism until 1999.

Since the mid-1940s, when practicing psychotherapy in the Army as Chief of Neuropsychiatry at Camp Lee, VA, Sokoloff believed that there was a physiologi-

Louis Sokoloff. (*Lasker Award Archives / NLM*)

cal and biochemical component to mental illness. A pioneer in functional imaging of the brain, Sokoloff and his team used a radioactive analogue to glucose to measure brain blood flow and metabolism and to develop images of brain activity using a positron emission tomography (PET) scanner.

In 1981, Sokoloff received the Lasker Award for Clinical Medical Research for his role in developing vivid color images that map brain function. As the Lasker Foundation noted, Sokoloff's PET technique measured the metabolism of its primary fuel, glucose, through a radioactive substitute that, unlike glucose, lingers long enough to undergo chemical analysis. Moreover, "the Sokoloff method has facilitated the diagnosis, understanding and possible future treatment of such disorders of the brain as schizophrenia, epilepsy, brain changes due to drug addiction, and senile dementia."[45]

Today, PET scanning also has major applications in general clinical medicine, becoming an important imaging modality for the diagnosis of diseases throughout the body.

---

## Swick, Moses (USA, 1900–1985)

Born Moses Goldstein in New York City, the son of Lithuanian immigrants, Swick received an undergraduate degree from Columbia University. Because medical schools at the time had strict quotas for Jewish students, he changed his surname to Swick, presumably to escape from these quotas. After being accepted into medical school at Columbia and earning his degree, Swick was awarded a fellowship to pursue postgraduate training at Hamburg University in Germany.

At the time, contrast imaging of the genitourinary tract was in its infancy. Sodium iodide had been injected intravenously, but this produced poor images unless given in large doses, which were associated with frequent reactions. Arthur Binz, a Berlin biochemist, had developed a new iodinated compound called Selectan-neutral, which was less toxic than simple sodium iodide, to treat urinary tract infections of the liver and kidney, and this material was being tested on the medical service in Hamburg where Swick was assigned. He noted that this new iodinated compound was preferentially excreted by the kidney and wondered whether it could be transformed from a potential therapeutic agent to one of possible diagnostic value.

Swick worked to modify the structure of the compound to lessen the side effects of vomiting, nausea, and headache, moving to the large urological hospital in Berlin under the direction of the famed Alexander von Lichtenberg. By replacing the methyl radical in the compound with a sodium acetate radical, Swick was able to lower the toxicity of the compound and increased its solubility to allow for more iodine content. The result was Uroselectan, which when injected intravenously was excreted by the kidney and provided distinct images on radiographs. This 1929 discovery led to a new era in urologic diagnosis, because the excretory urogram, or intravenous pyelogram (IVP), allowed physicians to image stones, cysts, and tumors with a material that was reasonably non-toxic.

---

45. Speert H, *Essays in eponymy. Obstetrics and Gynecologic Milestones*. (NY: The MacMillan Co., 1958), 279-283.

Excited by his discovery, Swick cabled Emanuel Libman, his mentor at Mount Sinai Hospital, asking that he inform von Lichtenberg, who was speaking at a urologic convention in New York. Controversy ensued when plans were made to present the new compound at the upcoming meeting of the German Urologic Society in Munich. Von Lichtenberg argued that he should be the principal author, since he was an internationally renowned urologist and director of the institution where the work had been performed. He thought that Swick should be relegated to a minor role in the presentation. Swick's mentor in New York arranged a compromise, whereby Swick would make the first presentation alone, but only concerning the developmental work done on animals and humans, mostly in Hamburg. The second presentation on clinical applications was offered by von Lichtenberg and Swick. However, Swick was soon ushered into the background. The next year, von Lichtenberg gave the first American lecture on intravenous pyelography, mentioning Swick only once as an afterthought. For the next 35 years, Swick did not get the recognition he deserved, even in his own country. Only after careful investigations by Victor Marshall of the Urology Section of the New York Academy of Medicine were Swick's vital contributions to iodinated contrast material rewarded with the distinguished Valentine Medal, following introductory remarks referring to the many unkind years of heartache and oblivion he had suffered.

Prior to the Nazi rise to power in Germany, Swick returned to New York and spent the rest of his academic career at Mount Sinai Medical Center.

## NEUROLOGY, NEUROSURGERY, NEUROPSYCHOLOGY

Jewish physicians have been heavily involved in all aspects of the study of the brain and peripheral nervous system. Remak described what became known as the autonomic nervous system, which controls the movement of involuntary muscles and the secretion of hormones throughout the body. The founder of modern neuroanatomy, Edinger described the ventral and dorsal spinocerebellar tracts. Auerbach identified the network of nerves consisting of ganglion cells ("Auerbach's" or myenteric plexus), located between the layers of the intestinal muscles, which control the movements of the gastrointestinal tract via the autonomic nervous system. Boshes, Bychowski, Goldflam, Halpern, and Oppenheim made major contributions to understanding such neuromuscular conditions as multiple sclerosis, myasthenia gravis, traumatic epilepsy, and tabes dorsalis, and the effects of drugs on the tremor of Parkinson's disease. Alpers described a progressive and ultimately fatal degenerative disease of the central nervous system, which occurs mostly in infants and children and bears his name, and Pick described an eponymous neurodegenerative condition characterized by the build-up of tau proteins in neurons. Romberg is universally known for the sign that bears his name, a loss of sensory proprioception secondary to dysfunction of the posterior columns of the spinal cord caused by tabes dorsalis, the disease caused by syphilis.

Cooper developed cryogenic techniques for treating the painful and crippling childhood disorder of dystonia and the brain damage suffered by victims of stroke, as well as deep brain stimulation to treat movement disorders. Elsberg was the first to surgically remove a tumor within the spinal cord. Davidoff invented a one-way silicon valve that expedites drainage of excessive cerebrospinal fluid from the ventricular system of patients with hydrocephalus. He also wrote the first textbook on pneumoencephalography, which for years was the most sophisticated technique for imaging the brain. Prusiner was awarded the Nobel Prize for discovering prions and proposing that these agents were the cause of "mad cow" disease.

Believing that sport was a superb method of therapy for injured military personnel, helping them build up physical strength and self-respect, Guttmann organized the first Stoke Mandeville Games for disabled persons, which developed into the Paralympic Games. Together with an ophthalmologist, Sachs made the most comprehensive description of the familial nature of a fatal condition that primary occurs in Ashkenazic Jews from Eastern Europe and now bears their names.

Goldstein was a pioneer in modern neuropsychology, creating a holistic theory of the organism based on Gestalt thought. He coined the phrase "self-actualization" for the motive to realize one's full potential, a concept that greatly influenced Abraham Maslow's idea of "hierarchy of needs."

---

**Alpers, Bernard Jacob**                    (USA, 1900–1981)

---

Born in Salem, Massachusetts, Bernard Alpers graduated from Harvard Medical School and went to Europe for advanced training in neuropathology. After several years in the Department of Neurosurgery at the University of Pennsylvania, in 1939 Alpers became Head of the Department of Nervous and Mental Disease at Jefferson Medical College, where he soon established an independent Department of Neurology. Alpers published a series of pioneering studies on brain tumors and on the pediatric neuropathology. Alpers' disease is a progressive and ultimately fatal degenerative disease of the central nervous system that occurs mostly in infants and children, which is inherited as an autosomal recessive disorder.

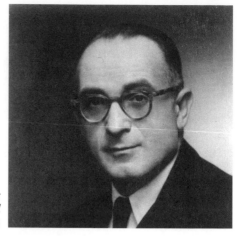

Bernard Jacob Alpers. (*NLM / Thomas Jefferson University, Archives & Special Collections*)

## Auerbach, Leopold                    (Germany, 1828–1897)

Born in Breslau, Leopold Auerbach studied medicine in Breslau, Berlin, and Leipzig. He was a practicing physician, specializing in neurology. Limited by his Jewish religion from an academic career in a university laboratory, he never could achieve a rank higher than *privatdozent* (private lecturer).

One of the first to diagnose the nervous system using histological staining methods, Auerbach published multiple papers on neuro-pathological and muscle-related disorders. He is best known for discovering the network of nerves consisting of ganglion cells ("Auerbach's" or myenteric plexus), located between the layers of the in-

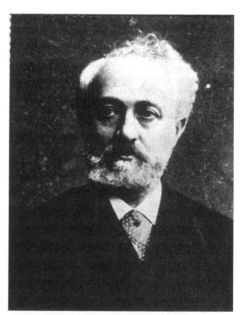

Leopold Auerbach. (*NLM*)

testinal muscles, which control the movements of the gastrointestinal tract (via the autonomic nervous system). Auerbach also performed microscopic studies demonstrating the process of division of the nucleus in the fertilized egg and showing that the walls of capillaries are composed of flat nucleated cells and that the amoeba is a single-celled creature.

## Boshes, Benjamin (USA, 1907–1984)

Born in Chicago, Benjamin Boshes received his medical degree and doctorate from Northwestern University. After graduation, Boshes joined the faculty at his alma mater, eventually becoming Chairman of the Department of Neurology and Psychiatry. During World War II, Boshes was Chief of Neurology and Psychiatry for the Fifth Army in the Mediterranean theater. After studying the effects of flight on brain activity, Boshes was credited with discovering the mechanism by which dive bomber pilots "blacked out," and he devised a method by which the fliers could be protected as they lost altitude rapidly. An authority on the effects of aging on the brain, Boshes performed extensive studies on Par-

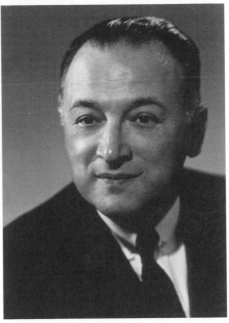

Benjamin Boshes. (*NLM / Northwestern University, Feinberg School of Medicine, Galter Health Sciences Library & Learning Center, Chicago, IL, USA*)

kinson's disease, Alzheimer's disease, and multiple sclerosis. Appointed as Chair of the President's Committee on Brain Death, Boshes authored its 1975 report.

## Bychowski, Zygmunt (Poland, 1865–1934)

Born Schneur Zalman Bychowski in Korets, Zygmunt Bychowski received an extensive yeshiva education. Against the will of his parents, Bychowski learned secular subjects, passed his matriculation examinations, and crossed the border to Austria, where he studied natural sciences and philosophy at the University of Vienna. Returning to Warsaw, Bychowski received his medical degree from the Imperial University of Warsaw. Specializing in neurology and psychiatry, Bychowski worked at the Hospital of the Transfiguration in Warsaw, but in 1912 was dismissed from his post because of his Jewish origin. From 1923–1934, Bychowski directed the ministry of hospitality and public health and supply department of the Municipality of Warsaw.

A prominent neurologist and the author of about 100 works in four languages, Bychowski pursued investigations in traumatic epilepsy and multiple sclerosis. Some of his writings concerned Jewish subjects, such as the hygiene of Jewish laws of slaughtering.

A member of the Lovers of Zion movement, Bychowski corresponded with Theodor Herzl, participated in the First Zionist Congress, and traveled several times to the Land of Israel. In 1905, Bychowski was imprisoned in Russia for Zionist activity.

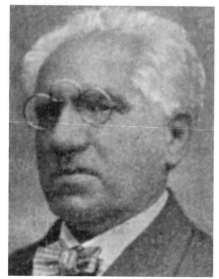

Zygmunt Bychowski. (*Wikimedia / Eufemiusz Herman: Neurolodzy polscy. Warszawa: Państwowy Zakład Wydawnictw Lekarskich, 1958 page 169*)

## Cooper, Irving S.                        (USA, 1922–1985)

Born in Atlantic City, New Jersey, Irving Cooper studied medicine at George Washington University. Specializing in neurosurgery at the Mayo Clinic, Cooper also received a doctorate in neurophysiology.

Cooper is known for developing successful techniques for treating Parkinson's disease and several other crippling neurological disorders. An operating room mistake led to his first breakthrough. While performing a routine operation to relieve some of the symptoms of Parkinson's disease, Cooper accidently cut an artery supplying blood to the thalamus, the part of the brain that controls

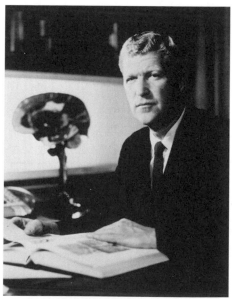

Irving S. Cooper. (*NLM*)

motor functions. When the patient awoke after the artery had been repaired, Cooper observed that the deprivation of blood had removed most of the muscular disorders associated with the disease. Consequently, Cooper perfected a technique that restored the muscular functions of thousands of victims of Parkinson's disease by destroying minute parts of the brain to cut off the blood supply to cells that were transmitting the disorder.

Cooper later developed other surgical techniques, one of which involved freezing tiny portions of the brain (cryosurgery), to treat various neurological disorders as well as the brain damage suffered by victims of stroke. Although drugs are now the standard treatment for Parkinson's disease, Cooper's technique for cryogenic surgery is still used in treating dystonia, a crippling and painful childhood neurological disorder.

Cooper devoted his career to surgically treating patients with the most painful and crippling neurological conditions, who others thought could not be successfully treated. To this end, Cooper developed a "pacemaker" brain implant (deep brain stimulation) to treat movement disorders. Delivering electrical impulses to the brain helped halt the seizures suffered by epileptics, relieve the spastic paralysis that often follows stroke, and reduce the spasms of victims of cerebral palsy.

---

## Davidoff, Leo Max                                      (Latvia, 1898–1975)

---

At age 8, Leo Davidoff immigrated with his family to the United States and settled in Salem, Massachusetts. After graduating from Harvard Medical School, Davidoff specialized in neurological surgery. The only Jewish neurosurgeon trained by the famed Harvey Cushing, Davidoff took time off from his training to travel as a surgeon with the Byrd-MacMillan Arctic Expedition in 1925. During his academic career, Davidoff was Chief of Surgery at the Jewish Hospital of Brooklyn and Beth Israel Hospital in New York, before becoming the Chair of the Department of Surgery in 1954 at the newly established Albert Einstein College of Medicine of Yeshiva University.

A prolific author, Davidoff published the first textbook on pneumoencephalography (1937), a common medical procedure in which most of the cerebrospinal fluid was drained from around the brain by means of a lumbar puncture and replaced with air, oxygen, or helium to allow the structures of the brain to show up more clearly on an X-ray image. In 1950, Davidoff published (with Bernard Epstein) *The Abnormal Pneumoencephalogram*, which established him as the father of neuroradiology.

Davidoff also was a co-developer of a one-way silicon valve that expedited drainage of excessive cerebrospinal fluid from the ventricular system of patients with hydrocephalus.

---

## Edinger, Ludwig                                    (Germany, 1855–1918)

---

Considered the founder of modern neuroanatomy, Ludwig Edinger was born in Worms and studied medicine at the universities of Heidelberg and Strasbourg. After specialty training in neurology, Edinger taught at the University of Giessen. In 1883, he established a private neurology practice in Frankfurt. Two years later, Edinger joined the prestigious Senckenberg Research Institute to pursue studies in brain anatomy. That same year, Edinger published *Twelve Lectures on the Structure of the Central Nervous System*, his most famous text on the topic based on presentations he had given before the Frankfurt Medical Society. In 1909, after a financial dispute with the Senck-

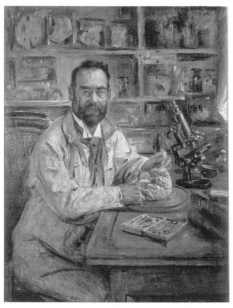

Ludwig Edinger in his anatomical laboratory with instruments and microscope. (*Wikimedia / Reprinted in: G. Mann. Das Porträt des Neuroanatomen Ludwig Edinger von Lovis Corinth, 1909*)

enberg Foundation, Edinger became the first Professor of Neurology at the University of Frankfurt. In this new position, Edinger was responsible for securing financing of the department, which presented little problem because of a large inheritance received by his wife, Anna Goldschmidt, the daughter of an old family of traditional Jewish bankers.

Edinger was the first to describe the ventral and dorsal spinocerebellar tracts and to distinguish the paleo-encephalon from the neo-encephalon and the paleo-cerebellum from the neo-cerebellum. He coined the terms "gnosis" and "praxis," which were later adopted in psychological descriptions of agnosia and apraxia. He identified what became known as the Edinger-Westphal nucleus and was the first to describe the syndrome of thalamic pain.

Edinger also was a renowned hypnotist and a gifted artist, delighting his students by simultaneously drawing the intricate structures of the brain with his left hand while writing their legend with his right.

A provision of Edinger's will directed that his brain be dissected in his own institute. It showed extraordinarily well-developed occipital lobes as well as other unusual features. The neurological department of the medicine faculty of the University of Frankfurt is named after him.

## Elsberg, Charles                                              (USA, 1871–1948)

Born in New York City, Charles Elsberg studied medicine at Columbia University. Joining the faculty at his alma mater, Elsberg climbed the academic ladder to become the first Chairman of Neurological Surgery at the Columbia Neurology Institute. A pioneer in spine surgery, Elsberg emphasized the importance of careful neurological examination and spinal manometric studies to localize blocks in the spinal canal. He described various types of spinal cord tumors and developed new surgical techniques.

Elsberg is renowned for being the first to surgically remove a tumor within the spinal cord. This type of operation had previously been avoided due to a very high morbidity, but Elsberg's "two-stage method of extrusion" for resecting intramedullary tumors was associated with a much lower complication rate.

## Goldflam, Samuel Wulfowicz                             (Poland, 1852–1932)

Born in Warsaw, Samuel Goldflam studied medicine at the University of Warsaw. Specializing in neurology, Goldflam pursued further training in Berlin and Paris before returning to Warsaw, where he opened an internal medicine and neurological clinic for the indigent that he ran for nearly 40 years. He worked as a volunteer in the Jewish Hospital and was the first president of the Warsaw Neurological Society. Goldflam collaborated with educator Janusz Korczak to reactivate the Jewish Children's Hospital, and he also established and directed a hospital for mentally ill patients of Jewish nationality. He was active in the Jewish Society for the Advancement of Fine Arts, a co-founder of the Friends of Hebrew University, and a delegate to the inauguration ceremony of the Hebrew University in Jerusalem. Known for his passion for classical music, especially the works of Wagner and Beethoven, Goldflam helped develop the careers of many artists, including Arthur Rubinstein.

A pioneer of contemporary neurology, Goldflam is best known for his description of myasthenia gravis. An excellent clinician with the ability to recognize small clues of illness that often escaped the attention of his colleagues, Goldflam devoted much of his research to the significance of reflexes and the neurologic aspects of syphilis. He described inequality of knee jerks and the decrease or disappearance of the Achilles tendon reflex in tabes dorsalis and sciatica, and compared tendon jerks in patients and healthy people both during sleep and wakefulness. Goldflam noted the antagonistic behavior of skin and tendon reflexes in advanced diabetes, with the tendon jerks often disappearing while the skin reflexes remain strong. He presented the first detailed clinical description and explanation of intermittent claudication, including

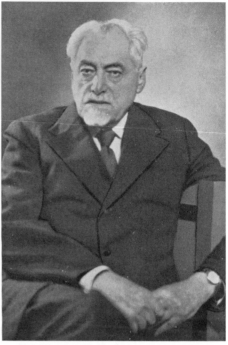

Samuel Wulfowicz Goldflam. (*Wikimedia / Pamięci Dra Samuela Goldflama 1852–1932. Warszawa: Tow. Przyjaciół Uniw. Hebr. w Jerozolimie, 1933*)

the causal role of habitual smoking and the paleness of the foot that occurs after active movement as a symptom of this disease (Goldflam–Oehler sign).

## Goldstein, Kurt                                        (Germany, 1878–1965)

Born in Katowice in Upper Silesia, now part of Poland, Kurt Goldstein received his medical degree from the University of Breslau. After postgraduate studies in neurology and psychiatry, Goldstein worked at a psychiatric clinic and was disappointed by how little real treatment the patients received. This inspired Goldstein to dedicate his career to the careful observation and treatment of individuals with psychiatric and neurological disorders. During World War I, Goldstein took advantage of the large number of traumatic brain injuries at the clinic and established The Institute for Research into the Consequences of Brain Injuries. After directing it until 1930, Goldstein accepted the Chair of the Neurology Clinic at the academic hospital Berlin Moabit. An institution with a large Jewish staff (70% of its physicians) and a socialist reputation, Moabit was an early target when the Nazis took power in 1933. As a Jew, Goldstein was imprisoned, but released within a week on the condition that he leave Germany. For a year, Goldstein was supported by the Rockefeller Foundation in Amsterdam, where he wrote his masterwork, *The Organism*. In 1935, Goldstein immigrated to the United States, working in various universities and clinics in New York and Boston until shortly before his death.

Goldstein described a woman whose hand started to strangle her in her sleep. Termed the "alien hand" syndrome, it is a condition in which the patient's hand leads an independent life that usually goes against the wishes of its owner. This disease was later called the "Doctor Strangelove Syndrome," in honor of the character from the 1963 film "Doctor Strangelove," directed by Stanley Kubrick, in which the doctor's arm involuntarily rises in a Nazi salute or tries to strangle its owner.

A pioneer in modern neuropsychology, Goldstein created a holistic theory of the organism based on Gestalt thought, which deeply influenced the development of Gestalt therapy. *The Organism* focused on patients with psychological disorders, especially schizophrenia and war trauma, and the ability of their bodies to readjust to substantial losses in central control. Based on his holistic approach to the human organism, Goldstein coined the phrase "self-actualization" for the motive to realize one's full potential. For Goldstein, self-actualization, which includes expressing one's creativity, quest for spiritual enlightenment, pursuit of knowledge, and the desire to give to society, constitutes the master motive and basic drive of the human organism. This concept greatly influenced Abraham Maslow's idea of "hierarchy of needs."

---

## Guttmann, Ludwig (Germany, 1899–1980)

---

Born in Tost (now Toszek, Poland), Ludwig Guttman studied medicine at universities of Breslau and Freiburg and became the pre-eminent neurosurgeon in Germany. However, when the Nazis assumed power, Jews were banned from practicing medicine and Guttmann was allowed to work only at the Jewish Hospital in Breslau,

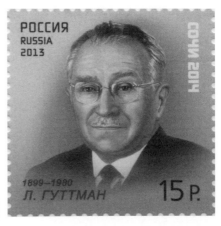

Ludwig Guttmann depicted on Russian stamp, 2013. (*Wikimedia*)

where he became hospital director. In early 1939, Guttmann received an opportunity for escape from Germany when the Nazis provided him with a visa and ordered him to travel to Portugal to treat a friend of the Portuguese dictator, Antonio de Oliveira Salazar. Scheduled to return to Germany via London, Guttmann and his family successfully obtained asylum in England.

In 1943, the British government asked Guttmann to establish the National Spinal Injuries Centre at Stoke Mandeville Hospital in Buckinghamshire. As director of the first specialist unit in England for treating spinal injuries, Guttmann's major concern was how to overcome the widely held belief, both within the medical profession and among the public, that paralyzed patients faced a pointless future and could never be reintegrated into society. He fervently believed that sport was a superb method of therapy for injured military personnel, helping them build up physical strength and self-respect. In 1948, Guttmann organized the first Stoke Mandeville Games for disabled persons, which began on July 28, the same day as the beginning of the London Summer Olympics in London. Guttmann termed his athletic contests the paraplegic games (later known as the Paralympic Games) to encourage his patients to take part. In 1961, Guttmann founded the British Sports Association for the Disabled and became the first President of the International Medical Society of Paraplegia (now the International Spinal Cord Society).

**Halpern, Lipman**                                    (Poland, 1902–1968)

Born in Bialystok and the son and great-grandson of two Chief Rabbis of the city, Lipman Halpern fell victim to the notorious anti-Jewish quota (*numerus clausus*) practiced in Poland and was forced to study medicine at the University of Konigsberg in Germany. Halpern served as an assistant in the Department of Psychiatry in Königsberg and later in the Psychiatric Clinic in Berlin. With the rise of Nazism in Germany, in 1933 Halpern escaped to Zurich and worked for a year at the Institute for Brain Research. One year later, Halpern immigrated to Mandatory Palestine, where he initiated the first epidemiological study of psychiatric disorders among Jews and Arabs in order to create a much-needed plan for Jerusalem's hospitals and clinics. A founder of the Hadassah Hospital in Jerusalem and first director of its academic neurological department, Halpern was the first winner of the Israel Prize in medicine in 1953.

Halpern performed research on a broad range of subjects, including the electrophysiology of muscles and peripheral nerves, the effect of drugs on the tremor of Parkinson's disease, frontal lobe injuries causing oculomotor disturbances, classification of epilepsy, and disturbances of the sense of position in various brain lesions. To mark the first graduating class of the Medical School at the Hebrew University, Halpern was asked to compose a new oath for physicians in Hebrew, which would combine ancient Jewish culture and heritage with the spirit and vision of a modern Faculty of Medicine. To this day, all medical school graduates in Israel take this oath.

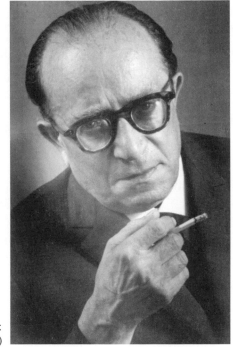

Lipman Halpern, 1965. (*Courtesy of Dr. Halpern's family*)

## Koreff, David Ferdinand (Germany, 1783–1851)

Born in Breslau, David Ferdinand Koreff was the personal physician Prince Karl August von Hardenberg and a student of homeopathy with Samuel Hahnemann. A follower of Antoine Mesmer's concept of animal magnetism, in 1817 Koreff was appointed as one of two professors (the other was Wilhelm von Humboldt) of animal magnetism established at the University of Berlin. At that time in Prussia, almost no unbaptized Jews were admitted to teaching posts. Consequently, Prince von Hardenberg neglected to mention Koreff's religion to King Friederich Wilhelm III. When the medical faculty in

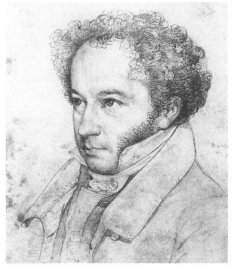

Drawing of David Koreff by Wilhelm Hensel. (*Wikimedia / Klaus Günzel: Die deutschen Romantiker. Artemis, Zürich, 1995*)

Berlin brought this fact to the monarch's attention, Koreff had no choice but to agree to hastily convert to Christianity in an "overnight baptism" to retain his professorial chair.

A personal friend of poet E.T.A. Hoffmann and a member of his literary club, Koreff was immortalized in *The Tales of Hoffmann*, an opera by the Jewish composer, Jacques Offenbach. A year after Hoffmann's death in 1822, Koreff moved to Paris to become a celebrated authority on animal magnetism for the French literary world.

## Oppenheim, Hermann                                          (Germany, 1858–1919)

Born in Warburg, Westphalia, Hermann Oppenheim studied medicine at the universities of Berlin, Göttingen, and Bonn, before beginning his career as a neurologist at the Charité Hospital in Berlin. Although responsible for directing the clinic during the protracted terminal illness of its section head, Oppenheim was not rewarded with the chair because official government anti-Semitism overruled the university's nomination of him as professor. Consequently, Oppenheim established a successful private hospital in Berlin, which produced so many publications of high scientific value that it became recognized as an international center for neurology.

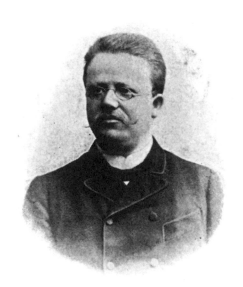

Hermann Oppenheim, 1901. (*Wikimedia/ Biographisches Lexikon hervorragender Ärzte des neunzehnten Jahrhunderts Berlin, Wien 1901*)

In 1894, Oppenheim authored a textbook on nervous diseases entitled *Lehrbuch der Nervenkrankheiten für Ärzte und Studierende* (Textbook of Nervous Disorders for Physicians and Students), which soon became a standard work in the specialty and is considered one of the best textbooks on neurology ever written. He also published significant works on tabes dorsalis, alcoholism, anterior poliomyelitis, syphilis, and multiple sclerosis. Oppenheim's treatise on traumatic neurosis was harshly criticized by eminent neurologists because of his assertion that psychological trauma was a physical reaction to fright and a cause of molecular changes that perpetuated psychic neuroses.

Oppenheim coined the term "dystonia musculorum deformans" for a type of childhood torsion disease, and another name for amyotonia congenita is "Oppenheim's disease."

---

## Pick, Arnold (Moravia, 1851–1924)

Graduating medical school from the University of Vienna and specializing in neurology, Arnold Pick moved to Prague to become *privatdozent* in neurology and psychiatry at the University of Prague. He later was appointed professor in these disciplines and head of the psychiatric clinic at the German University in the city.

Pick undertook extensive pathological studies of patients with neuropsychiatric diseases, concentrating on the cortical localization of speech disturbances and other functions of the brain. In 1892, Pick described a man who had presented with progressive loss of speech and dementia. When the man died, examination of the brain showed atrophy due to the death

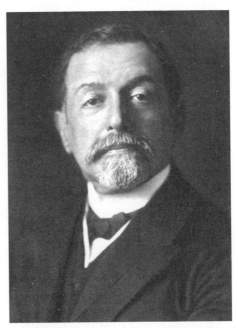

Arnold Pick, circa 1920. (*Wikimedia / Zeitschrift für die gesamte Neurologie und Psychiatrie 76, H. 1-2, 1922*)

of brain cells. Unlike the generalized atrophy in Alzheimer's disease, this patient had more localized atrophy involving the frontal and temporal lobes. This rare neurodegenerative condition, which became known as Pick's disease, is characterized by the build-up of tau proteins in neurons, which accumulate into silver-staining, spherical aggregations known as "Pick bodies."

A prolific writer, Pick wrote a textbook on the pathology of the nervous system.

## Prusiner, Stanley Benjamin                                    (USA, 1942–)

Born in Des Moines, Iowa, Stanley Prusiner studied medicine at the University of Pennsylvania. After several years at the National Institutes of Health, Prusiner completed a residency in neurology at the University of California, San Francisco, and joined the faculty. He eventually became a Professor of Neurology and Biochemistry at UCSF and head of the research laboratory at its Institute for Neurodegenerative Diseases

Prusiner received the 1997 Nobel Prize in Physiology or Medicine for his discovery of prions (the term he coined from the words "proteinaceous" and "infectious"), a class of infectious self-reproducing agents composed

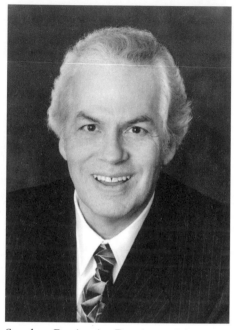

Stanley Benjamin Prusiner. (*American Academy of Neurology*)

of protein. He proposed that these agents were the cause of bovine spongiform encephalopathy ("mad cow disease") and its human equivalent, Creutzfeldt-Jakob disease. Prusiner had received the 1984 Lasker Award in Basic Medical Research for "prions as a cause of chronic neurodegenerative diseases."

## Remak, Robert                                             (Poland, 1815–1865)

Born in Posen (Posnan), Robert Remak came from an Orthodox Jewish family. He was a direct descendant of the 16th century Rabbi Moses ben Jacob Cordovero, known from his Hebrew initials as the ReMak, whose classic book on the concepts of kabbalah influenced the philosophical thought of Spinoza. While studying medicine in Berlin, Remak engaged in research work in the microscopic laboratory under Johannes Müller, the famed Professor of Anatomy and Physiology. Specializing in neurology and establishing a clinical practice in that area, Remak continued his research activities as an unpaid assistant in Müller's laboratory.

Combining microscopic studies of various nerve fibers with his clinical observations, Remak described what became known as the autonomic nervous system, which controls the movement of involuntary muscles and the secretion of hormones throughout the body. He established that nerves were composed of extremely fine fibrils within the axis cylinder, contrary to the common belief that the inside of nerves was either empty or filled with fluid. Remak is best known for being the first to state that there are three germ layers in the early embryo – ectoderm, mesoderm, and endoderm. He also discovered the presence of nerve cells in the heart, called Remak's ganglia, and was a pioneer in the use of electrotherapy for the treatment of nervous diseases.

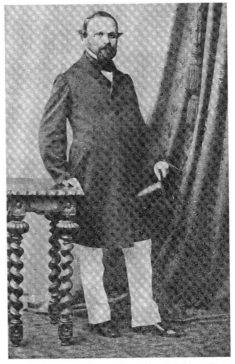

Portrait of Robert Remak. (*Wikimedia / Welcome Trust*)

Remak played a major role in the development of modern cell theory. In a series of observations, Remak showed that all cells arise from the division of pre-existing cells. This applied to embryonic development starting from the division of a single fertilized cell, malignant tumors (cancer) arising only from other body cells and never spontaneously outside the cells, and even to microorganisms and all other life forms.

According to Prussian law, Jews were explicitly prohibited from holding university teaching posts. Remak adamantly refused to reject his Jewish identity and submit to baptism. Consequently, despite his vast accomplishments, Remak was repeatedly denied professorial status or even the position of university lectureship. Only through the efforts of Alexander von Humboldt and Johann Lukas Schonlein, physician to the king, was Remak granted a minor university appointment. His first lecture was a major news event, since it was the first time that a Jew had taught at the University of Berlin.

## Romberg, Moritz Heinrich

(Germany, 1795–1873)

Born in Meiningen, Moritz Romberg studied medicine in Berlin, writing his doctoral thesis on rachitis, in which he provided the classic description of achondroplasia ("congenital rickets"). After further studies on neurology in Vienna, Romberg returned to Berlin to become medical officer for the indigent in the city. In 1830, Romberg was appointed *privatdozent* of special pathology and therapy. As the first position established in this specialty, Romberg can be considered the first clinical neurologist.

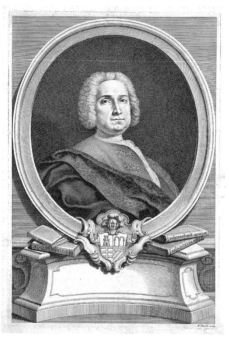

Lithograph of Moritz Heinrich Romberg by Wildt after J. Schlesinger. (*Wikimedia/ Wellcome Trust*)

Today, Romberg is universally known for the sign that bears his name. In his original account of tabes dorsalis, the disease caused by syphilis that produces dysfunction of the posterior columns of the spinal cord, patients experience a loss of sensory proprioception. This sensory ataxia reflects loss of position in the legs and feet, which is normally compensated for by a patient using vision to provide that information. With the eyes closed, however, the patient experiences an inability to maintain a steady standing posture. Once synonymous with tabes dorsalis, this sign later became recognized as common to all proprioceptive disorders of the legs.

Romberg revolutionized European neurology with the publication of his classic *Lehrbuch der Nervenkrankheiten des Menschen* (Manual of the Nervous Diseases of Man), the first systematic and comprehensive textbook in the specialty. Published separately in three volumes (1840–1846), it was written while Romberg was Director of the University Hospital in Berlin. Romberg also translated famous English neurology textbooks by Andrew Marshall and Charles Bell into German.

A dedicated teacher, Romberg stressed the importance of a careful physical examination to make a correct diagnosis, using patients from both his private and indigent practices.

## Sachs, Bernard (USA, 1858–1944)

The son of immigrants from Germany, Bernard Sachs initially studied classics at Harvard. In a class with the noted psychologist and philosopher, William James, who was having trouble with his eyes, Sachs volunteered to read to his classmates a chapter from Wilhelm Wundt's *Psychology*. This aroused his interest in the study of mental disorders, and Sachs left for Europe to study medicine in Strasbourg, Vienna, and Berlin. After receiving his degree in 1882 with fellow student Sigmund Freud, Sachs remained to continue postgraduate studies in cerebral anatomy and neuropsychiatry.

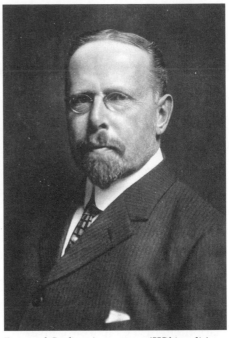

Bernard Sachs, circa 1900. (*Wikimedia*)

Returning to the United States, Sachs established a private practice in New York for the treatment of mental and nervous diseases and became one of America's leading clinical neurologists. Sachs is best known for his role is describing Tay-Sachs disease. Although ophthalmologist Warren Tay had earlier (1881) described the characteristic cherry red spot on the retina, six years later Sachs (unaware of Tay's work) provided a more comprehensive description of the disease and noted its familial nature, with a higher occurrence in Ashkenazi Jews from Eastern Europe.

Among Sachs' many publications were *Nervous and Mental Disorders from Birth through Adolescence*, a reference work for professionals, and *The Normal Child*, a popular manual on child rearing intended for the general public, both published in 1926. In the latter book, Sachs advocated a common-sense approach to parenting and rejection of psychological theories, especially those of Freud. Sachs was the publisher of the *Journal of Nervous and Mental Disease* (1886–1911) and president of the American Neurological Association (1894–1932).

## Wechsler, Israel S.           (Romania, 1886–1962)

Brought from Romania to the United States as a young child, Israel Wechsler studied medicine at New York University. Wechsler joined the faculty at Columbia University and later became Chief of Neurology at Mount Sinai Hospital. An eminent neurologist and psychiatrist, Wechsler was internationally recognized as one of the foremost physicians and teachers in his field. A prolific writer, Wechler's *Textbook of Clinical Neurology* (1927) was one of the first systematic books in the field and became a standard text in multiple editions.

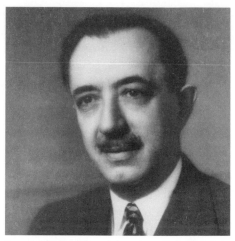

Israel S. Wechler. (*American Friends of the Hebrew University Photo Archive*)

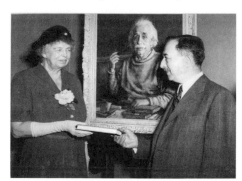

Israel S. Wechler with Eleanor Roosevelt and an image of Albert Einstein. (*American Friends of the Hebrew University Photo Archive*)

Wechsler was devoted to the development of the Hebrew University of Jerusalem, a pioneer of the American Jewish Physicians Committee (founded in 1921), and for many years a major leader of the American Friends of the Hebrew University. In 1959, the Chair of Neurology at the Hebrew University-Hadassah Medical School was named in his honor.

## OBSTETRICS/GYNECOLOGY

Rubin developed an eponymous, non-operative office procedure for tubal insufflation to check for patency of the fallopian tubes in women with infertility and was one of the first to use hysterosalpingography, an x-ray imaging study in which contrast material is injected into the uterus for the diagnosis of tubal and uterine disorders. Freund performed the first total abdominal hysterectomy for uterine cancer. DeLee championed the early use of mechanical intervention (such as forceps delivery and episiotomy) to prevent the poor outcomes that sometimes resulted from childbirth at the time. Henschel was an early proponent of asepsis during childbirth, believing that infection was the major problem leading to poor outcomes in hospital maternity wards. Aschheim and Zondek developed the first reliable pregnancy test, known by their names.

## Aschheim, Selmar (Germany, 1878–1965)

Born in Berlin, Selmar Aschheim studied medicine at the universities of Berlin and Freiburg and specialized in gynecology. Aschheim became the director of the laboratory of the *Universitäts-Frauenklinik* at the Berlin Charité Hospital, and in 1930 he was appointed as the Chair of Biological Research in Gynecology at the University of Berlin. With the rise of the Nazis to power in 1933, Aschheim fled to Paris, where he worked at the national center for medical research at the Hôpital Beaujon.

With Bernhard Zondek, Aschheim discovered a substance in the urine of pregnant women, later identified as human chorionic gonadotropin (hCG), which when injected into an immature laboratory mouse caused the rodent to go into heat and show characteristic ovarian changes in the ovary after being sacrificed. This was the basis for what became known as the Aschheim-Zondek (A-Z) test for pregnancy. At the time, Aschheim and Zodek believed that the gonadotrophin was produced by the anterior pituitary, but further research demonstrated that it was elaborated by the placenta.

The Aschheim-Zondek text was extremely reliable, with almost 99% accuracy for detecting whether a woman was pregnant. Later variations on this test used amphibians or rabbits, leading to the phrase "the rabbit died" as meaning that the woman was pregnant. An important step in the development of modern pregnancy test kits, the Aschheim-Zondek test passed into oblivion with the introduction in 1960 of an immunoassay for pregnancy testing, which was more convenient and did not require animal sacrifice.

---

## DeLee, Joseph Bolivar                                    (USA, 1869–1942)

---

The son of Jewish immigrants from Poland, Joseph DeLee was born in Cold Springs, New York. Despite his father's wishes that DeLee become a rabbi, Joseph decided to pursue a medical career, earning a degree from Chicago Medical College and specializing in obstetrics.

Noting that obstetric care in Chicago was often inadequate and after consulting with Jane Addams, DeLee opened a clinic on Maxwell Street that provided prenatal care to women in the neighborhood. Initially, almost all the babies were delivered by midwives, but over time an increasing number preferred that DeLee deliver

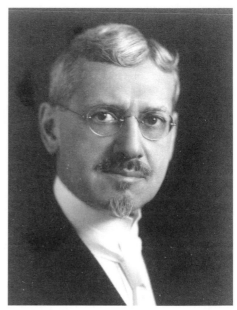

Joseph Bolivar DeLee. (*University of Chicago*)

their children. In 1899, DeLee opened the Chicago Lying-in Hospital, which offered a larger space and focused on providing obstetrical care and the training of doctors and nurses. DeLee spoke out against the use of midwives in childbirth, asserting that his goal was to have obstetric practice dominated by specialist physicians.

Observing the high frequency of obstetric complications and deaths in the early 20th century, DeLee was a leader of a movement that changed the view of childbirth from a normal physiologic process to a pathologic one. He also believed that mechanical intervention (such as forceps delivery and episiotomy) could prevent the poor outcomes that sometimes resulted from childbirth at the time. DeLee argued that the early use of forceps would avoid pressure from the pelvic bones against a baby's head, thus preventing such complications as epilepsy and cerebral palsy. He advocated episiotomy to prevent perineal tears, which could lead to uterine prolapse and vesicovaginal fistula. DeLee's championing of these active techniques is sometimes blamed for the rise in mechanical interventions during childbirth that persists to this day.

DeLee was an early proponent of asepsis during childbirth. Although by 1933 hospital births had become increasingly popular, maternal complications and deaths were increasing. DeLee believed that infection was the major problem leading to poor outcomes in hospital maternity wards. Consequently, DeLee called for hospitals to construct maternity wards in separate buildings, with their own staff members and laundry. However, such proposals were met with great criticism by influential physicians, who accused DeLee's precautions as verging on "infectio-phobia."

DeLee authored several editions of *Principles and Practice of Obstetrics*, and he created *Our Baby's First Seven Years*, a book that offered advice on child care and could be used by parents to record various milestones of infancy and childhood.

---

### Freund, Wilhelm Alexander                                     (Germany, 1833–1917)

Born in Krappitz in Silesia, Wilhelm Freund earned his medical degree at the University of Breslau and specialized in gynecology. In 1874, Freund was appointed Associate Professor at his alma mater, and five years later became Professor of Gynecology and Obstetrics at the University of Strasbourg.

In 1878, Freund performed the first total abdominal hysterectomy for uterine cancer ("Freund operation"). The eponymous "Freund's anomaly" is a narrowing of the upper thoracic aperture caused by shortening of the first rib and its associated cartilage.

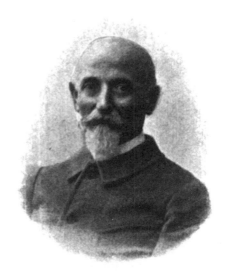

Wilhelm Alexander Freund. (*Wikimedia / Pagel: Biographisches Lexikon hervorragender Ärzte des neunzehnten Jahrhunderts. Berlin, Wien 1901, Sp. 545–546*)

## Henschel, Elias                                    (Germany, 1755–1839)

Born in Breslau, Elias Henschel graduated from medical school at the University of Halle and became a pioneer in modern obstetrics. Despite his thriving private practice, Henschel devoted much of his time serving as an obstetrician in the hospital for the Jewish poor. He rendered his services during a cholera epidemic, writing a book about his experiences. Henshel even took charge of a lazaretto (quarantine station for maritime travelers) when the need arose, and he was a patron of local painters.

## Kristeller, Samuel                                  (Germany, 1820–1900)

After completing his medical studies at the University of Berlin, Samuel Kristleller was appointed physician to the Board of Health in Gnesen. A year later, he returned to Berlin, where he practiced medicine until his death. In 1855, Kristeller opened a private gynecologic hospital, and five years later he was admitted to the medical faculty at Berlin University.

One of the founders of the Medical and Gynecological Society of Berlin, Kristeller was active in Jewish communal affairs. He was a patron of Jewish emancipation and a member of societies devoted to helping Romanian and Russian Jews and the promotion of handicrafts. Kristeller even translated some Hebrew poems into German.

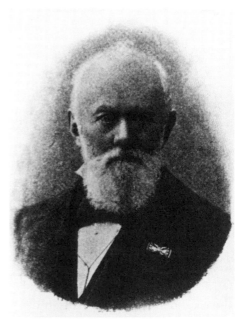

Samuel Kristeller. (*Wikimedia / Pagel: Biographisches Lexikon hervorragender Ärzte des neunzehnten Jahrhunderts. Berlin, Wien 1901, Sp. 914–915*)

Kristeller introduced an obstetrical procedure of pushing out the fetus, which bears his name. It consists of strengthening uterine contractions during labor by massaging the uterus and pressing it many times briefly, towards the long axis of the birth canal. However, it is now rarely used because of the danger of intrauterine fetal anoxia and other complications.

## Landau, Leopold

(Poland, 1848–1920)

Born in Warsaw, Leopold Landau studied medicine at the universities of Breslau, Würzburg, and Berlin, serving as an assistant surgeon during the Franco-Prussian War. After four years as a Lecturer in Gynecology at the University of Breslau, Landau returned to the University of Berlin.

In 1892, Leopold and his brother Theodor opened a successful private gynecological hospital, which became well known throughout Germany. Landau is most famous for his vaginal radical operation, which was the subject of a 1892 book that he wrote with his brother. Active in civic and political affairs in Berlin, Landau was an alderman and a member of

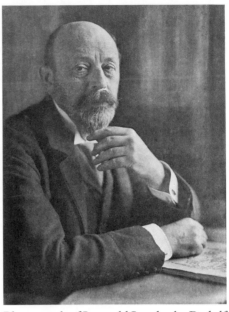

Photograph of Leopold Landau by Rudolf Duhrkoop. (*Wikimedia / National Library of Israel, Schwadron collection*)

the city board of hospitals. He participated in the Zionist movement and was one of the founders of the Berlin Academy for Jewish Studies (*Wissenschaft des Judentums*).

## Rubin, Isidor Clinton

(Germany, 1883–1958)

Born in Prussia, Isidor Rubin was brought to America at a young age and studied medicine at Columbia University. Specializing in obstetrics and gynecology, Rubin established a practice in New York City and served as a staff member at various area hospitals.

Rubin is best known for the tubal insufflation test that bears his name. This non-operative office procedure is performed to check for patency of the fallopian tubes in women with infertility. The Rubin test, first performed at Mount Sinai Hospital in 1919, consists of introducing gas under pressure into the uterine cavity. Rubin initially used oxygen, but later changed to carbon dioxide, a gas that is quickly absorbed, less painful, and safer. Blockage of the fallopian tubes, which causes sterility, could be

diagnosed if no gas could be detected within the abdominal cavity, even after the pressure in the
uterus was increased to a thresh-
old level. The Rubin test reduced
the number of surgical procedures
needed to diagnose and treat sterility in women, and in some cases
even appeared to have therapeutic value by facilitating conception. Although this test has been
supplanted by newer techniques,
especially laparoscopy, one prominent obstetrician wrote that "many
gynecologists regard it as the 20th
century's most important contribution to the clinical study of female
infertility."[46]

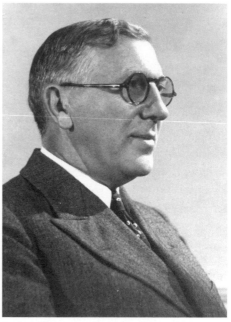

Isidor Clinton Rubin. (*Wikimedia / The Arthur H. Aufses, Jr. MD Archives, Icahn School
of Medicine at Mount Sinai*)

Rubin was among the first to use
hysterosalpingography, an x-ray
study in which contrast material
is injected into the uterus for the diagnosis of tubal and uterine disorders.
He also made important studies related to carcinoma of the cervix, uterine
endoscopy, and ectopic pregnancy.

---

## Zondek, Bernhard                                    (Germany, 1891–1966)

---

Born into a family of physicians in Wronke, Bernhard Zondek studied
medicine at the University of Berlin and specialized in obstetrics and gynecology. He served as an assistant in the women's clinic of the Charité
Hospital, rising to Chair of the Department of Obstetrics and Gynecology at the University of Berlin in 1929. After the Nazis came to power in
1933, Zondek was dismissed from his posts and left Germany for Sweden.
A year later, he moved to Jerusalem to become a Professor at the Hebrew
University and later Head of the Department of Obstetrics and Gynecology at the Hadassah Medical School.

In experiments on mice, Zondek discovered the existence of trophic or
"feedback" hormones, demonstrating that the anterior lobe of the pituitary

---

46. http://www.washingtonpost.com/wp-dyn/content/article/2010/03/12/AR2010031203970.html.

drives the reproductive system by producing hormonotrophin, which induces the ovaries to secrete estrogen which, in turn, regulates the activity of the pituitary gland. This led to the formulation of a fundamental new concept in modern endocrinology – that the endocrine glands do not function independently but instead are interdependent under the control of a "master regulator," the pituitary gland.

A pioneer in reproductive endocrinology, Benhard Zondek is best known for developing (with Selmar Aschheim) the first reliable pregnancy test in 1928. This was based on the observation that the chorionic tissue of the placenta possesses endocrine capacity. The Aschheim-Zondek (A-Z) test for

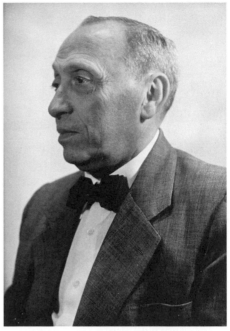

Bernhard Zondek. (*The David dan Collection of Digital Images from the Central Zionist Archives, via Harvard University Library*)

pregnancy (see under Aschheim) became the most widely used and accurate pregnancy test, serving as the basis for modern chemical pregnancy tests. In addition to its application in reproductive health, the finding that chorionic tissue has endocrine capacity led to the development of important diagnostic techniques for diagnosing and treating hydatiform mole, chorionic carcinoma, and ectopic pregnancy.

In 1958, Zondek was awarded the Israel Prize in medicine.

## OPHTHALMOLOGY

Virtually excluded from entering careers in general surgery, Jews interested in performing surgical procedures often pursued further specialty training in ophthalmology and achieved great academic success. Jews were appointed chairs of ophthalmology departments throughout Germany and Austria (even Berlin and Vienna). In the United States, Jews were major figures in the development of the Wills Eye Hospital in Philadelphia.

Kelman developed techniques for the removal of cataracts still used today and pioneered the use of freezing for the repair of retinal detachments. Patz conducted early research into the use of lasers to treat retinal disorders and participated in developing one of the first argon laser photocoagulators. Hirschberg was the first to use an electrical hand magnet for the extraction of metallic foreign bodies from the eye, Blum developed laser technology that was the foundation for LASIK (laser in situ keratomileusis) eye surgery, and Koller demonstrated the clinical use of cocaine as a local anesthetic for eye surgery. Igersheimer established eye clinics in Turkey; Friedenwald traveled to numerous agricultural settlements in the Land of Israel treating thousands of cases of trachoma, a contagious bacterial infection of the eye; Michaelson led efforts to eradicate trachoma and river blindness from Israel, set up eye clinics in several African countries, and trained local doctors and assistants to run them; and Igersheimer developed a medical treatment for optical syphilis. Hays published the first study of non-congenital color blindness, reported the first case of astigmatism in America, and devised a needle knife for cataract surgery. Patz was the first to show that treating premature infants with high levels of oxygen led to the development of blindness resulting from severe retrolental fibroplasia.

---

**Blum, Samuel E.**                                      (USA, 1920–2013)

---

Born in New York City, Samuel Blum received a doctoral degree in physics from Rutgers University. Working with chemist Rangaswamy Srinivasan and physicist James J. Wynne at IBM's Watson Research Center, Blum developed the ultraviolet excimer laser for use in surgical and dental procedures. This demonstrated the value of the laser technology that was the foundation for LASIK (laser in situ keratomileusis) eye surgery.

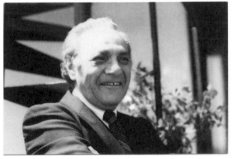

Samuel E. Blum. (*Courtesy of Dr. Blum's Family*)

Up until that time, lasers had been used to create scar tissue when needed for therapeutic value. However, the excimer laser made it possible to perform more delicate surgeries, in which scar tissue was neither required nor desired. In LASIK, the shape of the cornea is permanently changed using the excimer laser. Adjustments can be made for nearsightedness, farsightedness, and astigmatism. Since its invention, LASIK surgery has brought 20/20 vision and freedom from eyeglasses and contact lenses to millions of people.

## Friedenwald, Harry                                    (USA, 1864–1950)

Born in Baltimore and the son of an ophthalmologist, Harry Friedenwald received his medical degree from Johns Hopkins University. He specialized in ophthalmology in Berlin before opening a practice at Baltimore's Eye, Ear, and Throat Hospital and becoming an Associate Professor of Ophthalmology at the College of Physicians and Surgeons in the city.

Friedenwald is best known as a historian of Jewish medicine. In 1944, he published *The Jews and Medicine*, a classic reference work on the subject. A passionate book collector, Friedenwald's vast collection of works dealing with the history of Jews and medicine was donated to the Jewish National and University Library in Jerusalem.

Friedenwald was a fervent Zionist and one of the founders of the movement in the United States. A personal friend and colleague of Theodor Herzl, Friedenwald served as the second President of the Zionist Federation of America. After his first visit to the Land of Israel, Friedenwald suggested to Henrietta Szold, his lifelong friend, that it would be helpful if trained American nurses could be sent to Jerusalem. It appears that he was the first person to seriously suggest that Hadassah build a hospital. Friedenwald was present at the cornerstone laying of the Hebrew University on Mount Scopus, and his son Jonas was one of the founding fathers of its medical school. In 1914, Friedenwald spent two months traveling to numerous agricultural settlements in the Land of Israel, treating thousands of cases of trachoma, a contagious bacterial infection of the eye.

## Hays, Isaac                                           (USA, 1796–1879)

Born in Philadelphia to a wealthy merchant family and a nephew of educator and philanthropist Rebecca Gratz, Isaac Hays studied medicine at the University of Pennsylvania. Specializing in ophthalmology, Hays practiced at several hospitals in Philadelphia before joining the staff of the newly opened Wills Hospital for the Relief of the Indigent Blind and Lame (now Wills Eye Hospital) in 1834, remaining there for 20 years. While at Wills, Hays published the first study of non-congenital color blindness, reported the first case of astigmatism in America, and devised a needle-knife for cataract surgery.

Among the founders of the American Medical Association and credited with the authorship of the AMA's first Code of Ethics, Hays was especially well-known as an editor. From 1827, Hays spent 52 years as editor or co-editor of *The American Journal of the Medical Sciences*, the leading medical publication of its day. As the medical bibliographer John Shaw Billings wrote, everything of consequence in the American medicine of that generation was found in the pages of Hays' journal. He made certain to include ophthalmology articles in the publication, since this specialty did not have its own journal until 1862.

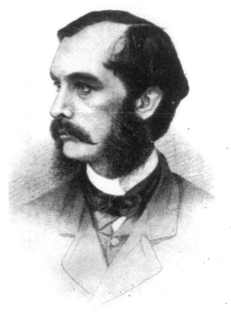

Isaac Hayes. (*NLM*)

Hays was the first president of the Philadelphia Ophthalmological Society (1870) and participated actively in a variety of non-medical organizations, including the Philadelphia Academy of Natural Sciences, the Boston Academy of Arts and Sciences, the American Philosophical Society, and the Franklin Institute.

He was joined by his son, Isaac Minis Hays (1847–1925), as an ophthalmologist at Wills Eye Hospital and together served as editors of two major textbooks – *Ophthalmic Surgery* and *Diseases of the Eye*.

---

### Hirschberg, Julius (Germany, 1843–1925)

---

Born in Berlin, Julius Hirschberg was considered one of the most brilliant ophthalmologists of his time. Hirschberg was the first to use an electrical hand magnet for the extraction of metallic foreign bodies from the eye. He developed the Hirschberg test for measuring strabismus and coined the term "campimetry" for the measurement of the visual field on a flat surface (tangent screen test). Hirschberg investigated many other areas of clinical ophthalmology, including the ocular manifestations of general diseases such as diabetes.

As the editor of the journal *Centralblatt für praktische Augenheilkunde* (Central Publication for Practical Ophthalmology; 1877–1919), Hirschberg developed a world-wide reputation. His major achievement was a nine-volume history of ophthalmology, written between 1899 and 1917, which traced treatment of eye disease from the ancient Egyptians until has own time.

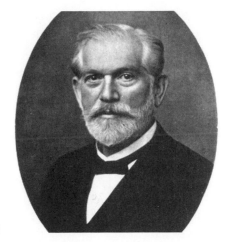

Julius Hirschberg. (*NLM*)

## Igersheimer, Joseph (Germany, 1879–1965)

After medical studies in Heidelberg, Berlin, Strasbourg, and Tubingen, Joseph Igersheimer specialized in ophthalmology, rising to the rank of Professor of Ophthalmology at Heidelberg University. A pioneer in writing about the impact of syphilis and tuberculosis on eyesight, Igersheimer was the first to use arsphenamine to treat syphilis of the eye and the first to operate on retinal detachment by closing the holes. Forced to flee Germany in 1933 to escape the Nazis, he was cognizant of the restrictive immigration laws and economic depression in the United States. Therefore, Igersheimer decided to join other Jewish intellectuals moving to Turkey, which had a need to modernize its society. He became the architect of modern ophthalmology in his adopted country by building a modern eye clinic, training medical residents (without a common language), and writing scientific articles in the field. However, fearful of increasing German pressure on Turkey to not renew contracts with its new Jewish physicians, Igersheimer searched for a position in the United States. He finally received a visa in 1939 to

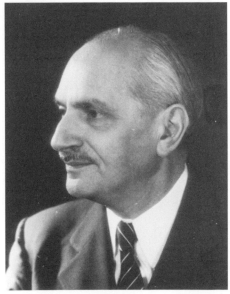

Joseph Igersheimer. (*NLM*)

join the faculty of Tufts University Medical School, where he became a major contributor to ophthalmology in America.

---

## Kelman, Charles                                                    (USA, 1930–2004)

---

Born in Brooklyn, Charles Kelman earned his undergraduate degree at Tufts University and his medical degree from the University of Geneva. After a residency in ophthalmology at Wills Eye Hospital in Philadelphia, Kelman set up a private practice in New York City, specializing in cataract surgery.

In 1962, Kelman devised the cryoprobe, a freezing instrument for the extraction of cataracts within their capsules. This became the most widely used method for cataract removal in the world until about 1978, when Kelman introduced the technique of extracapsular cataract extraction with irrigation and aspiration that is still the procedure used by most cataract surgeons today.

In 1967, Kelman introduced the technique of phacoemulsification, which has dramatically reduced the recovery period from cataract surgery from a 10-day hospital stay to the outpatient surgery of today. Instead of making a large incision in the eye and removing the lens, the ophthalmologist could make a tiny one and insert an ultrasonic tip, which vibrates thousands of times a second and can break up cataracts as that they can be suctioned out through a small needle without damaging the surrounding tissue. This procedure allows the patient to immediately return to activity, greatly improving the results of cataract surgery and resulting in huge savings in healthcare costs.

Kelman pioneered the use of freezing for the repair of retinal detachments, which remains a frequent part of retinal surgery more than 50 years later. Among his many scientific works, Kelman wrote a lay book on cataracts and an autobiography entitled *Through My Eyes* (1985).

Kelman was a recipient of both the US National Medal of Technology (1992) and the Lasker Award for Clinical Medical Research (2004, posthumously).

---

## Koller, Karl                                                    (Austria, 1857–1944)

---

Born in Schüttenhofen, now part of the Czech Republic, Karl Koller began his medical career as a house surgeon at the Vienna General Hospital, specializing in ophthalmology. His research was focused on a search for a procedure or agent to use during eye operations, which often required the patient to be awake and aware. In the absence of appropriate anesthesia, eye operations were very difficult for the surgeon because of the involuntary reflex motions of the eye in response to the slightest stimuli. Koller had tested solutions such as chloral hydrate, bromide, and morphine as anesthetics in the eyes of laboratory animals without success. In 1884, his colleague, the future psychoanalyst Sigmund Freud, suggested he consider cocaine, derived from chewing coca leaves, which had known pain-killing properties. Recognizing that the tissue-numbing prop-

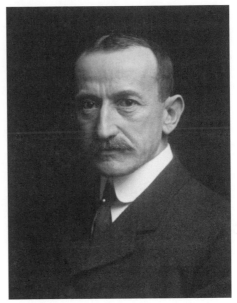

Karl Koller, circa 1900. (*NLM / Alman Co., New York*)

erties of cocaine did not have to be an unwanted side-effect of its use, Koller demonstrated the clinical potential of a few drops of cocaine as a local anesthetic for eye surgery.

In 1888, Koller moved to the United States to practice ophthalmology in New York. Scholars debate whether this was the direct result of a nasty anti-Semitic incident in Vienna. After his colleague, surgeon Fritz Zinner, called him a *saujud* (Jewish swine) in public in front of fellow hospital physicians, Koller reacted by hitting the man in the face. Zinner immediately challenged Koller to a duel with heavy sabers, a practice that was already strictly forbidden but still occurred. Koller was unharmed, but his opponent received two deep gashes. However, this incident probably dashed Koller's hope for a promising academic career in Vienna.

Koller received many distinctions in his career, including being honored in 1922 by the American Ophthalmological Society as the first recipient of the Lucien Howe Medal, awarded to physicians in recognition of outstanding achievements in ophthalmology.

## Mandelstamm, Max Emmanuel (Russia, 1838–1912)

Born in Žagarė, Lithuania, Max Mandelstamm had a typical *cheder* education supplemented by lessons in French and German and four years of gymnasium in Vilna. Mandelstamm was among the first Russian Jews to study in a Russian high school, but he received his main education at the German University of Dorpat (Estonia). After completing his medical degree at Kharkov University, Mandelstamm continued his studies in ophthalmology in Berlin. In 1868, Mandelstamm was appointed a *privatdozent* in ophthalmology at the University of Kiev, but was three times rejected for a full professorship because of his Judaism. Therefore, in 1880 Mandelstamm was the founding director of a private ophthalmologic hospital in the city.

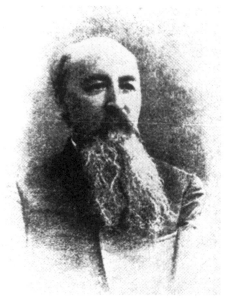

Max Emmanuel Mandelstamm, circa 1900. (*NLM / Jewish Academy of Medicine*)

A founder of the Lovers of Zion movement in Russia, Mandelstamm became an associate of Theodor Herzl and the Zionist Organization representative for the Kiev district. After Herzl's death, Mandelstamm participated in the Founding Conference of the Jewish Territorial Organization. He became head of the office established by the Territorialists in Kiev to organize the emigration of Jews to Galveston, Texas.

---

## Michaelson, Isaac                                    (Scotland, 1903–1982)

---

Born in Edinburgh, Isaac Michaelson studied ophthalmology at the universities of Glasgow and Edinburgh. During World War II, Michaelson served in Egypt as an advisor to the British Army on ophthalmology and later immigrated to the Land of Israel, where he was an advisor to the Israel Defense Forces and worked as an eye surgeon.

In 1949, Michaelson was named Director of Ophthalmology at Rambam Hospital in Haifa. Five years later, he took a similar position at Hadassah University Hospital in Jerusalem. Michaelson established and managed the Ophthalmology Research Center at Hadassah Hospital, which has set up eye clinics in several African countries and trained local doctors and medical assistants to run them.

Michaelson was among the first to recognize the importance of angiogenesis (formation of new blood vessels) in retinal disease. He led efforts to eradicate trachoma and river blindness from Israel, and in the 1960s his procedures were introduced by Israeli doctors in many African countries. Michaelson is the author of *Circulation of the Inner Eye in Man and Animals* (1952) and co-author of *Textbook of Diseases of the Eye* (1970). In 1960, Michaelson was awarded the Israel Prize for medicine.

---

**Patz, Arnall**                                                    (USA, 1920–2010)

Born into the only Jewish family in rural Elberton, Georgia, the son of an immigrant father from Lithuania, Arnall Patz received his medical degree from Emory University in Atlanta and specialized in ophthalmology. During residency, Patz observed more than 20 premature infants who had developed severe retrolental fibroplasia (then known as "retinopathy of pregnancy") after receiving the standard treatment of high levels of oxygen to help them breathe. During the 1940s and early 1950s, there was an epidemic of blindness affecting about 10,000 premature babies in the United States. Patz

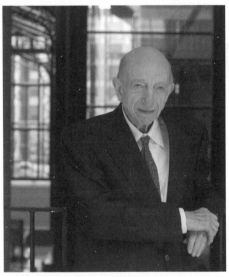

Arnall Patz. (*American Printing House for the Blind, Louisville, KY*)

determined that the cause was oxygen therapy, which led to overgrowth of blood vessels in the eye and irreversible damage to the retina. Patz proposed a clinical study to test his hypothesis, but the National Institutes of Health refused to provide funding on ethical grounds, fearing the study would "kill a lot of babies by anoxia to test a wild idea."[47] Unable to obtain a grant, Patz borrowed money from his family to conduct the first controlled clinical trial in ophthalmology, which produced data that proved his suspicion. After Patz's findings became known, the use of high-dose oxygen therapy was limited, leading to an immediate 60% reduction in childhood blindness in the United States.

---

47. Obituary of Arnall Patz, written by Emma Brown in the Washington Post http://www .washingtonpost.com/wp-dyn/content/article/2010/03/12/AR2010031203970.html.

Patz later conducted pioneering research into the use of lasers in the treatment of retinal disorders, collaborating with the Johns Hopkins Applied Physics Laboratory in developing one of the first argon laser photocoagulators. These can seal leaks and stop the growth of retinal blood vessels that develop in many eye diseases, and this procedure is now a standard treatment for macular degeneration and for certain eye disorders occurring in patients with diabetes.

Patz received the 1956 Lasker Award for Clinical Medical Research in 1956 for demonstrating "excessive oxygen as the cause of blindness in premature infants" and the 2004 Presidential Medal of Freedom for his lifetime of work in the field of ophthalmology.

## Zamenhof, Ludwig Lazar                                    (Poland, 1859–1917)

Born in Bialystok, Ludwig Zamenhof studied medicine in Moscow and completed his degree in Warsaw, specializing in ophthalmology. Intent on solving the problem of national conflicts, Zamenhof sought to develop a simple international language that would not eliminate other languages but instead serve as a second language to advance relations and mutual understanding between nations. In 1878, Zamenhof completed writing the first pamphlet detailing the fundamentals of the new language, which used all the letters of the Roman alphabet except Q, W, X, and Y. It contained only 90 root words and a grammar with 16 rules. The work was published under the title *Lingvo Internacia* (International Language) in 1887, the year considered the beginning of the movement. Zamenhof signed the pamphlet with the pseudonym "Doktoro Esperanto" (Dr. Hopeful), which became the name of the language. Esperanto is spelled as pronounced, its rules have no exceptions, and its guiding principle is to use roots common to the main languages of Europe. At first,

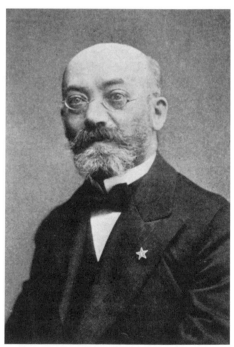

Ludwig Lazar Zamenhof. (*NLM*)

Zamenhof encountered opposition and mockery; however, he succeeded in gaining numerous enthusiastic supporters in every country and more than 10,000 publications have appeared in Esperanto.

In his pamphlets, Zamenhof termed his plan "Hillelism," a reference to the revered sage who is famed for his statement: "What is hateful to you, do not do to your neighbor. This is the entire Torah. All the rest is commentary." As he wrote, "This plan [which I call Hillelism] involves the creation of a moral bridge by which to unify in brotherhood all peoples and religions, without creating any newly formulate dogmas and without the need for any people to throw out their traditional origins." All too familiar with the intense anti-Semitism of the majority of the Polish Christians among whom he lived, Zamenhof added that Hillelism offered "the possibility of avoiding all untruths and antagonisms in the principles of his national religion and of communicating with people of all languages and religions on a basis that is neutrally human, on principles of common brotherhood, equality, and justice."[48]

Zamenhof's son Adam (Poland, 1888–1940) also became a specialist in ophthalmology, inventing a device to check blind spots in the visual field. Appointed as Chair of Ophthalmology and later Chief of the Orthodox Jewish Hospital in Warsaw, Adam Zamenhof was active in the leadership of the Bialystok-Warsaw Chamber of Medical Doctors, but perished during the Shoah.

## OTOLARYNGOLOGY

Politzer was the first to describe otosclerosis and made major contributions to understanding the pathology of cholesteatoma, serous otitis media, labyrinthitis, congenital deafness, and the intracranial complications of otitis media. Bárány developed a caloric reaction making possible the surgical treatment of vestibular organ disease causing vertigo and nystagmus (involuntary eye movement). Solis-Cohen, the father of laryngoscopy in America, performed the first laryngectomy for laryngeal cancer. Politzer developed new techniques in nasal and laryngeal surgery and for the treatment of internal ear diseases by insufflating the middle ear through the Eustachian tube, precluding the need for the difficult procedure of catheterizing it. Rosen serendipitously developed the delicate

---

48. Aleksander Korzhenkov, *Zamenhof: The Life, Works and Ideas of the Author of Esperanto* (New York: Mondial Books, 2009).

stapes mobilization operation to restore hearing to partly deaf people. Schiff championed efforts to curb excessively loud music and other causes of noise pollution, which can result in irreversible hearing loss and other serious medical disorders. Hajek authored the fundamental work on the pathology and therapy of inflammatory diseases of the sinuses and the nose. Politzer published a self-illustrated atlas of the tympanic membrane in health and disease and established the first clinic in the world devoted to the treatment of ear diseases. Sherman was the first otolaryngologist in the Land of Israel, and served as Editor-in-Chief of *Harefu'ah*, the official journal of Israel Medical Association.

## Bárány, Róbert                                              (Austria, 1876–1936)

Born in Vienna to Hungarian Jewish parents, Robert Bárány studied medicine at the University of Vienna. Specializing in diseases of the ear, Bárány joined the University of Vienna ear clinic under Adam Politzer, the founder of otology in Austria.

When syringing fluid into the inner ear of a patient to relieve dizziness, Bárány noted that the patient experienced vertigo and nystagmus (involuntary eye movement) when the injected fluid was too cold; but when he warmed the fluid, the patient had nystagmus in the opposite direction. Bárány theorized that the endolymph in the vestibular apparatus was sinking when it was cool and rising when

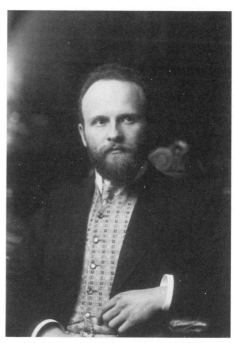

Róbert Bárány. (*Wikimedia / NLM*)

it was warm, so that the direction of flow of the endolymph was providing the proprioceptive signal to the vestibular organ. Consequently, he tested what he termed the "caloric reaction" in a series of experiments and analyzed the factors controlling labyrinthine nystagmus. These findings made possible the surgical treatment of vestibular organ disease. Bárány also investigated other aspects of equilibrium control, including the function of the cerebellum in integrating sensory perception. For his work on the physiology and pathology of the vestibular apparatus of the inner ear, which helps to provide balance, Bárány was awarded the 1914 Nobel Prize for Physiology or Medicine. Ironically, Bárány learned of the award while a prisoner of war, after being captured by the Russian Army while serving as a civilian surgeon in the Austrian army during World War I. Following diplomatic negotiations with Russia conducted by Prince Carl of Sweden and the Red Cross, Bárány was released in time to receive his award at the Nobel Prize ceremony in 1915.

Bárány was criticized by his colleagues in Vienna because of issues of priority in his observations, especially after he admitted witnessing a demonstration of labyrinthine nystagmus in experimental animals conducted by Alexander Spitzer. Therefore, he left his native city to accept a professorship at an Otological Institute in Uppsala, Sweden.

---

## Hajek, Markus (Hungary, 1861–1941)

A graduate of the medical school at the University of Vienna, Markus Hajek was one of the leading authorities in the field of rhinology of his time. The developer of new techniques in nasal and laryngeal surgery, Hajek rose through the academic ranks to become Professor and Chair of Otolaryngology in Vienna. Hajek authored a popular textbook on diseases of the paranasal sinuses (1899), and in 1926 wrote his fundamental work on the pathology and therapy of inflammatory diseases of the sinuses and the nose. With the Nazi occupation of Austria, Hajek immigrated to England.

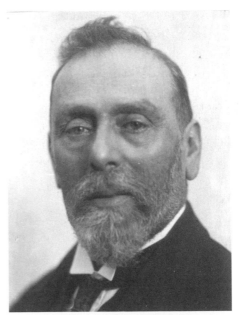

Photograph of Markus Hajek by Max Schneider, Wien. (*Wikimedia*)

---

## Politzer, Adam (Hungarian, 1835–1920)

Born into a wealthy Jewish family living near Budapest, Adam Politzer studied medicine at the University of Vienna. Working on the physics of

the auditory system in the laboratory of Carl Ludwig, Politzer was
the first to demonstrate physiologically that the innervation of the
tensor tympani muscle was by the
trigeminal nerve, while that of the
stapedial muscle was by the facial
nerve. By connecting two manom-
eters, one placed in the external
auditory canal meatus and another
in the pharynx, Politzer studied the
movements of air through the Eustachian tube. This led to his development of a new technique to
treat internal ear diseases by insufflating the middle ear through the
Eustachian tube, precluding the
need for the difficult procedure of
catheterizing it. Widely adopted
throughout the world, this technique became known as "politzerisation."

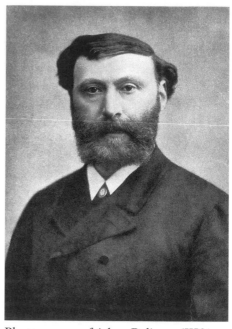

Photogravure of Adam Politzer. (*Wikimedia / Wellcome Trust*)

After a year of traveling to multiple academic centers to increase his
practical training, in 1861 Politzer returned to Vienna to become Professor
of Otology at the University of Vienna, a post he held for 40 years. Later
he established the first clinic in the world devoted to the treatment of ear
diseases. In addition to his hospital and university duties, Politzer attended
his private clinic, which attracted patients from all over the world. To obtain more material for study, Politzer persuaded the mayor of Vienna to
allow him to treat indigent ear patients at the charity hospital, as well as
those living at the local home for the elderly.

A prolific inventor of new medical devices for the diagnosis and treatment of ear diseases, Politzer developed the head mirror and several surgical instruments for operating on structures of the outer and inner ear, as
well as an apparatus for examining the outer ear canal and tympanic membrane, which became known as Politzer's otoscope. Politzer also developed
an acoumeter for measuring hearing acuity and two acoustical hearing aids.

Politzer developed the first illustrated atlas of the tympanic membrane
in health and disease, with color drawings that he made himself. In 1878,
Politzer wrote *Lehrbuch der Ohrenheilkunde* (Textbook of Otology), one
of the most outstanding and authoritative textbooks on otology of the
century. He also was a co-founder of *Archiv für Ohrenheilkunde*, the first

journal dedicated to ear disorders, and wrote a comprehensive book on the history of otology in 1893. Politzer was the first to describe otosclerosis, and he also made major contributions to understanding the pathology of cholesteatoma, serous otitis media, labyrinthitis, congenital deafness, and intracranial complications of otitis media.

Generally considered the greatest otologist of the 19th century, the International Society of Otology bears his name. Politzer donated his remarkable collection of specimens to the *Anatomy and Pathology Museum* of Vienna.

## Rosen, Samuel (USA, 1897–1981)

Born in Syracuse, Samuel Rosen studied medicine at Syracuse University and completed a residency in otolaryngology. He is best known for developing the Rosen stapes mobilization operation to restore hearing to partly deaf people, an extremely delicate procedure on the smallest bone in the body (measuring slightly more than a tenth of an inch). A patient suffering from otosclerosis, a disease in which sound waves are unable to reach the auditory nerve, was on the operating table when Rosen accidentally jarred loose the small, stirrup-shaped stapes in the middle ear. When the patient regained his hearing immediately, Rosen concluded that freeing the stapes had restored the bone's ability to vibrate and transmit sound energy from the eardrum to nerve endings in the inner ear.

Rosen subsequently taught this technique to other otolaryngologists and personally performed the operation on hundreds of thousands of patients around the world.

## Schiff, Maurice (USA, 1917–1993)

Born in Boston to immigrants from Lithuania, Maurice Schiff attended Boston Medical School and specialized in otolaryngology. While serving in Italy as a career officer in the Navy, Schiff became the personal physician of Ambassador Claire Booth Luce after diagnosing the cause of her serious illness as lead poisoning from the dust particles falling from the ancient painted ceilings in her bedroom villa and later writing a docudrama about the episode. After retiring from the Navy with the rank of Captain, Schiff moved to La Jolla, where he started and headed the first ENT Head and Neck department at the medical school of the University of California San Diego. A passionate lover of music, Schiff designed and taught a course entitled "The Voice of Authority and How to Maintain It" for performers at the Santa Fe Opera, and he cared for the vocal health of opera stars of the San Francisco and San Diego Operas.

Schiff championed efforts to curb excessively loud music and other causes of noise pollution, which can result in irreversible hearing loss and other serious medical disorders. He demonstrated the value of heparin and ACTH for treating sudden deafness. This therapy was based on the fact that both of these medications prevent or ameliorate vasculitis, inhibit hypercoagulation, and

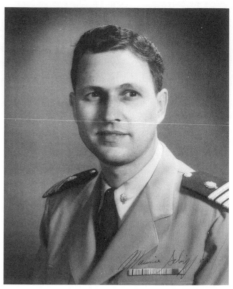

Maurice Schiff. (*Courtesy of Dr. Schiff's family*)

decrease hyperlipidemia, the various possible etiologists for this condition. Schiff played a major role in understanding the pathogenesis of calcification of the ear drum (tympanosclerosis). Demonstrating that tympanosclerosis can be prevented in its early but treatable stage, he stressed the responsibility of otolaryngologists to educate pediatricians and general practitioners about the initial appearance of this condition.

## Semon, Sir Felix                              (1849–1921)

Born in Danzig and moving to Berlin as a young child, Felix Semon studied medicine in Heidelberg and Berlin and pursued advanced training in Vienna and Paris. Influenced by the recent introduction of the laryngoscope, Semon decided to specialize in diseases of the throat.

Settling in London in 1874, Semon became a physician at the

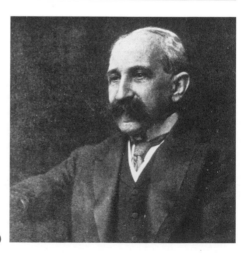

Sir Felix Semon. (*NLM*)

Golden Square Throat Hospital and then assumed similar posts at St. Thomas's Hospital and the National Hospital for Epilepsy, Queen Square.

A distinguished figure in the early development of laryngology, Semon's scientific interests included complications after thyroid surgery, as well as cancer, tuberculosis, motor innervation, and movement disorders of the larynx. In 1893, Semon founded the Laryngological Society of London. Four years later, he was knighted by King Edward VII.

## Sherman, Moshe                    (Russia, 1881–1969)

Born in Nikolayev, Moshe Sherman studied medicine in Odessa and Berlin before graduating from the University of Dorpat (Estonia) and pursuing postgraduate studies in otolaryngology at Moscow University. In 1911, Sherman settled in Jaffa as the first otolaryngologist in the Land of Israel, setting up a private practice and soon becoming a famous specialist. Sherman volunteered at Sha'ar Zion, the Jewish hospital in Jaffa, and twice a year spent several weeks in Jerusalem seeing patients and performing small operations. In 1912, Sherman joined five other physicians to lay the foundation for the first doctors' organization in Israel. Long a consultant of the Hadassah Hospital in Tel Aviv, in 1932 he directed the newly established department for ear, nose and throat diseases. A prolific write of articles in his specialty and on the history of Jewish organizations in the country, Sherman served as Editor-in-Chief of *Harefu'ah*, the official journal of Israel Medical Association.

## Solis-Cohen, Jacob da Silva                    (USA, 1838–1927)

Born in New York of distinguish Spanish and Portuguese ancestry, Jacob Solis-Cohen studied medicine at Jefferson Medical College and the University of Pennsylvania. Solis-Cohen was trained as a general surgeon and, without formal training, taught himself the art of laryngoscopy. Considered the father of this surgical specialty in America, Solis-Cohen gained much technical expertise while serving in the Union Army during the Civil War. In 1867, Solis-Cohen performed the first laryngectomy for laryngeal cancer.

Solis-Cohen's *Diseases of the Throat and Nasal Passages* (1872) became a standard textbook in the field and among the classics of laryngology. His monograph on "Croup in its Relations to Tracheotomy" (1874) was based on the study of 5,000 recorded cases. Solis-Cohen taught physiology and hygiene of the voice at the National School of Elocution and Oratory in Philadelphia, incorporating material from these classes into his *The Throat and the Voice* (1879).

In 1866, Solis-Cohen began the first series of regular lectures on laryngology in the United States. Four years later, Solis-Cohen was appointed lecturer on laryngoscopy and diseases of the throat and chest at Jefferson Medical College, and two years later was promoted to Professor of Laryngology. One of the founders of the *Archives of Laryngology*, for many years Solis-Cohen edited the laryngological department of the *American*

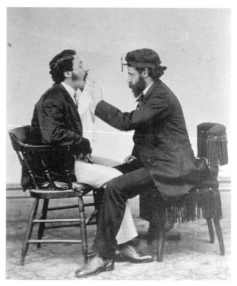

Jacob Solis-Cohen examining a patient, circa 1868. (*Thomas Jefferson University, Archives & Special Collections*)

*Journal of the Medical Sciences.* He was a founder of the American Laryngological Association and its second president.

## PATHOLOGY

Jewish pathologists made fundamental observations that enhanced understanding of basic disease processes. Henle demonstrated the role of microscopic living organisms as causative agents of many diseases. Cohnheim showed that occlusion of terminal arteries caused infarction of such organs as the heart and kidney; and he proved that acute inflammation was the result of a collection of white blood cells to produce what had long been termed "pus." Weigert made important contributions to anatomy and histology, staining bacteria to demonstrate their presence in tissue sections and pioneering the now-universal method of freezing fresh pathological objects for examination; developing histological techniques permitting visualization of the fine structure of the brain, spinal cord, and remainder of the nervous system. Liebow produced the first histologic classification of interstitial lung disease. Klemperer coined the term "diffuse collagen disease" to describe changes in connective tissue in patients with scleroderma, lupus, rheumatoid arthritis, and polyarteritis nodosa, laying the foundation for what are now known as multi-system autoimmune diseases. In the cardiovascular system, Cohnheim detailed the pathophysiology of pericardial effusion and the relationship of coronary embolism and severe coronary atherosclerosis to sudden death from myocardial necrosis. Disorders named for the Jewish pathologists who first described them include Buerger's disease (thromboangitis obliterans) and Castleman's disease (angiofollicular lymphoid dysplasia), and Hamman-Rich syndrome (an idiopathic acute interstitial pneumonia).

---

## Buerger, Leo (Austria, 1879–1943)

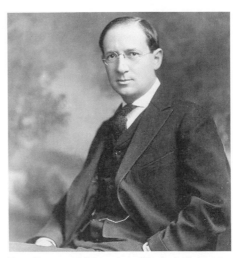

Born in Vienna, Leo Buerger and his family immigrated to the United States when he was one year old. Buerger studied medicine at Columbia University and specialized in urologic surgery and pathology. He developed a form of radium therapy for malignant tumors of the bladder and was the co-inventor of a new type of cystoscope.

Buerger is best known for his 1908 article that provided the first accurate pathological description of thromboangiitis obliterans, popularly known as Buerger's disease. This circulatory system disorder is a progressive inflammation and clotting of small and medium arteries and veins of the hands and feet that is strongly associated with the use of tobacco products, primarily smoking. Unless an affected person ceases smoking, Buerger's disease requires amputations of fingers or toes and eventually of entire limbs.

Leo Buerger. (*American Urological Association William P. Didusch Center for Urologic History*)

---

## Castleman, Benjamin (USA, 1906–1982)

Born in Everett, Massachusetts, Benjamin Castleman studied medicine at Yale University and worked for many years at the Massachusetts General Hospital in Boston, serving as Chief of Anatomic Pathology and as

Professor of Pathology at Harvard Medical School.

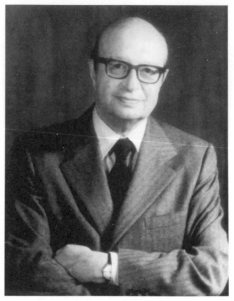

Castleman is best known for his 1956 description of angiofollicular lymphoid hyperplasia, a group of uncommon lymphoproliferative disorders that share common histological features that may be localized to a single lymph node (unicentric) or occur systemically (multicentric). Now bearing his name, Castleman's disease is not officially a cancer, though the multicentric form acts very much like lymphoma. Many people with this disease eventually develop lymphoma, which ironically was pathologist Castleman's cause of death.

Benjamin Castleman. *(Harvard Medical School, Department of Pathology, Massachusetts General Hospital)*

An expert on diseases of the parathyroid gland, Castleman was an author of the first case series on pulmonary alveolar proteinosis (1958), and he wrote important papers on diseases of the thymus and mediastinum. Castleman also was an editor of the clinicopathological case presentation series in the New England Journal of Medicine.

---

## Cohnheim, Julius Friedrich                                    (Germany, 1839–1884)

---

Born in Pomerania, Julius Cohnheim studied at multiple institutions before receiving his medical degree from the University of Berlin. After practicing medicine there for several years and a brief stint as a military surgeon, Cohnheim joined the Pathological Institute of Berlin University under Rudolf Virchow. Focusing his research on the mechanism of inflammation, Cohnheim performed a series of

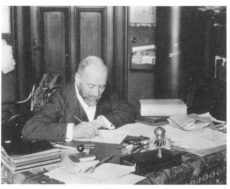

Julius Friedrich Cohnheim. *(NLM)*

animal experiments showing that acute inflammation was the result of leukocytes that circulated to the site of injury and then migrated through capillary walls to form collections of white blood cells that contributed to what had long been termed "pus" – challenging the incorrect theory of his mentor. After relatively short stays at universities in Kiel and Breslau, Cohnheim accepted the Chair of Pathology at the University of Leipzig, where he remained until his death.

Cohnheim demonstrated that infarction of various organs such as the heart and kidney occurred as a result of occlusion of terminal arteries. In the cardiovascular system, Cohnheim detailed the pathophysiology of pericardial effusion, the relationship of coronary embolism and severe coronary atherosclerosis to sudden death and left ventricular dysfunction (as a result of myocardial necrosis), the causes and consequences of ventricular hypertrophy, and the pathophysiology of thrombosis and embolism and arteriosclerosis.[49] He also was the first to use the now universal method of freezing fresh pathological objects for examination.

He also was the first to demonstrate the termination of nerves in what are called "Cohnheim's areas," polygonal areas indicating the cut ends of muscle columns when seen in the cross-sections of striated muscle fibers. Cohnheim's pioneering in the field of pathological circulation and the causes of embolism led to new approaches to medical treatment.

---

## Henle, Friedrich Gustav Jakob      (Germany, 1809–1885)

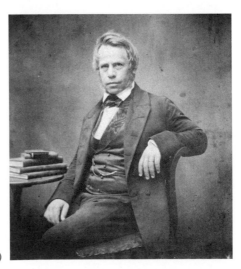

Born in Bavaria and grandson of a rabbi on his mother's side, Jakob Henle qualified as a physician after medical studies at the universities of Heidelberg and Bonn. As with many ambitious German Jews at the time, Henle had been baptized to permit his academic advancement. Henle became prosector in the Anatomical Institute of Johannes Müller, who had recently been appointed Chair of Anatomy

Friedrich Gustav Jakob Henle. (*NLM*)

---

49. Fye, WB. Julius Friedrich Cornheim. Clin. Cardiol. 2002; 25, 575–577.

and Physiology in Berlin. Henle soon became editor of *Zeitschrift für rationelle Medizin*, a journal whose name indicated the goal of relating normal and pathologic processes to the physical and chemical events underlying them. In 1840, Henle accepted the Chair of Anatomy at Zurich; four years later, he returned to Heidelberg to teach anatomy, physiology, and pathology. In 1848, Henle became a chair at Gottingen University in the state of Hannover, where he remained for almost four decades until his death.

In his first major work, *Pathologische Untersuchungen* (Pathological Research), Henle made a major contribution to medical science in the first chapter, *Von den Miasman und Kontagien* (Concerning Miasmata and Contagions). This was the most convincing description of the concept that microscopic living organisms (which he termed *contagia animata*) were the causative agents of many diseases, especially those that occurred in epidemic form. Henle argued that, in communicable diseases, an increase in morbid matter develops in the host only after a period of incubation, which must correspond to the reproductive period of the agent – setting the stage for the general acceptance of the germ theory. Henle observed that "organic substances can neither ferment nor putrefy, nor become moldy, even in atmospheric air, if they are *boiled*."[50] He also noted the disinfecting power of strong acids in combating post-surgical infection, which Pasteur later showed was the result of contamination by micro-organisms.

Henle wrote a *Handbook of Rational Pathology*, which described diseased organs in relation to their normal physiological functions and represents the beginning of modern pathology. He also was the author of *Systematic Human Anatomy*, a three-volume work released over 16 years. Regarded as the most complete and comprehensive work of its kind, it was replete with a large number of excellent illustrations demonstrating the minute anatomy of the blood vessels, central nervous system, eye, kidney, and other organs. Many anatomical structures now bear his name, such as the loop of Henle, ascending and descending structures of the uriniferous tubule that are central to understanding function of the kidney.

---

**Klemperer, Paul**  (Austria, 1887–1964)

---

Born in Vienna, Paul Klemperer was a young law student in his native Vienna when he attended a lecture by Sigmund Freud and became one of his followers. However, Klemperer soon concluded that psychiatry had too many limitations and he turned to pathology, receiving his medical degree

---

50. Frank Heynick, *Jews in Medicine: An Epic Saga* (NJ: KTAV Publishing House, 2002).

from the University of Vienna. After serving as an army pathologist during World War I, Klemperer immigrated to the United States in 1921, initially working at Loyola University in Chicago before coming to New York. Named Director of Pathology at Mount Sinai Hospital in 1926, Klemperer served in that position for almost 30 years.

Klemperer was widely known as a teacher and for his research on the pathology of connective tissue diseases. Realizing that vascular connective tissue served more than a merely supportive function, Klemperer performed extensive

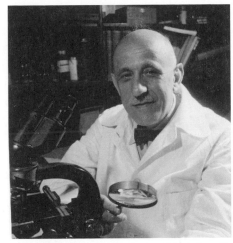

Paul Klemperer. (*The Arthur H. Aufses, Jr. MD Archives, Icahn School of Medicine at Mount Sinai*)

pathological research in the late 1930s and developed the term "diffuse collagen disease" to describe changes in connective tissue (tendons, joints, ligaments, cartilage) in patients with scleroderma, lupus, rheumatoid arthritis, and polyarteritis nodosa. This laid the foundation for what are now known as multi-system autoimmune diseases.

## Liebow, Averill Abraham (Austria, 1911–1978)

Immigrating to the United States at a young age, Averill Liebow studied medicine at Yale University and remained on the faculty as a pathologist for many years. In 1968, Liebow moved to the University of California School of Medicine, San Diego, where he served for 7 years as Professor and Chairman of the Department of Pathology.

Liebow is best known for the first histologic classification of the interstitial lung diseases. Considered the "founding father" of pulmonary pathology, Liebow authored many classic studies of lung disease in sclerosing pneumocytoma, pulmonary alveolar proteinosis, meningothelial-like nodules, pulmonary hypertension, pulmonary veno-occlusive disease, lymphomatoid granulomatosis, and pulmonary Langerhans cell histiocytosis. He also published several seminal books on pulmonary diseases.

As a lieutenant in the US Army in World War II, Liebow was a member of commission that studied the effects of the atomic bombs on Hiroshima and Nagasaki.

## Rich, Arnold Rice                                                      (1893–1968)

Born in Birmingham, Alabama, Rich studied medicine at Johns Hopkins University, where he remained for the rest of his career. Rich was appointed Chairman of Pathology and Pathologist-in-Chief of the Johns Hopkins Hospital in 1944, serving in this position until his retirement.

Rich concluded that bile pigment in the liver derived from destroyed red blood cells. He showed that bile pigments originate solely in the reticuloendothelial cells of the liver, especially the Kupffer cells, with the epithelial liver cells playing a role only in their excretion, but not the formation of bile pigment. Rich classified the major types of jaundice; studied the relationship between hypersensitivity and immunity, especially in tuberculosis; and discovered the phagocytic function of the Gaucher cell that is characteristic of this connective tissue disease. Rich is best known for the eponymous Hamman-Rich syndrome, an idiopathic, acute interstitial pneumonia that is a rapidly progressive and, at times, fatal form of interstitial lung disease.

## Weigert, Karl                                              (Germany, 1845–1904)

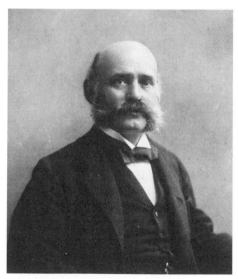

Born in Muensterberg in Silesia, Karl Weigert studied medicine at universities in Berlin, Vienna, and Breslau. Specializing in pathology, Weigert became an assistant to Julius Cohnheim and followed him to Leipzig. He later became Head of the Pathological Institute in Frankfurt.

Weigert's first major project focused on the eruption of smallpox on the skin, in which he opened a new area of research in pathological anatomy – the demonstration of the primary damage of cells and tissues by external influences. In 1871, Weigert was the first to

Karl Weigert, circa 1900. (*NLM*)

stain bacteria and demonstrate their presence in tissue sections, a scientific advance that was very important for the subsequent work of Robert

Koch. He developed histological techniques that made it possible for researchers to gain fundamental insights into the fine structure of the brain, spinal cord, and remainder of the nervous system. Weigert's experiments on the staining of fibrin were also important for general pathology, exerting a lasting influence on the study of inflammation and on the theory of thrombosis.

## PEDIATRICS

Koplik identified a sign diagnostic of measles, which occurs a few days before the characteristic skin rash appears and before infectivity reaches its maximum, thus allowing children incubating the disease to be isolated and helping to prevent epidemics. Alfred Hess determined that rickets could be prevented by cod liver oil or exposure to ultraviolet light and that irradiated ergosterol (vitamin D) could prevent the disease. Hirschsprung described a surgically curable cause of neonatal colonic obstruction related to failure of a segment of the distal bowel to relax due to a lack of ganglion cells in its wall. Krugman developed the first vaccine against rubella, and Schick introduced a test to detect exposure to the organism causing diphtheria. Nadas established the first American pediatric cardiology program at Children's Hospital in Boston, specializing in congenital heart disease. Jacobi introduced the method of bedside clinical teaching on medical wards and establishing first outpatient pediatric clinics. Julius Hess invented an infant incubator that could regulate the temperature and humidity and set up the first premature infant station (nursery) in the country. Rosen investigated the pathogenesis of primary pediatric immune deficiencies, developing bone marrow transplantation as a treatment for these congenital defects. Shwachman developed a program for the diagnosis and treatment of cystic fibrosis that dramatically extended the lives of children affected with this disease. During the Holocaust, Korczak was director of an orphanage in the Warsaw Ghetto, who refused an offer of safe passage and courageously accompanied his children to their deaths.

## Abt, Isaac Arthur                                         (USA, 1867–1955)

Born in Wilmington, Illinois, to immigrants from Germany, Isaac Abt earned his medical degree from Chicago Medical College. One of the first

American physicians to specialize in pediatrics, Abt was a professor at Northwestern University, where he had a particular interest in nutrition. Abt was the first President of the American Academy of Pediatrics and the author of *The Baby's Food: Recipes for the Preparation of Food for Infants and Children*, an influential book published in 1917.

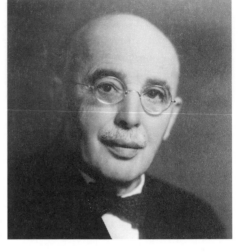

Isaac Arthur Abt. (*Pediatric History Center, American Academy of Pediatrics*)

---

**Baginsky, Adolf Aron**                                      (Germany, 1843–1918)

---

Born in Ratibor in Silesia, Baginsky studied medicine in Berlin and Vienna. Specializing in diseases of children, in 1892 Baginsky founded and became Director of the Kaiser und Kaiserin Friedrich Kinderkrankenhaus, the children's hospital of Berlin. Generally considered the founder of modern pediatrics, Baginsky also founded and served as Editor-in-Chief of the *Archives of Pediatrics*.

Baginsky's major contributions to pediatrics related to infectious diseases, the study of milk, and hygiene. His works included a standard textbook of pediatrics, a manual on school hygiene, a book entitled *Practical Contributions to Pediatrics*, and numerous articles

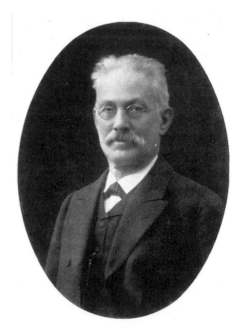

Adolf Aron Baginsky. (*NLM / Munich. Galerie Hervorr. ärzte: J.F. Lehmann*)

such as "The care of healthy and sick children" and "The life of women."

Sigmund Freud spent the month of March 1886 at the Baginsky clinic to become better versed in children's diseases before becoming "sector head" in the first public institution for childhood diseases in Vienna.

In recognition of his leading role in the movement for the promotion of child welfare, Baginsky received orders and decorations from many governments. In addition to medical care for sick children, Baginsky supported initiatives for preventive actions such as open air schools, educational medicine, and milk distribution.

Baginsky was an active member of the Jewish community, even though this may have hampered his academic career. He was a member of several associations and committees formed in Berlin for the purpose of curbing anti-Semitism in Germany. In an essay, Baginsky discussed the significance of hygiene in Mosaic legislation and expressed admiration for biblical laws on the subject. Baginsky was an opponent of the Reform plan to hold Sunday services in Berlin synagogues.

## Diamond, Louis Klein (Russia, 1902–1999)

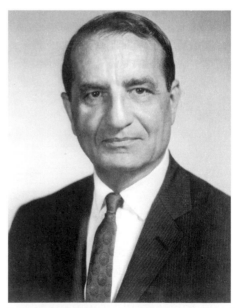

Born in Kishinev, now in the Ukraine, Louis Diamond was brought to the United States at age 2 after the pogrom in his home town. Attending Harvard College and Medical School, Diamond specialized in pediatrics at Boston Children's Hospital.

Known as the "father of pediatric hematology," Diamond established one of the first pediatric hematology research centers in the United States at Children's, serving as Chair of Pediatrics in the 1960s. Focusing on childhood anemias, he identified thalassemia, a hereditary anemia affecting children of Italian and Greek ancestry.

Louis Klein Diamond. (*American Society of Hematology*)

With Sidney Farber, Diamond developed modern chemotherapeutic techniques to treat childhood leukemia and produced important studies on Rh disorders relating to transfusion reactions. Diamond collaborated with his mentor, Kenneth Blackfan, in identifying erythroblastosis fetalis, later called hemolytic anemia of the newborn, which at the time was a significant condition in this age range.

---

## Henoch, Edward Heinrich                              (Germany, 1820–1910)

Born in Berlin, Edward Henoch obtained a medical degree in his native city and specialized in diseases of children. After several years at the university, Henoch became Director of the Department of Pediatrics at the Charité Hospital.

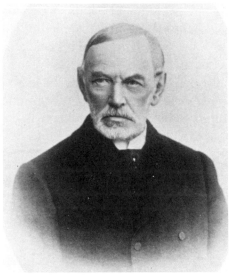

Henoch is remembered for his 1868 description of the association of colic, bloody diarrhea, painful joints, and allergic non-thrombocytopenic purpural rash, a vasculitis that is known today as Henoch-Schönlein purpura. Henoch also authored books entitled *Lectures on Diseases of Children* and *Lectures on Diseases of Children: A Handbook for Physicians and Students.*

Edward Heinrich Henoch. (*NLM / München.: J.F. Lehmann, 1910*)

---

## Hess, Alfred Fabian                                  (USA, 1875–1933)

Born in New York City, Alfred Hess studied medicine at Columbia University. He served as a pediatrician at Rockefeller University before going into private practice. Hess also worked at the Beth Israel Hospital and the Hebrew Infant Asylum in New York, where he helped modernize that institution and was able to study the nutrition of patients who were admitted for long periods.

Independently wealthy, for 25 years Hess financed his own research on the nutritional deficiencies of children at several laboratories in the city. Hess showed that the missing factor in scurvy was present in citrus fruits and tomatoes, as well as some dried milk preparations, and that pasteurization reduced this effect in fresh milk. In experiments on infants that today would be considered unethical, Hess proved the etiology of scurvy by withholding orange juice from institutionalized infants until they developed hemorrhages as a result of the disease. After conducting similar studies on the cause and cure of rickets, Hess concluded that the disease could be prevented with cod liver oil or exposure to ultraviolet light. Collaborating with Adolph Windaus of Germany, Hess demonstrated that irradiated ergosterol (vitamin D) plus ultraviolet light could cure the disease. For this discovery, Windaus received the 1929 Nobel Prize in Chemistry, giving credit to Hess for his part in the work and sharing the monetary award with him.

In a major 1921 lecture, Hess stated that the process of food manufacture and preservation should aim to maintain the nutritional value of fresh food, a concept widely recognized today.

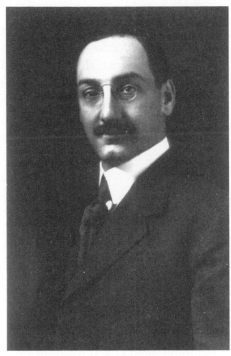

Alfred Fabian Hess. (*NLM*)

## Hess, Julius (USA, 1876–1955)

Born in Ottawa, Illinois, Julius Hess studied medicine at Northwestern University and specialized in pediatrics. Often considered the father of American neonatology, in 1922 Hess published the first textbook dealing with the care of prematurity and birth defects in infants. In the same year, Hess and nurse Evelyn Lundeen created the first premature infant station (nursery) in the United States, recognizing the importance of intensive nursing care and temperature management in optimizing the

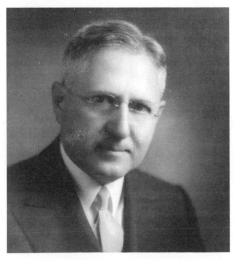

Julius Hess. (*NLM*)

care of preterm babies. Other important aspects of care included special feeding techniques, the provision of breast milk, strict procedures for the prevention of infection, and minimal handling.

While working at Michael Reese Hospital in Chicago, Hess created a form of an infant incubator, which contained a double water jacket with insulation to prevent heat loss and an electric heating plate with rheostat control to regulate the temperature and humidity. This later was converted into a chamber that provided a 40% concentration of oxygen. Hess also invented an incubator designed for the transport of infants.

---

**Hirschsprung, Harald**                                    (Denmark, 1830–1916)

---

Born in Copenhagen, the son of a German-Jewish immigrant who became a tobacco magnate, Harold Hirschsprung chose to become a doctor rather than taking over his father's factory. He studied medicine at the University of Copenhagen, writing his doctoral thesis on the subject of atresia of the esophagus and small bowel. This interest in rare conditions, especially of the gastrointestinal tract, continued throughout his life, resulting in a large number of publications in this field.

In 1870, Hirschsprung became the first Danish pediatrician when he was appointed to a hospital for neonates. He was made the Chief Physician at the Queen Louisa Hospital for Children when it opened in 1879. Hirschsprung provided free health care for poor children, while requiring more affluent patients to pay. Contrary to the wishes of the queen, for whom the hospital was named, Hirschsprung insisted that pictures of animals, rather than biblical texts, be placed above each child's bed.

Hirschsprung published on many areas of pediatrics, including pyloric stenosis, intussusception, rickets, and rheumatic nodules, but he is most famous for the disease that bears his name. In 1886, at the Berlin Congress for Children's Diseases, Hirschsprung gave a lecture describing two infants who had died from constipation associated with dilatation and hypertrophy of the colon. He stated that this condition, now known as Hirschsprung's disease, developed in utero, but erroneously believed that the proximal, dilated bowel was diseased. It is now known that the diseased segment of the colon is the distal portion (down to the rectum), which lacks ganglion cells so that the muscles in its wall cannot relax. This prevents the passage of stools and causes intestinal obstruction and constipation. Early recognition and surgical correction of Hirschsprung disease prevents affected infants from developing devastating enterocolitis and debilitating constipation.

## Jacobi, Abraham                              (Germany, 1830–1919)

Born in Westphalia to a family of limited means, Abraham Jacobi studied medicine at several universities before graduating in Bonn. An active participant in the 1848 revolutionary movement in Germany, Jacobi was convicted of treason and imprisoned. Released in 1853, Jacobi joined the millions of immigrants fleeing to the United States from Europe in search of the freedom that they were denied when the revolution collapsed. En route he lived in England, where he stayed with both Karl Marx and Friederich Engels, with whom he remained in contact.

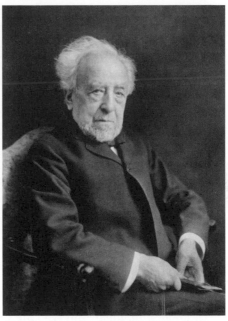

Arriving in New York in 1853, Jacobi practiced general medicine, surgery, and obstetrics. In 1860, he

Abraham Jacobi. (*NLM / Alman & Company*)

became the first Chair of Childhood Diseases at New York Medical College (not connected with the modern medical school of the same name), launching pediatrics as a medical and academic discipline in the United States. Considered the founder of American pediatrics, Jacobi introduced the method of bedside clinical teaching on medical wards. Later Jacobi worked at almost every teaching hospital in New York, but spent most of his time at Jews Hospital (later Mount Sinai Hospital), where he established the first outpatient pediatric clinic. By 1878, Jews Hospital had the first department of pediatrics in an American general hospital.

A prolific writer on various aspects of pediatrics, Jacobi was the head of several professional societies, including the American Medical Association.

## Koplik, Henry                                    (USA, 1858–1927)

Born in New York City, Henry Koplik studied medicine at Columbia University. Specializing in pediatrics and taking postgraduate courses at the universities of Leipzig, Prague, and Vienna, Koplik returned to the

United States and worked at several hospitals in New York. For 25 years, Koplik was on the staff at Mount Sinai Hospital, where he established a children's pavilion and also established the first free distribution center for sterilized milk for poor infants and children in the United States.

In 1896, Koplik was the first to describe an important and early diagnostic sign of measles, now known as "Koplik's spots." Considered pathognomonic of measles, these clustered, white lesions on the buccal mucosa occur a few days before the characteristic skin rash appears and before infectivity reaches its maximum. This allows children incubating the disease to

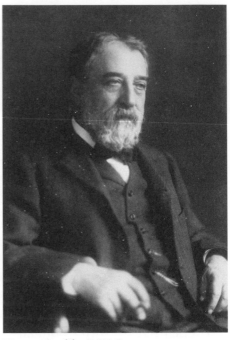

Henry Koplik. (*NLM*)

be isolated, which helps to control measles epidemics. Koplik also discovered the bacterium *Bordetella pertussis*, the organism that causes whooping cough. One of the founders of the American Society of Pediatrics, in 1902, Koplik published his *Diseases of Infancy and Childhood*.

---

## Korczak, Janusz                                    (Poland, 1878–1942)

Born Henryk Goldsmit in Warsaw, Janusz Korczak (his pen name) studied medicine and specialized in pediatrics. A champion for human rights and bringing happiness to impoverished children by improving their living conditions, Korczak was well regarded as a writer of juvenile novels dealing with children in need. In 1912, he became director of *Dom Sierot* in

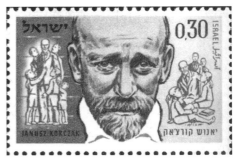

Janusz Korczak depicted on an Israel stamp, 1962. (*Author's private collection*)

Warsaw, an orphanage that he designed for Jewish children complete with its own small parliament, court, and newspaper.

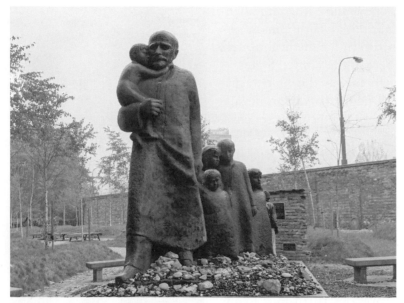

Photograph of Janusz Korczak monument at Jewish Cemetery in Warsaw by Jolanta Dyr. (*Wikimedia*)

Between 1934–1936, Korczak traveled yearly to Mandatory Palestine, visiting kibbutzim and being inspired by them. Korczak is best remembered for his selfless act during World War II. When the Germans occupied Poland, his orphanage was forced to move to the Warsaw Ghetto. In 1942, German soldiers came to collect the almost 200 orphans for transport to the Treblinka extermination camp. According to a popular legend, when the group of orphans reached the site for deportation, an SS officer recognized Korczak as the author of one of his favorite children's books and offered to help him escape. In another version, the officer was acting in an official capacity, offering Korczak the "special treatment" afforded to some prominent Jews with international reputations by sending them to the "show-camp" of Theresienstadt. Regardless of the precise details, Korczak refused and courageously accompanied his children to their deaths.

## Krugman, Saul (USA, 1911–1995)

The son of Russian-Jewish immigrants, Saul Krugman was born in New York and received a degree from the Medical College of Virginia. After four years as a flight surgeon during World War II, Krugman joined the medical faculty of New York University in 1946, where he remained for 47 years and served as Chair of Pediatrics from 1960–1975. Krugman established one of the first comprehensive children's health clinics, setting a pattern for medical centers elsewhere in the United States.

Krugman was the first to distinguish hepatitis A from hepatitis B, describing the different characteristics and behaviors of these two diseases. He discovered that heating blood containing hepatitis B would kill the virus, while preserving an antibody response when used as a vaccine.

From 1958–1964, Krugman pursued a controversial study at the Willowbrook State School in New York, described by a fellow specialist in vaccines as "the most unethical medical experiments ever performed on children in the

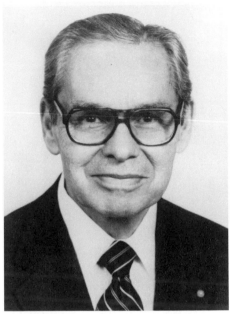

Saul Krugman. (*NYU Health Sciences Library*)

United Sates."[51] He injected mentally retarded children with live hepatitis virus to develop a vaccine to be used to protect United States military personnel from this chronic, and often fatal, disease. Poor families were often coerced into allowing their children to be included in these "treatments" as a prerequisite for admission into the state school, which was the only option for working-class families needing care for a child suffering from mental retardation or other disability. Many of the staff at Willowbrook quit in disagreement or disgust over the experiments. In this study, Krugman proved that "infectious" (type A) hepatitis, transmitted by the fecal-oral route, and the more serious "serum" (type B) hepatitis, transmitted by blood, body secretions, and sexual contact, were caused by two immunologically distinct viruses.

In 1969, Krugman and colleagues developed the first vaccine against rubella. Usually only a mild disease, then known as German measles, rubella can cause severe brain damage and other disabilities in a fetus. In the United States, this vaccine has virtually eliminated birth defects due to rubella. Krugman also played a major role in conducting tests that gained

---

51. Paul A. Offit, *Vaccinated: One Man's Quest to Defeat the World's Deadliest Diseases* (New York: Smithsonian Books/Collins, 2007), p. 27.

approval for the widespread use of the first vaccine against measles, which once was a threat to all children but now rarely occurs.

Krugman received the 1983 Lasker Award for Public Service for "vaccines for hepatitis B and other infectious diseases," He also was a co-author of the classic textbook, *Infectious Diseases of Children* (1958).

## Nadas, Alexander Sandor (Hungary, 1913–2000)

Born in Budapest, Alexander Nadas attended medical school in his native city and immigrated to the United States in 1938 as war clouds loomed in Europe. After further training in several American cities, Nadas received a medical degree from Wayne State University. Specializing in pediatrics, in 1950 Nadas became a staff member at the Children's Hospital of Boston and established the first pediatric cardiology program in the United States, building the department's national and international renown for the care of children with heart disease.

Nadas's research centered on cardiovascular physiology, especially in children with congenital heart disease. The author of hundreds of clinical research papers, including the first description of hypoplastic left heart syndrome, Nadas wrote four editions of *Pediatric Cardiology*, a textbook for medical students. With dramatic improvement in surgical techniques, including open heart surgery to treat congenital cardiac defects, patients flocked to Children's Hospital to take advantage of Nadas's clinical knowledge in diagnosing and understanding congenital heart disease.

## Rosen, Fred S. (USA, 1930– 2005)

Born in Newark, New Jersey, Fred Rosen studied medicine at Case Western Reserve University and completed a residency in pediatrics. A world leader in pediatric immunology, Rosen was Chief of the Division of Immunology at Children's Hospital in Boston and later became President of the Center for Blood Research Institute for Biomedical Research.

Rosen focused his research on the pathogenesis of primary immune deficiencies that afflict children, developing bone marrow transplantation as a treatment for these congenital defects. He was instrumental in defining and understanding the molecular basis of several of the primary immunodeficiency diseases and pioneered methods of treating them, including the use of intravenous gamma globulin therapy.

## Schick, Béla                                    (Hungary, 1877–1967)

Raised in Graz, Austria, Béla Schick attended medical school in that city. Quoting the Talmudic phrase, "The world is kept alive by the breath of children" (Shab. 119b), Schick succeeded in persuading his father to allow him to pursue continued education in pediatrics, rather than join the family grain merchant business. Schick became an assistant at the Children's Clinic in Vienna and later Professor of Pediatrics at Vienna University. In 1923, he moved to the United States to become Director of the Pediatrics Department at Mount Sinai Hospital in New York. Also serving as professor at Columbia University, after 1950 Schick headed the Pediatric Department of Beth-El Hospital in Brooklyn.

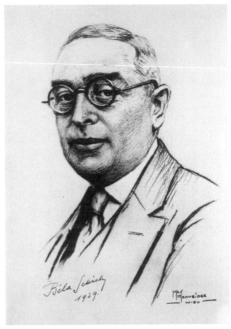

Bela Schick, 1929. (*NLM*)

Considered the leading pediatrician of his time, Schick performed important research dealing with scarlet fever, tuberculosis, and infant nutrition. However, his international fame rests on his 1913 development of the Schick test, which detected exposure to the organism causing diphtheria, an often deadly disease affecting large numbers of children in the early 20th century. Although an antiotoxin to diphtheria had been developed, it had such serious side effects that it was important to determine those children who were susceptible to contracting the disease. The Schick test consisted of injecting a tiny amount of the diluted toxin into the arm. If there was no reaction, the patient had already been exposed to diphtheria toxin and thus was immune from contracting the disease again. However, if the spot turned red and swollen, the patient had not previously suffered from the disease. Lacking the toxin-neutralizing antibodies, the patient would be treated with an antitoxin. Within a decade, a diphtheria antitoxin without side effects was developed and given to babies during their first year of life. A massive five-year campaign, coordinated by Schick, virtually eliminated this dreaded disease. In future years, the Schick test was used to determine whether immunity persisted. It eventually was also employed to treat people with allergies, using the same technique of injecting small doses of an antitoxin.

Schick also formulated and publicized child care theories that were advanced for his day. In his popular book, *Child Care Today* (1932), Schick expounded his progressive beliefs about how children should be raised, arguing against corporal punishment in early childhood, because it often has an adverse lasting effect.

---

**Shwachman, Harry** (USA, 1910–1986)

---

Born in Boston, Harry Shwachman received his medical degree from Johns Hopkins University and specialized in pediatrics. Joining the faculty at Children's Hospital in Boston, Shwachman directed its Clinical Laboratories for 25 years and eventually became Chief of the Division of Clinical Nutrition. For more than four decades, Shwachman focused his clinical and research activities on understanding cystic fibrosis, developing a program of diagnosis and treatment that dramatically extended the lives of children affected with this disease. Indeed, during his academic career, Children's Hospital became the largest cystic fibrosis center in the world.

Shwachman discovered a less invasive screening procedure for cystic fibrosis than the intubation technique used previously. He and his colleagues identified pulmonary involvement to be the primary manifestation of cystic fibrosis, and he was a pioneer in establishing the autosomal recessive genetic pattern of the disease. Shwachman introduced new methods for treating cystic fibrosis, including antibiotics, a new pancreatic enzyme replacement, and chest physical therapy. Shwachman developed the first reproducible sweat test and helped establish the Cystic Fibrosis Foundation.

---

**Zaizov, Rina** (Israel, 1932–2005)

---

Receiving her degree from Hadassah Medical School of the Hebrew University of Jerusalem and specializing in pediatrics in the United States, Rina Zaizov returned to the Beilinson Medical Center in Petaḥ Tikvah. In 1973, Zaizov established the Hematology-Oncology Division for treatment and research in blood disorders and malignant diseases at the Schneider Children's Medical Center, which she headed for more than 25 years. In 2005, Zaizov was awarded the Israel Prize for Medicine.

Zaizov made major contributions to clinical, laboratory, and epidemi-

ological research programs concerning genetic disorders of blood
production, leukemia, lymphomas,
bone tumors, tumors of the nervous system, and the genetic disorder Gaucher's disease. From 1998,
Zaizov chaired the Kupat Holim
program for services in pediatric
hematology and oncology.

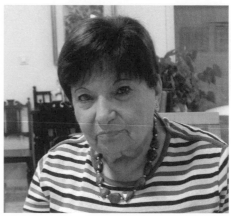

Photograph of Rina Zaizov by
Timrac11. (*Wikimedia*)

## PSYCHIATRY, PSYCHOLOGY

An area of medicine that attracted few Gentiles, the development of psychiatry as a specialty depended to a great degree on Jewish physicians in
Austria and Germany. For example, of the original 13 members of Sigmund
Freud's circle in Vienna, only one (Carl Jung) was not Jewish. Breuer described the "cathartic method" or "talking cure," formulating many of the
key concepts that laid the foundation of psychoanalysis, as developed by
his protégé Sigmund Freud. Freud's daughter Anna applied psychoanalytic
teachings to children. Beck developed cognitive behavioral therapy, Adler
championed individual psychology, and Maslow developed the discipline of
humanistic psychology. Rank developed a concept of the will as the guiding force in personality development, arguing that it could be channeled
into a path toward direct self-discovery and development.

Kety demonstrated the physiological and chemical problems that lay
behind mental disease, thus transforming modern psychiatry into a rigorous branch of medicine by applying basic science to the study of human
behavior in health and disease. Kline developed tranquilizers and antidepressants, the two major treatments for psychiatric illness, paving the way
for many people suffering from mental illness to be cared for as outpatients
and lead productive lives.

Erikson described a theory of development through the entire lifespan
from birth until death, grouped into eight key stages. Klein posited that
children's play was a symbolic way of controlling anxiety. Frankl founded
logotherapy, an existential analysis maintaining that human nature is motivated by the search for life purpose and meaning.

## Adler, Alfred

Born just outside Vienna, Alfred Adler attended medical school at the University of Vienna and began his career as an ophthalmologist, but soon switched to general practice. Although marrying a Jewess, he converted to Protestantism and embraced socialism, establishing a practice to provide care to the underprivileged workers in the city.

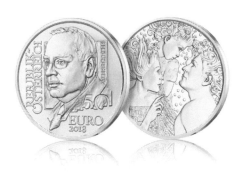

Alfred Adler depicted on second of Austrian Vienna Psychotherapy trilogy gold coin (front and back, 3D version), 2018. *(Austrian Mint / Michael Stelzhammer)*

Adler joined Sigmund Freud, Rudolf Reitler, and Wilhelm Stekel in weekly meetings that eventually grew into the Vienna Psychoanalytic Society, of which Adler was the first president. In 1907, Adler published a book entitled *A Study of Organic Inferiority and Its Psychical Compensation*, an alternate model of the mind that emphasized the importance of feelings of inferiority (inferiority complex) with a compensatory upward striving as playing a key role in personality development. Considering human beings in a holistic way as an indivisible whole, Adler founded the independent school of individual psychology in 1912, thus becoming the first major figure to break away from psychoanalysis. Instead of the Freudian approach, which focused on the unconscious and a distant therapist, Adler developed the therapeutic strategy of face-to-face meetings between a patient and psychiatrist sitting on two chairs to create a sense of equality between them (rather than the analytic couch). The role of the therapist was to uncover the hidden purpose of symptoms and use the therapeutic functions of insight and meaning, simply pointing things out to the patient rather than depending on years of free association. Adler often wrote for the lay public, espousing a pragmatic, task-oriented approach. He also focused attention on the role of family dynamics, specifically the relationship among parents and children, as a way to prevent possible future psychological problems.

In the early 1930s, most of Adler's Austrian clinics were closed due to his Jewish heritage, despite his conversion to Christianity. Consequently, Adler left Austria for a professorship at the Long Island College of Medicine in the United States. In 1952, one of his followers, Rudolf Dreikurs, founded the Institute of Adlerian Psychology, now known as the Adler School of Professional Psychology. As the oldest independent psychology school in North America, Adler University continues the pioneering work of Alfred Adler by graduating socially responsible practitioners, engaging communities, and advancing social justice.

## Beck, Aaron Temkin                                    (USA, 1921–)

Born to Russian Jewish immigrants in Providence, Rhode Island, Aaron Beck attended medical school at Yale University and spent most of his career in the Department of Psychiatry at the University of Pennsylvania. Beck is regarded as the father of cognitive behavioral therapy (CBT), and his pioneering theories are widely used in the treatment of clinical depression and a host of other psychological problems.

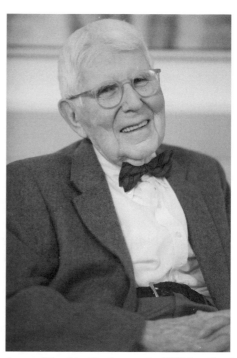

CBT is a talking therapy, provided either in individual or group settings, which focuses on having the patient understand how past negative thought patterns affect present behaviors and thoughts. Rather than reliving past traumas or exploring childhood issues,

Aaron Temkin Beck, 2016. (*Wikimedia / Slicata*)

CBT aims to transform learned reactions that cause current problems into healthy reactions that result in positive, constructive behaviors. Thus, CBT does not necessarily require that a person discover why a certain negative thought pattern exists, but rather stresses the importance of recognizing and understanding the thought process and stopping it before it starts.

Beck was the founder of the non-profit Beck Institute for Cognitive Therapy and Research, and the director of the Psychopathology Research Unit (PRU), which is the parent organization of the Center for the Treatment and Prevention of Suicide. He developed the Beck Depression Inventory (BDI), one of the most widely used models to measuring the severity of depression. He also devised the Beck Hopelessness Scale, a series of

20 statements with which a person can agree or disagree, which measures feelings about the future and is sometimes used to evaluate suicide risk.

Beck received the 2006 Lasker Award for Clinical Medical Research "for the development of cognitive therapy, which has transformed the understanding and treatment of many psychiatric conditions, including depression, suicidal behavior, generalized anxiety, panic attacks, and eating disorders."

## Breuer, Josef (Austria, 1842–1925)

Born in Vienna, Josef Breuer received his medical degree from the University of Vienna. Breuer is best known for his work with Anna O, the pseudonym of Bertha Pappenheim, a woman suffering from "paralysis of her limbs, and anesthesias, as well as disturbances of vision and speech."[52] Over two years (1880–1882), Breuer observed that Anna's symptoms reduced or disappeared as she described them to him. Breuer described this form of therapy as the "cathartic method" or "talking cure," formulating many of the key concepts that laid the foundation of psychoanalysis, as developed by his protégé Sigmund Freud. Freud and Breuer documented their discussions of Anna O. and other case studies in their classic 1895 book, *Studies in Hysteria*, which is considered the founding text of psychoanalysis.

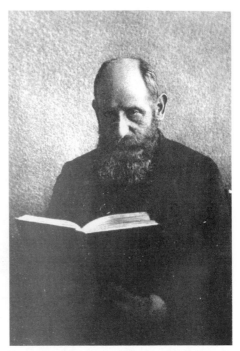

Josef Breuer, 1905. (*Wikimedia / Albrecht Hirschmüller: Physiologie und Psychoanalyse im Leben und Werk Josef Breuers. Jahrbuch der Psychoanalyse, Beiheft Nr. 4. Verlag Hans Huber, Bern 1978*)

Breuer's theory differs with Freud's formulation of psychoanalysis in three major respects. For Breuer, psychic trauma was the primary cause of psychopathology, whereas for Freud it was sexual conflict. Breuer con-

---

52. Dusan I. Bjelic, *Intoxication, Modernity, and Colonialism: Freud's Industrial Unconscious* (New York, Palgrave Macmillan, 2016), p. 122.

sidered hypnoid states (dissociation) as the primary mechanism, whereas for Freud it was repression (defense). Finally, Breuer believed that emotional expression (catharsis) was the primary means of recovery, while for Freud it was interpretation (analysis). On each of these differences, the modern view of psychotherapy increasingly favors Breuers. Understanding the effects of trauma is now a major focus of medical research to discover effective treatment for PTSD (post-traumatic stress disorder), and Breuer's concept of the hypnoid state is similar to such modern techniques as mindfulness, focusing, and neurofeedback.

The publication of *Studies on Hysteria* marked the end of the collaboration between Breuer and Freud, in view of the essential differences in their views of the underlying basis of psychiatric disease and its preferred treatment.

---

## Erikson, Erik                                      (Germany, 1902–1994)

Born in Frankfurt, Erik Erikson was born to a young unmarried Jewish mother (Karla Abrahamsen), who raised him for many years until she married a physician, Theodor Homberger. When Erikson finally was told the truth about his biological father, he was plagued by confusion about who he really was, which sparked a strong interest in the formation of identity that led him to focus on questions of identity throughout his career. Although Erikson did not even have a bachelor's degree, he received a certificate in psychoanalysis from

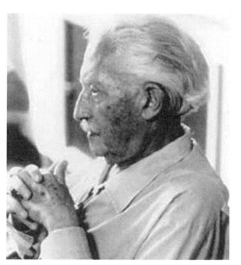

Erik Erikson. (*WPClipart /Wikimedia*)

the Vienna Psychoanalytic Institute and studied the Montessori Method of education, focusing on child development and sexual stages. As a developmental psychologist and psychoanalyst, Erikson became known for his theory of the psychological development of human beings and was famous for coining the phrase "identity crisis." Despite his lack of academic credentials, after moving to the United States in 1933, Erikson served as a professor in such major American institutions as Harvard, Yale, and Berkeley.

While Freud's theory of psychosexual development essentially ends at early adulthood, Erikson's theory described development through the entire lifespan from birth until death, grouped into eight key stages:

1. Trust vs. Mistrust (birth–2 years): development of a sense of trust in caregivers and the world. If receiving responsive care, the child is able to develop the psychological quality of hope.
2. Autonomy vs. Shame and Doubt (ages 2–3): gaining a sense of independence and personal control. If successful, this allows a person to develop will and determination.
3. Initiative vs. Guilt (ages 3–6): the time when a child begins to explore the environment and exert more control over choices. Successful completion of this stage enables the child to develop a sense of purpose.
4. Industry vs. Inferiority (ages 5–11): developing a sense of personal pride and accomplishment, which leads to the development of a sense of competence.
5. Identity vs. Confusion (teens): a time of personal exploration, which if successful enables a child to develop a healthy identity and a sense of fidelity. Failure to complete this stage may result in a child feeling confused about his/her role and place in life.
6. Intimacy vs. Isolation (early adulthood): the stage at which a person develops healthy relationships with others. Success during this period leads to the ability to form committed, lasting, and nurturing relationships with others.
7. Generativity vs. Stagnation (middle adulthood): the period when a person becomes concerned with contributing something to society and leaving a mark on the world, with raising a family and having a career being the two key major activities that contribute to success during this stage.
8. Integrity vs. Despair (late adulthood): the final stage, in which a person reflects back on life. Feeling a sense of satisfaction fosters a sense of integrity and wisdom, whereas feeling regrets may trigger bitterness and despair.

---

**Frankl, Viktor Emil** (Austria, 1905–1997)

---

Born in Vienna into a Jewish family of civil servants, Victor Frankl studied medicine at the University of Vienna and specialized in neurology and psychiatry, concentrating on the topics of depression and suicide. With the Nazi takeover of Austria in 1938, Frankl was prohibited from treating "Aryan" patients due to his Jewish identity. Two years later, he became the head of neurology at the Rothschild Hospital, the only facility in Vienna to which Jews were still admitted. His medical opinions, which included deliberately false diagnoses, saved several patients from being killed in the Nazi euthanasia program. Deported to Theresienstadt in 1942, where he worked as a general practitioner, Frankl was transported to Auschwitz two years later, where he worked as a slave laborer for five months. Frankl then was moved to Dachau, where he served as a physician until being liberated by the American army.

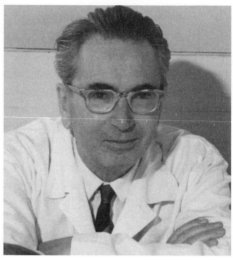

Victor Frankl, 1965. (*Prof. Dr. Franz Vesely / Wikimedia*)

Returning to Vienna, Frankl developed and lectured about his own approach to psychological healing. Believing that people are primarily driven by a striving to find meaning, Frankl wrote that it is this sense of meaning that enables people to overcome painful experiences such as the horrors of the death camps. Frankl was the founder of logotherapy, a form of existential analysis positing that human nature is motivated by the search for life purpose, which has been termed the "Third Viennese School of Psychotherapy."

Frankl is best known for his 1946 book in German, *Saying Yes to Life in Spite of Everything: A Psychologist Experiences the Concentration Camp*, which became a best-seller in English with the title *Man's Search for Meaning*. Frankl related his experiences as a concentration camp inmate, leading him to conclude that even in the most absurd, painful, and dehumanized situation, life has potential meaning, and thus even suffering is meaningful. He concluded that those without a meaning in their life are prone to aggression, depression and addiction.

As Frankl wrote, "We can discover this meaning in life in three different ways: (1) by creating a work or doing a deed; (2) by experiencing something or encountering someone; and (3) by the attitude we take toward unavoidable suffering," concluding that "everything can be taken from a man but one thing: the last of the human freedoms – to choose one's attitude in any given set of circumstances."[53]

---

53. Victor Frankl Institute of Logotherapy, Austin, Texas (www.logotherapyinstitute.org/About_Logotherapy.html)

# Freud, Anna                                          (Austria, 1895–1982)

Born in Vienna, the youngest
daughter of famed psychoanalyst
Sigmund Freud, Anna Freud was
devoted to her father and enjoyed
an intimate association with the
developing psychoanalytic theory
and practice. The founder of child
psychoanalysis and one of its foremost practitioners, Anna Freud
made fundamental contributions
to understanding how the ego, or
consciousness, functions in avert-
ing painful ideas, impulses, and
feelings.

Freud's daily observation of
children while teaching elementary school led her to develop an
interest in child psychology. *An In-*
*troduction to the Technique of Child*
*Analysis* (1927), which outlined her
approach to child psychoanalysis,
was published during her term as
Chair of the Vienna Psychoanalytic Society. Freud organized the
lectures she gave to teachers and
caretakers of young children in
Vienna in *An Introduction to Psy-*
*choanalysis: Lectures for Child Ana-*
*lysts and Teachers 1922–1935.* In *Ego*
*and Mechanisms of Defense* (1936),
Freud stressed that the principal
defense mechanism is repression,
an unconscious process that develops as the young child learns
that some impulses, if acted upon,
could prove dangerous to herself.
A pioneering work in the development of adolescent psychology,

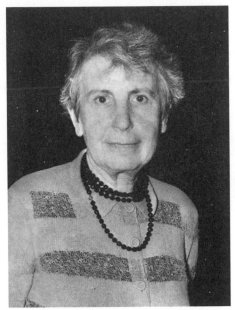

Anna Freud, 1957. (*Wikimedia / Dutch Na-*
*tional Archives, The Hague*)

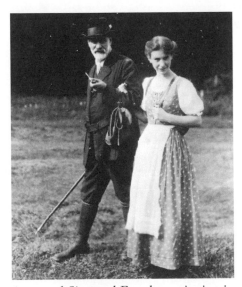

Anna and Sigmund Freud vacationing in
the Italian Dolomites, 1913. (*Wikimedia /*
*United States Library of Congress Prints and*
*Photographs Division*)

Freud described other defense mechanisms, such as the projection of one's own feeling on another, directing aggressive impulses against the self (with suicide as the most extreme example), identifying an overpowering aggressor, and separating ideas from feelings. Freud saw play as the adaptation of a child to reality, not necessarily as a revelation of unconscious conflicts.

With the Nazi takeover of Austria in 1938, Anna Freud and her father escaped to London. She founded the Hampstead Child Therapy Course and Clinic in 1947, serving as its director for three decades (1952–1982). During this time, Freud published *Normality and Pathology in Childhood* (1965), which summarized "the use of developmental lines charting theoretical normal growth from dependency to emotional self-reliance."[54]

---

### Freud, Sigmund                                                    (Moravia, 1856–1939)

Born Sigismund Schlomo Freud in Freiberg, now the Czech Republic, Sigmund Freud initially studied law before embarking on a career in medical research. He studied medicine at the University of Vienna and began investigations on the central nervous system and the possibility of cocaine as a general curative for various disorders.

After establishing a private practice, Freud was consulted on the case of Anna O (real name, Bertha Pappenheim), which marked a turning point in his career. Anna suffered from hysteria, demonstrating a host of

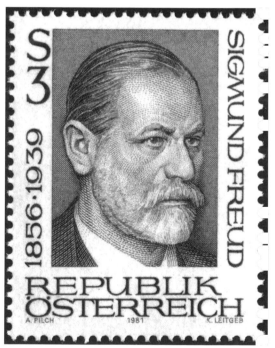

Sigmund Freud depicted on an Austrian stamp, 1981. (*Author's private collection*)

symptoms (paralysis, convulsions, hallucinations, loss of speech) without an apparent physical cause. After her doctor, Josef Breuer, succeeded in

---

54. Freud, Anna: Her Life and Work. (London, *Freud Museum Publications*, 1993), p. 5. Also cited in Wikipedia article – https://en.wikipedia.org/wiki/Anna_Freud.

treating Anna by helping her to recall forgotten memories of traumatic events, Freud developed the general concept that physical symptoms are often the surface manifestations of deeply repressed conflicts, which he put forth in his *Studies in Hysteria*. (1895)

This revelation led Freud to postulate the existence of three levels of the mind. The surface level is the consciousness, which he described as the tip of the iceberg. Beneath this lay the preconscious, which consists of everything that can be retrieved from memory. The third and most significant region is

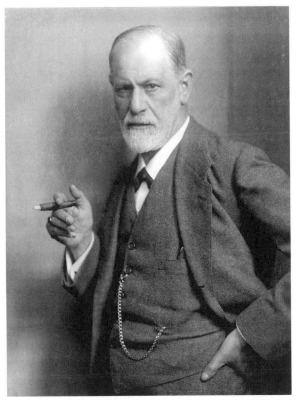

Portrait of Sigmund Freud by Max Halberstadt. (*Wikimedia*)

the unconscious, which is responsible for the underlying cause of most behavior and consists of a set of primitive wishes and impulses kept under control by the preconscious area. The contents of the unconscious could be so threatening and painful that a person needs to lock it away from any conscious thought, via the process of repression and other defense mechanisms.

In 1923, Freud developed a more structural model of the mind – composed of the id, ego, and superego – which represent hypothetical conceptions of mental functions rather than specific physical areas within the brain. The id operates at an unconscious level according to the pleasure principle of gaining gratification from satisfying basic instincts. The ego, which develops from the id during infancy, is designed to satisfy the demands of the id, but in a safe and socially acceptable way. The superego develops during early childhood and is responsible for ensuring that moral standards are followed so that the person can behave in a socially correct manner. The interaction between these three very different components of the mind inevitably leads to inner conflict.

When there is conflict between the goals of the id and superego, the ego must act as a referee and mediate this conflict. The ego can develop various defense mechanisms to prevent it from becoming overwhelmed by anxiety and guilt.

Although initially using hypnosis in his practice, Freud decided that a more effective approach was to encourage his patients to talk freely (on his famous couch) about whatever ideas or memories occurred to them, a technique he termed "free association." He also noted that an analysis of the dreams of his patients could reveal the complex structure of their unconscious minds and demonstrate how repression led to the formation of their symptoms. In 1899, Freud published *The Interpretation of Dreams*, which he considered the most important of his books.

The term psychoanalysis is used to describe the set of Freud's psychological and psychotherapeutic theories and associated techniques. The weekly Wednesday meetings at his home, where colleagues discussed Freud's discoveries and theories, led to the emergence of the Viennese Association of Psychoanalysis in 1908. Over time, some of Freud's colleagues and students, most notably Alfred Adler and Carl Jung, broke away to develop their own independent approaches.

## Kety, Seymour S. (USA, 1915–2000)

Born in Philadelphia, Seymour Kety studied medicine at the University of Pennsylvania. During internship, Kety became aware of an increase in children developing lead poisoning from chewing on cribs that were coated in paint containing lead. He developed the concept of chelation, the use of citrate to help flush the lead out of children's systems, which became the treatment for heavy metal intoxication.

After internship, Kety left clinical medicine to pursue a research career. As the first scientific director of the new National Institute of Mental Health in the early 1950s,

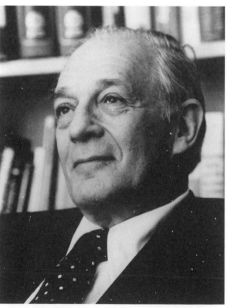

Seymour S. Kety. (*Lasker Foundation*)

Kety played a major role in shifting the direction of psychiatric research, putting much greater emphasis on the biological bases of mental illness. At the time, psychoanalysis dominated most academic psychiatry departments, but Kety believed that there were physiological and chemical problems that lay behind mental disease. Consequently, Kety has been credited with transforming modern psychiatry in a rigorous branch of medicine by applying basic science to the study of human behavior in health and disease.

Kety spent much of his life studying schizophrenia. Using Danish national birth registries to track the transmission of the illness in people separated at birth from their biological families, Kety was the first to provide strong evidence that the illness ran in families, with heredity playing a significant role. This helped overturn the prevailing wisdom that schizophrenia was caused by bad parenting. However, Kety believed that schizophrenia is not entirely genetic, with environmental stressors (not yet completely understood) appearing to trigger the illness in those with a genetic vulnerability.

---

## Klein, Melanie Reizes (Austria, 1882–1960)

Born in Vienna, Melanie Reizes Klein was educated at the gymnasium, but was unable to attend medical school because of the collapse of her family's wealth. She married Arthur Klein, an industrial chemist, and began to raise a family. After moving to Budapest in 1910, Klein began a course of psychoanalysis with Sandor Ferencz (a close associate of Sigmund Freud), who encouraged her to psychoanalyze her own children. Without any formal guidance, Klein developed a technique of child analysis that is still used today. In her "play technique," the play activity of a child is considered as a meaningful

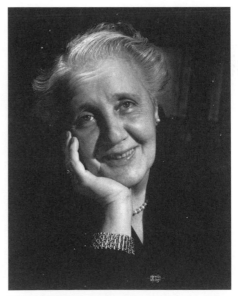

Melanie Reizes Klein, 1952. (*Douglas Glass, Wellcome Images / Wikimedia*)

symbol of unconscious material and is interpreted in the same way that dreams and free associations are used in the analysis of adults.

In 1926, Klein moved to London to join the British Psycho-Analytical Society. Her landmark book, *The Psychoanalysis of Children* (1932), presents her observations and theory of child analysis. Believing children's play to be a symbolic way of controlling anxiety, she observed free play with toys as a means of determining the psychological impulses and ideas associated with the early years of life. Her "object-relation" theory related the development of the ego during this period to the experience of various "drive objects," physical objects that were associated with psychic drives. She posited that in early development, a child relates to parts rather than to complete objects, such as to the breast rather than to the mother. Klein termed this unstable and primitive mode of identification the "paranoid-schizoid position." The next development phase is the "depressive position," in which the infant comes to relate to whole objects, such as the mother or father. This phase is marked by the infant's recognition of ambivalent feelings toward objects, and thus the moderation of internal conflicts about them. Klein believed that the anxiety in the paranoid-schizoid position was persecutory, threatening the annihilation of the self. The anxiety of the second and later position was depressive, related to fear of the harm done to loved objects by the infant's own destructive impulses.

---

## Kline, Nathan Schellenberg                              (USA, 1916–1983)

---

Born in Philadelphia, Nathan Kline studied medicine at New York University. Kline was the founder and initial director of the Rockland Research Institute in Orangeburg, New York, where he introduced the use of tranquilizers and antidepressant drugs in the treatment of mental illnesses despite widespread skepticism among his colleagues. Kline took the unusual step of investigating reserpine, used in the Unites States to treat high blood pressure, as a treatment for psychiatric disease. In a two-year trial on hospitalized patients, Kline found that about 70% of those suffering from

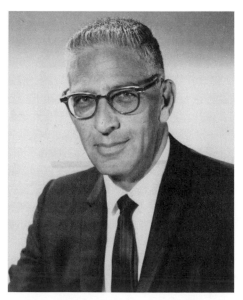

Nathan Schellenberg Kline. (*NYU Health Sciences Library*)

schizophrenia demonstrated marked relief of their symptoms. For this work, Kline received the first of his Lasker Awards for Clinical Medical Research in 1957.

Encouraged by his success with this tranquilizer, Kline investigated the properties of antidepressants, demonstrating that iproniazid, a monoamine oxidase inhibitor widely used at the time to fight tuberculosis, was a valuable treatment for severe depression. This resulted in Kline winning a second Lasker Award in 1964 (the only two-time winner), though the drug was later withdrawn from the United States market for causing liver damage in some patients.

Kline's development of tranquilizers and antidepressants, the two major treatments for psychiatric illness, made possible the treatment of many patients formerly considered untreatable. This paved the way for many people suffering from mental illness to be cared for as outpatients and lead productive lives. Kline's work is generally acknowledged as opening the new field of psychopharmacology.

After his death, the Rockland Research Institute was renamed the Nathan Kline Institute for Psychiatric Research, part of the New York State Office of Mental Health.

---

## Lombroso, Cesare (Italy, 1835–1909)

Born into a wealthy Jewish family in Verona, Cesare Lombroso studied at Pavia, Padua, and Vienna and earned degrees in medicine and surgery. While at the University of Vienna, Lombroso studied psychology and psychiatry, as well as the anatomy and physiology of the brain. After four years of military service as a surgeon in the Italian army, Lombroso worked as a doctor at Pavia, Pesaro, and Regio Emilia. Lombroso then taught legal medicine and public hygiene at Turin University and was appointed professor of psychiatry in 1896. Ten years later, a chair in the new "science" of criminal anthropology was especially created for him.

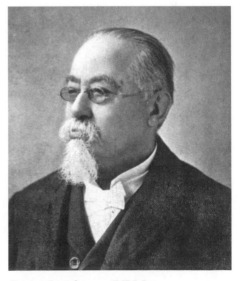

Cesare Lombroso. (*NLM*)

While in the army, Lombroso made systematic measurements of physical differences among soldiers from various regions of Italy, as well as of differences between well-disciplined and aggressive or criminal soldiers. He later compared physical and psychological characteristics of mentally ill and sane people, and criminals and law-abiding citizens, to search for differences that could affect their behavior. Influenced by French positivism and by Darwinian evolutionary theories, Lombroso concluded that there is a degenerate class of human beings, distinguished by anatomical and psychical characteristics, who are born with criminal instincts and who represent a reversion to a primitive form of humanity. Signs of "born criminals" included sloping forehead, ears of unusual size, asymmetry of the face, prognathism, excessive length of the arms, and asymmetry of the cranium. Convinced that various types of criminals, such as thieves, rapists, and murderers, could be distinguished by specific characteristics, Lombroso published this controversial theory in his *L'Uomo Delinquente* (The Criminal Man, 1876).

Over time, Lombroso gradually admitted the existence of acquired criminogenic pathological or environmental factors, though he continued to maintain that the true criminal was a subspecies of man of atavistic origin. Although the concept of the "born criminal" is no longer accepted, Lombroso remains an important figure in the history of the behavioral sciences for shifting the emphasis in criminology from the crime itself to the criminal and his origins.

In the field of penology Lombroso supported such reformist ideas as the compensation of the victims of crime from the prison work of the malefactor. Despite his views on inherited delinquency, Lombroso rejected capital punishment and favored rehabilitation of the criminal so that his work potential could be used for the benefit of society.

In his *The Man of Genius/The Gifted Man* (1888), Lombroso analyzed the "genius," another type of what he considered "deviant" from general society. To support his claim that artistic genius was a form of hereditary insanity, Lombroso amassed a large collection of "psychiatric art," from which he identified 13 typical features of the "art of the insane."

His friendship with Max Nordau led Lombroso to support Zionism. He published a monograph on anti-Semitism in which he stressed that those who espoused this view represented an anthropological degeneration similar to that of the criminal.

## Maslow, Abraham Harold (USA, 1908–1970)

Born in Brooklyn to immigrants who fled czarist persecution in Russia, Abraham Maslow received a doctorate in psychology from the University of Wisconsin. After academic appointments at Columbia University and Brooklyn College, Maslow served as chair of the psychology department at Brandeis University (1951–1969). There he met Kurt Goldstein, who had originated the idea of self-actualization in his famous book, *The Organism* (1934). This influenced Maslow to develop his concept of "hierarchy of needs" and the discipline of humanistic psychology.

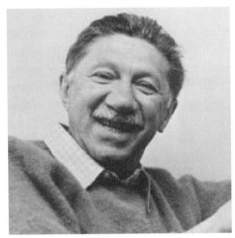

Abraham Harold Maslow. (*Wikimedia*)

The hierarchy of needs is Maslow's theory that psychological health is predicated on fulfilling innate human needs in a prescribed order, culminating in self-actualization. Envisioning a pyramid, Maslow described five basic categories leading to psychological health. At the bottom of the hierarchy are the basic/physiological needs of a human being, such as food, water, sleep, and sex. The next level consists of the safety needs of security, order, and stability. These first two levels are essential to the physical survival of the person, and once satisfied an individual can attempt to accomplish more. The third level is love and belonging, the psychological need to share oneself with others, such as family and friends. The fourth level is esteem, when individuals feel comfortable with what they have accomplished. This is the need to be competent and recognized, such as through status and success. It also includes the cognitive level, in which individuals intellectually stimulate themselves and explore, and the aesthetic level, which reflects the need for harmony, order, and beauty. At the top of the pyramid is the need for self-actualization, which occurs when individuals reach a state of harmony and understanding because they are engaged in achieving their full potential. At this stage, people focus on themselves to build their own image, which may reflect such feelings as self-confidence or accomplishing a set goal.

Humanistic psychology emerged during the 1950s as a reaction to psychoanalysis and behaviorism, which dominated psychology at the time.

Psychoanalysis was focused on understanding the unconscious motivations that drive behavior, while behaviorism studied the conditioning processes that produce behavior. Humanistic psychology posited that both psychoanalysis and behaviorism were too pessimistic, either focusing on the most tragic of emotions or failing to take into account the role of personal choice.

The fundamental belief of humanistic psychology is that people are innately good and that mental and social problems result from deviations from this natural tendency. It also stresses that people have free will that enables them to help achieve their full potential as human beings, and that this need for fulfillment and personal growth is a key motivator of all behavior. In 1961, Maslow and others officially established the American Association for Humanistic Psychology, and he and Tony Sutich founded the *Journal of Humanistic Psychology*.

---

## Rank, Otto                                            (Austria, 1884–1939)

Born Otto Rosenfeld in Vienna, reading Sigmund Freud's *The Interpretation of Dreams* inspired him to write *Der Künstler* (The Artist; 1907), an attempt to explain art by using psychoanalytic principles. After reading this short manuscript, Freud assisted Rank (his legally adopted pen name) to enter the University of Vienna, where he received a doctoral degree in philosophy. Rank joined the Vienna Psychoanalytic Society, serving as its secretary, and for more than a decade (1912–1924) he edited the International Journal of Psychoanalysis. In 1924, Rank published *The Trauma of Birth*, which posited that the transition from the womb to the outside world causes severe psychological trauma in the infant, which may persist as anxiety neurosis into adulthood. Many

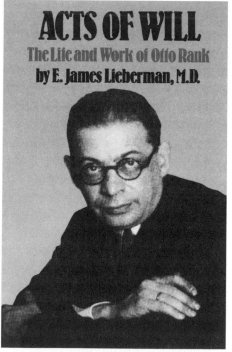

Otto Rank, 1922. (*Wikimedia / Becker & Maass, Berlin; United States Library of Congress, Prints and Photographs Division*)

members of the Viennese society viewed this thesis as conflicting with the concepts of psychoanalysis, and Rank was expelled from membership in the group. Nevertheless, Rank continued to extend psychoanalytic theory to the study of legend, myth, art, and creativity.

Leaving Vienna soon afterward, Rank subsequently taught and practiced as a therapist in Paris, before moving to New York in 1936. During this time, Rank developed a concept of the will as the guiding force in personality development, arguing that it could be a positive tool for controlling and using a person's instinctual drives, which Freud believed to be the motivating factors in human behavior. Rather than regard patient resistance during psychoanalysis as a negative factor, Rank thought that this was a manifestation of the will. Consequently, Rank believed that instead of wearing down such resistance, as would be the goal of a Freudian analyst, the will could be channeled into a path toward direct self-discovery and development.

## PUBLIC HEALTH, PRIZES, MEDICAL EDUCATION AND MEDICAL ADMINISTRATION

Baruch was a major advocate for free public baths for tenement dwellers, stressing the hygienic benefits of regular bathing or showering. He championed hydrotherapy and stressed natural remedies (water, fresh air, and diet) to strengthen the body's natural healing powers. A pioneer of modern sanitary engineering, Wolman invented the basic technique used worldwide for the controlled chlorination of drinking water supplies that kills pathogens but does not harm the people who drink the water. Rosenau developed a technique for slow pasteurization of milk at low temperature, which preserves its taste while eliminating pathogens.

The only Jewish general of the Second French Empire and head of the military health services, Lévy served as permanent director and inspector of the Army Health Service of Eastern Turkey and the Crimea, where he established a hygiene program to combat a cholera epidemic. Goldberger showed that pellagra was related to a diet heavily based on corn (cornbread and molasses), to the virtual exclusion of other foods, which was common among impoverished individuals in the South. Wynder co-authored the first major scientific publication identifying smoking as a contributory cause of lung cancer.

Lasker endowed yearly awards for Basic and Clinical Medical Research, while Wolf established a foundation in Israel that awards annual prizes for medicine.

Abraham Flexner published a scathing attack on medical education, which sparked a dramatic reform in medical education in the United States and Canada and led to the closing of a majority of the medical schools in North America. Simon Flexner was the first director of the Rockefeller Institute for Medical Research and instrumental in shaping the research goals and priorities for the new institution.

---

## Baruch, Simon                                    (Germany, 1840–1921)

---

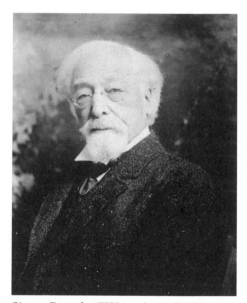

Emigrating from Prussia to the United States at age 15, Simon Baruch attended the Medical College of South Carolina. When South Carolina became the first state to secede from the Union at the onset of the Civil War, the medical school temporarily closed its doors. Consequently, Baruch was forced to complete his education at the Medical College of Virginia, in the Confederate capital of Richmond. Baruch served the Confederacy as a surgeon for three years, briefly captured and imprisoned twice. During the conflict, Baruch gained extensive experience that helped him later in civilian life

Simon Baruch. (*Wikimedia / NLM*)

as a specialist in surgery of diseases of the eye, ear, and throat. Returning to South Carolina during Reconstruction, Baruch assisted in reactivating the State Medical Association and served as president of the State Board of Health.

Moving north with many other southern physicians, Baruch settled in New York in 1881, where he soon made a name for himself by diagnosing a case of perforated appendix that was successfully treated surgically, one of the first operations of its kind. Baruch became a major advocate for free public baths for tenement dwellers, stressing the hygienic benefits of regular bathing or showering. Baruch championed hydrotherapy and stressed natural remedies (water, fresh air, and diet) to strengthen the body's natural healing powers. This put Baruch at odds with his medical colleagues, who were increasingly relying on surgical and pharmacological interventions. Although a controversial figure, Baruch became one of the most prominent physicians in New York.

Baruch wrote several books arguing the rational, scientific basis for the beneficial physiological effects of water treatments. In 1907, Baruch was appointed Professor of Hydrotherapy at Columbia College of Physicians and Surgeons. However, he resigned six years later when hydrotherapy was changed from a required to an elective subject.

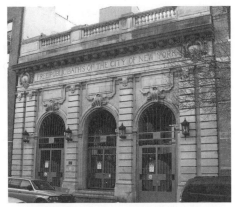

Free Public Baths in the East Village neighborhood of Manhattan, New York City, 1904–5. (*Wikimedia / Beyond My Ken*)

Baruch may be best remembered as the father of Bernard Baruch, the famed financier and adviser to multiple presidents of the United States.

## Flexner, Abraham                                             (USA, 1866–1959)

The elder brother of Simon, Abraham Flexner was born in Lexington, Kentucky. After completing a degree in Classics from Johns Hopkins University in only two years, Flexner pursued graduate studies at Harvard University and at the University of Berlin, but did not complete an advanced degree at either institution. Returning to Louisville, Flexner taught Greek, Latin, physiology, and algebra at his former high school, copying the Hopkins emphasis on scholarship and knowledge for its own sake rather than professional training. Flexner then started his own college preparatory school, where pupils received individualized attention. His goal was to attain excellence, refusing to allow mediocrity

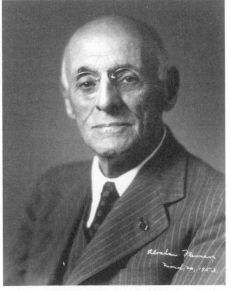

Portrait of Abraham Flexner by W.M. Hollinger, 1910. (*Wikimedia / The World's Work*)

to set the standard. Flexner designed his educational program so that the best students could receive their degrees from top colleges at an age when graduates from other prep schools were only just entering them.

In 1906, Flexner visited Berlin to observe the German educational system, especially the elite gymnasia. He was impressed by their devotion to excellence, but not their rigid standardization and tests that required rote answers rather than original thought. Returning to the United States, in 1908 Flexner wrote *The American College*, a highly critical assessment of the state of the American educational system. His work encouraged the Carnegie Foundation to commission an in-depth evaluation of the 155 medical schools across the United States and Canada, many of which were for-profit enterprises. The resulting *Flexner Report*, published in 1910, was a scathing attack on medical education, which described an appalling lack of entrance requirements, low-quality teaching, and inadequate practical training in clinical practice, even among medical schools associated with universities. The only medical school that Flexner deemed adequate was Johns Hopkins, where the curriculum included basic medical sciences and lab work, encouraged pure research, and was closely tied to an excellent teaching hospital. Unusual for its time, Johns Hopkins also required that every student admitted to its medical school already have a college degree, which included pre-med and language courses. The *Flexner Report* sparked a dramatic reform in medical education in the United States and Canada. It led to the closing of a majority of the medical schools in North America, especially in rural areas, including six of the seven medical schools in his native city of Louisville.

In the 1930s, the Bambergers, heirs to a department store fortune, were determined to fund a new medical school in Newark, New Jersey. This would give preference in admission to Jewish applicants to fight the rampant prejudice against Jews in the medical profession existing at that time. Flexner informed them that a successful medical school also required a teaching hospital and other faculties, eventually persuading the Bamberger siblings and their representatives to fund instead the development of an Institute for Advanced Study in Princeton. This unique facility brought together some of the greatest minds in history to collaborate on intellectual discovery and research in an unstructured environment that supported the pursuit of pure knowledge with no formal teaching responsibilities. Ironically, the establishment of the Institute for Advanced Study helped bring a host of brilliant scientists from Europe to the United States, including many Jews such as Albert Einstein who would have been persecuted or even killed by the rising fascist government in Germany.

## Flexner, Simon                                    (USA, 1863–1946)

Born in Louisville, Simon Flexner was the younger brother of Abraham Flexner. After surviving a serious case of typhoid fever, Flexner took night courses at the Louisville College of Pharmacy, graduating at the top of his class. He then enrolled at the Medical Institute of the University of Louisville, at the time a local two-year diploma mill. After graduating in 1889, Flexner returned to college, getting his medical degree from Louisville Medical College. Despite his dubious degree, in 1890 Flexner was invited to do postgraduate work in

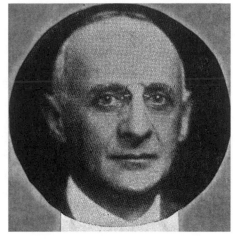

Portrait of Simon Flexner by Elias Goldensky. (*Wikimedia / The World's Work*)

pathology at the new Johns Hopkins University Medical School, where he developed a particular interest in the fields of pathology and bacteriology and the study of meningitis. Remaining on the staff and rising to the rank of professor, in 1899 he accepted the position of Professorship of Experimental Pathology at the venerable University of Pennsylvania.

At the turn of the century, John D. Rockefeller, the richest man in America, decided to donate the funds to develop a top-notch medical research institution on Manhattan Island. In 1901, Flexner became the first director of the Rockefeller Institute for Medical Research, a post he held for more than 30 years. Flexner was instrumental in shaping the research goals and priorities for the new institution, appointing an impressive staff of researchers. They were to be free of the burdens of classroom teaching, instead devoting all their efforts to pure investigation that would "cover the entire field of medical research in respect to both men and animals."[55] Flexner's own research also flourished at the Institute, where he developed an antiserum for the treatment of meningitis and assisted in identifying the viral causative agent of poliomyelitis.

---

55. Frank Heynick, *Jews in Medicine: An Epic Saga* (NJ: KTAV Publishing House, 2002).

## Goldberger, Joseph                                    (Hungary, 1874–1929)

Born in what is now the Czech Republic, as a young child Joseph Goldberger and his family immigrated to the United States, where they settled in New York City. He received his medical degree from Bellevue Hospital Medical College (now New York University Medical School). After a few boring years in private practice in rural Pennsylvania, in 1899 Goldberger joined the Marine Hospital Service, which was designed to care for merchant seamen who were sick and had as its main goal fighting epidemics. Renamed the U.S. Public Health Service in 1902, it steadily expanded to focus more on basic science and the investigation of human disease.

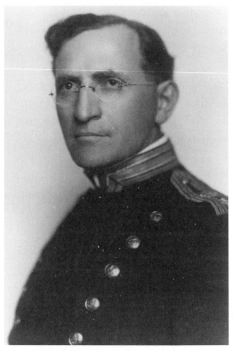

Joseph Goldberger as an epidemiologist member of the U.S. Public Health Service. (*CDC Public Health Image Library*)

After several years of energetically and successfully fighting tropical fevers, typhus, typhoid, and other infectious outbreaks throughout the United States and the Caribbean, Goldberger was appointed to tackle the crisis of pellagra, a disease recently reaching epidemic proportions in the South. Through extensive observation of healthy and pellagra-stricken people, Goldberger rejected the concept that pellagra was an infectious disease, instead theorizing that it was due to diet. After multiple experiments on prisoners, Goldberger showed that pellagra was related to a diet heavily based on corn (cornbread and molasses), to the virtual exclusion of other foods, which was common among impoverished individuals in the South.

Goldberger spent the rest of his career in a vain attempt to discover the missing dietary ingredient that resulted in pellagra. In pursuing his investigations, he angered many by the implied social criticism of a northerner pointing out flaws in southern society by linking the poverty of sharecroppers, tenant farmers, and mill workers to the deficient diet that caused the disease. It was only in the late 1930s that Conrad Elvehjem found that pellagra is caused by the dietary lack of nicotinic acid (the B vitamin niacin) and reduced levels of the essential amino acid tryptophan, which can easily be prevented by protein-rich food or small quantities of brewer's yeast.

## Hirsch, August                                              (Germany, 1817–1894)

Born in Danzig, August Hirsch studied medicine at the universities of Leipzig and Berlin before returning to his native city to practice. He was sent by the West Prussian authorities to investigate an epidemic of cerebrospinal meningitis and later to assess an outbreak of cholera.

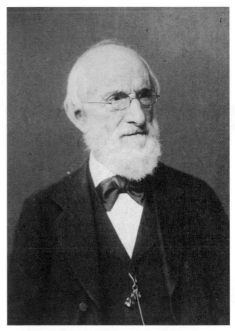

Chair of Medical History at the University of Berlin, Hirsch is most famous as a medical historian. Among his many works are *A Biographical Dictionary of Outstanding Doctors of All Time* and *Handbook of Geographical and Historical Pathology*, which is an indispensable text for military surgeons and practitioners in the tropics.

August Hirsch. (*Wikimedia / NLM*)

## Lasker, Albert Davis                                        (Germany, 1880–1952)

Born in Freiberg when his American parents were visiting their ancestral homeland, Albert Lasker was raised in Galveston, Texas. He made his fortune as a pioneer in modern advertising, exploiting the new medium of radio, introducing the concept of "salesmanship" into print advertising, and leading the shift in advertising from news to persuasion. Among Lasker's innovative ideas were the establishment of copy writing departments, the creation of soap operas to market products, and the application of advertising principles to Presidential campaigns. Under his leadership, the Chicago-based Lord and Thomas developed into the largest advertising agency in the United States.

Especially in combination with his third wife Mary, Lasker was a nationally prominent philanthropist. In addition to playing a major role in promoting and expanding the National Institutes of Health, in 1945 they founded and endowed the Lasker Awards, which are given annually to living persons who have made major contributions to basic or clinical medical science or who have performed public service on behalf of medicine. Administered by the Lasker Foundation, they are often referred to as the "American Nobel Prize."

Active in Jewish affairs, Lasker contributed to Hebrew Union College, was a Trustee of the Associated Jewish Charities of Chicago and a member of the Executive Committee of the American Jewish Committee.

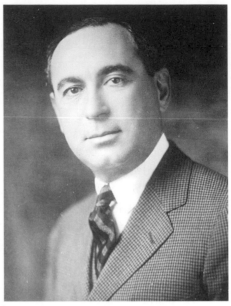

Albert Davis Lasker. (*Wikimedia / Bain News Service; Library of Congress*)

## Michel Lévy                                    (France, 1809–1872)

Born in Strasbourg and not following the suggestions of his grandfather who wanted him to become a rabbi, Michel Lévy decided to study medicine at the military training hospital in his native city. In 1836, Levy was appointed Professor of Hygiene and Legal Medicine at Val-de-Grâce in Paris. Nine years later, Lévy was named the first professor of pathology at the University in Metz. Returning to Val-de-Grâce two years later, Lévy became director of its Imperial School of Medicine and Pharmacy, a position he held until his death.

The consultant physician to Napoleon III, Lévy was the only Jewish general of the Second Empire and served as head of the military health services. He continually argued that military doctors are fully fledged officers and thus could benefit from training and continuing education, just like their civilian counterparts. During the Crimean War, Lévy served as permanent director and inspector of the Army Health Service of Eastern Turkey and the Crimea, where he established a hygiene program to combat a cholera epidemic. Long before Pasteur demonstrated microbial contagion, Michel Lévy practiced the basics of antisepsis, employing strict isolation measures, ventilation and disinfection contamination.

Lévy was the author of the monumental and widely acclaimed *Traite d'Hygiene Publique et Privee* (1845) and elected president of the French Academy of Medicine. For more than a half century, until the Nazi occupation of France, the Marseille military hospital was entitled "Michael Levy hospital."

## Rosenau, Milton Joseph (USA, 1869–1946)

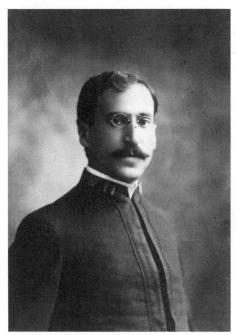

Born in Philadelphia, Milton Rosenau received his medical degree from the University of Pennsylvania and pursued additional training in Paris, Vienna and Berlin. Devoting his career to preventing the spread of infectious diseases, during his early professional years, Rosenau campaigned for the routine pasteurization of milk consumed in the United States. Because hot pasteurization gave milk an unpleasant "cooked" taste, as late as 1900, raw milk was the standard. To overcome this key obstacle to public acceptance of pasteurized milk, Rosenau developed a technique for slow pasteurization at low temperature (60° C for 20 minutes), which preserves the taste of milk while eliminating

Milton Joseph Rosenau wearing the uniform of the U.S. Public Health Service. (*NLM*)

pathogens. In 1890, Rosenau received a commission in the Marine Hospital Service, becoming director of the Hygienic Laboratory from 1899–1909.

From 1909 to 1935, Rosenau was the Chair of Preventive Medicine and Hygiene at Harvard Medical School. Early in his tenure, Rosenau joined two colleagues in developing a collaboration between Harvard and MIT that led to the founding of the Harvard University School of Public Health. After serving as Chief of the Division of Biologic Laboratories of the Massachusetts State Board of Health, Rosenau became Professor of

Epidemiology and Dean of the School of Public Health at the University of North Carolina.

## Wolf, Ricardo                                                    (Germany, 1887–1981)

Born Richard Wolf in Hannover, where his father was a pillar of the Jewish community, Ricardo Wolf immigrated to Cuba before World War I. The inventor of a technique for recovering iron from smelting process residue, its widespread use in steel factories all over the world brought him considerable wealth. A strong supporter of the Cuban revolution, in 1961 a grateful Fidel Castro fulfilled Wolf's request to be appointed as Ambassador to Israel. Wolf served in this position until 1973, when Cuba severed diplomatic ties, and he remained in Israel for the rest of his life.

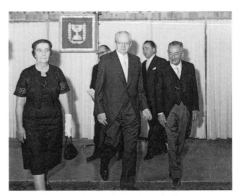

Ricardo Wolf, Cuban Ambassador to Israel, with Israeli Foreign Minister Golda Meir and President Yitzhak Ben-Zvi, after presenting his credentials in Jerusalem, 1960. (*Wikimedia / National Photo Collection of Israel*)

Wolf established a foundation in Israel, which since 1978 has awarded annual prizes in six fields – as Agriculture, Chemistry, Mathematics, Medicine, Physics, and an Arts prize that rotates annually between architecture, music, painting, and sculpture. In medicine, the Wolf Prize is generally considered the third most prestigious, after the Nobel Prize and the Lasker Award.

## Wolman, Abel                                                          (USA, 1892–1989)

Born in Baltimore, Abel Wolman received an engineering degree from Johns Hopkins University. From 1914, Wolman worked a quarter century for the Maryland State Department of Health, serving as Chief Engineer from 1922 to 1939. As a pioneer of modern sanitary engineering, Wolman, in cooperation with chemist Linn Enslow, invented the basic technique used worldwide for the controlled chlorination of drinking water supplies that kills pathogens but does not harm the people who drink the water. This resulted in a dramatic reduction in the incidence of such waterborne diseases as cholera, dysentery, and typhoid fever, and is considered by many the most important single contribution to public health in the 20th century. In the 1950's, Wolman served as the Chairman of the Advisory Council for planning the National Water Carrier Project in Israel.

An editor of the *Journal of the American Water Works Association* (AWWA), this group presents a yearly Abel Wolman Award of Excellence to recognize those whose careers in the water works industry exemplify vision, creativity, and excellent professional performance. Wolman received the 1960 Lasker Award for Public Service.

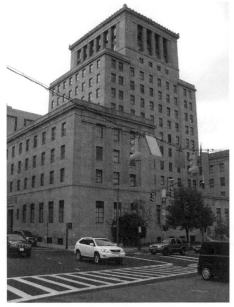

Abel Wolman Municipal Building, Baltimore, Maryland. (*Wikimedia*)

## Wynder, Ernst                                    (Germany, 1922–1999)

Born in Herford, Westphalia, Ernst Wynder and his family escaped Nazi rule and fled to the United States in 1938. After receiving his citizenship in 1943, Wynder joined the U.S. Army, and as a German-speaker became an intelligence officer assigned to monitor German newscasts. After the war, Wynder studied medicine at Washington University in St. Louis. In 1952, Wynder joined the Sloan-Kettering Institute for Cancer Research as an assistant researcher, eventually rising to Chief of Epidemiology.

As a medical student, Wynder became involved in cancer research with his professor and mentor, Evarts A. Graham. Together they authored the classic 1950 publication, "Tobacco Smoking as a Possible Etiologic Factor in Bronchogenic Carcinoma: A Study of 684 Proved Cases," which was the first major scientific publication identifying smoking as a contributory cause of lung cancer. They observed that "the enormous increase in the sale of cigarettes in this country approximately parallels the increase in [lung cancer]."[56] In a subsequent study of 605 men who had developed

---

56. Graham E Wynder EL, "Tobacco smoking as a possible etiologic factor in bronchiogenic carcinoma: a study of 684 proven cases" (*JAMA*, 1950), 143 (4): 329–36.

lung cancer, they determined that smoking was a common factor, with 97% of cases developing in heavy smokers. In a prospective study, published in 1960, Wynder showed that a condensate made from cigarette smoke, painted onto the backs of mice, caused malignant tumors. Four years later, the Surgeon General's office posted its first official warning that excessive smoking may cause lung cancer. Wynder later linked excessive tobacco use with cancers of the oral cavity, esophagus, larynx, pancreas, and bladder.

Despite the overwhelming evidence, as late as 1994, the heads of the major tobacco companies in the United States swore before a Congressional subcommittee that nicotine was not addictive and might not be a cause of cancer after all.

## SURGERY

Wölfler performed the first gastroenterostomy, Nissen introduced an eponymous fundoplication to treat reflux esophagitis, and Hamburger performed the first transplant in France. In the United States, Lilienthal performed the first successful pulmonary lobectomy for inflammatory disease of the lung, suprapubic prostatectomy, and colectomy for colitis. Cooper performed the first successful lung transplant in a patient dying from pulmonary fibrosis and was among the first to perform lung volume reduction surgery in patients with chronic obstructive pulmonary disease. Fisher showed that treating early-stage breast cancer by a simple lumpectomy – in combination with radiation therapy, chemotherapy, and/or hormonal therapy – was just as effective as disfiguring radical mastectomy. Greenfield developed an inferior vena cava filter to prevent pulmonary embolism, while Hamburger performed the first renal transplant in France and conducted pioneering research studies on the immunological basis of kidney disease and graft immunology. Immediately before World War II, Ravdin initiated studies on shock, especially the use of blood substitutes to treat war casualties. Heimlich developed a technique of abdominal thrusts to stop choking, a maneuver that bears his name, while Israel was the first to describe actinomycosis in humans, with the pathogen later named in his honor. Wolff established orthopaedics as a distinct discipline in medicine, while Thorek founded the International College of Surgeons.

## Cooper, Joel D.

(USA, 1939–)

A graduate of Harvard Medical School specializing in surgery, Joel Cooper joined the faculty of the University of Toronto in 1972 and eventually became the Head of the Division of Thoracic Surgery. In 1988, Cooper became Director of the Section of Thoracic Surgery in the Division of Cardiothoracic Surgery. Cooper later was Head of Thoracic Surgery at the Washington University School of Medicine in St. Louis, and in 2005 assumed a similar position at the University of Pennsylvania.

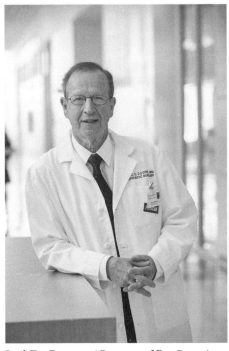

While in Toronto, in 1983 Cooper performed the world's first successful lung transplant on a patient dying from pulmonary fibrosis. Before this success, lung transplantation had been attempted 44 times

Joel D. Cooper. (*Courtesy of Dr. Cooper*)

worldwide, but all the patients died within a few weeks. Cooper himself had tried and repeatedly failed at lung transplantation, but decided to suspend further attempts until he was able to determine what was going wrong. After a series of experiments in dogs, Cooper realized that the problem was related to the steroid prednisone, which was routinely prescribed in high doses to transplant patients. Although prednisone prevented organ rejection, it also interfered with healing. Using cyclosporine, a more powerful anti-rejection drug that had recently become widely available, Cooper resumed human lung transplantation and had historic success. Several months after surgery, the patient returned to work and lived for seven years before dying of unrelated kidney failure. Three years later, Cooper performed the first successful double lung transplantation in a patient with alpha-1 anti-trypsin deficiency.

In the 1990s, Cooper was among the first surgeons to perform lung volume reduction surgery – removal of damaged portions of the lungs in patients with COPD (chronic obstructive pulmonary disease). In individuals with end-stage emphysema, reducing the size of the lungs is the only treatment (short of lung transplantation) that can restore lung function and permit patients to breathe more easily.

## Fisher, Bernard                                                                (USA, 1918–)

Born in Pittsburgh, Bernard Fisher obtained his medical degree from the University of Pittsburgh and specialized in surgery. Remaining on the staff, Fisher established and led the laboratory of surgical research. In 1957, Fisher accepted an invitation to join the Surgical Adjuvant Chemotherapy Breast Project of the NIH, where he was exposed to the novel concepts of using randomized clinical trials with biostatistics to obtain information and giving adjuvant therapy following surgery.

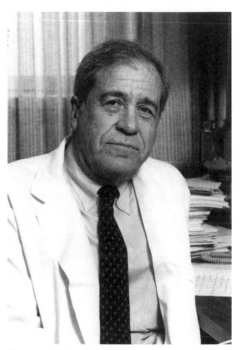

Fisher proved that treating early-stage breast cancer by a simple lumpectomy – in combination with radiation therapy, chemotherapy, and/or hormonal therapy – was just as effective as radical mastec-

Bernard Fisher. (*Wikimedia / National Cancer Institute*)

tomy, the traditional disfiguring therapy that had been used for more than 75 years. This totally transformed the surgical approach to breast cancer. In 1985, Fisher was awarded the Lasker Award for Clinical Medical Research "for his pioneering studies that have led to a dramatic improvement in survival and in the quality of life for women with breast cancer." Fisher also showed the value of the multicenter randomized clinical trial as a standard for the scientific evaluation of therapy for many other diseases.

## Folkman, (Moses) Judah                                            (USA, 1933–2008)

The son of a rabbi in Cleveland, Judah Folkman graduated from Harvard Medical School. A specialist in pediatric surgery, in 1967 Folkman was appointed Surgeon-in-Chief of Children's Hospital in Boston. At age 34, he was the youngest full professor in the history of Harvard Medical School.

Folkman is best known for his research on tumor angiogenesis. According to Folkman's concept, a tumor requires new blood vessels to nourish itself and sustain its existence. By cutting off this blood supply, a cancer could be starved into remission. Over the years, Folkman and a growing team of researchers succeeded in isolating the proteins and describing the processes that regulate angiogenesis, leading to the discovery of multiple therapies based on inhibiting or stimulating neovascularization.

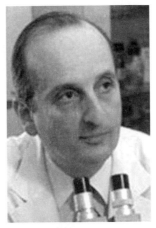

Judah Folkman, winner of the 1992 Wolf Foundation Prize in Medicine. (*Wolf Foundation*)

In 1961, Folkman was drafted into military service aboard a naval vessel. Assigned the task of determining whether blood could be dried and reconstituted, Folkman showed that a cultured rabbit thyroid gland bathed in the experimental blood thrived. Expanding this study to see whether the experimental blood could support new growth, Folkman injected the thyroid gland with fast-growing cancer cells. He observed that they grew into tiny tumors, but that all stopped growing at about 1 mm in size, a phenomenon that does not happen normally in living animals or humans. Concerned that the arrested rabbit thyroid tumor cells had died, Folkman injected them into mice and they grew rapidly. The mouse tumors had abundant blood vessel growth, whereas none was evident in cultured thyroid tumors. Folkman reasoned that the cancer cells in live animals were emitting some chemical signal that led to the development of the cancer's "own private blood supply," permitting it to survive and grow.

Folkman also inserted cancer cells in the cornea of rabbits, which normally is devoid of blood vessels. Much to his surprise, blood vessels began to shoot out from the limbus of the cornea in a direct line towards the cancer cells. Once they reached the tiny tumors, the cancers grew explosively.

After many years of effort, in 1983 Folkman and his colleagues isolated a protein from the urine of cancerous mice that, when placed as a pellet in rabbit cornea, triggered extensive blood vessel growth. This led Folkman to attempt to find a substance that could block the newly discovered angiogenic factor, believing that stopping blood vessel growth into a cancer would render it harmless. Eventually, Folkman discovered two anti-angiogenic molecules that he called angiostatin and endostatin. In one test, he injected 20 mice with cancer cells and treated half with angiostatin. At autopsy, the untreated mice had widespread cancer, whereas the treated mice were free of disease.

This discovery was hyped as a cure for cancer within a few years, and drug companies raced to be first to develop anti-angiogenesis agents. However, these molecules were much less successful in human clinical trials. Unexpectedly, Folkman's drive to cure cancer may contribute more to diseases other than malignant lesions. For example, anti-angiogenic agents are now used to save the vision of many patients with macular degeneration, and intensive studies are being performed to evaluate this technique for treating many other conditions.

## Greenfield, Lazar J.                                              (USA, 1934–)

Born in Houston, Texas, Lazar Greenfield graduated from the Baylor College of Medicine and pursued a surgical career, first at the University of Oklahoma Medical Center and later as Chair of Departments of Surgery at the Medical College of Virginia and then the University of Michigan. Greenfield is best known for developing an inferior vena cava filter that bears his name. This device is designed to limit stagnant flow, which may lead to clot propagation, thus preventing pulmonary embolism while maintaining caval blood flow. The Greenfield filter is used in patients who are particularly vulnerable to having venous emboli entering the pulmonary circulation, such as those with deep venous thrombosis and a contraindication to anticoagulation.

As an internationally recognized expert in vascular surgery and prolific writer, Greenfield was appointed as the editor of Surgery News, the official newsletter of the American College of Surgeons (ACS). However, after penning a strange sexist attempt at Valentine's Day humor, in which he implied that evolutionary biology shows that semen is a mood enhancer for women and in essence recommended unprotected sex on Valentine's Day as a better gift than chocolate, Greenfield was forced to resign his position as President-Elect of the ACS.

## Hamburger, Jean                                              (France, 1909–1992)

Born in Paris, Jean Hamburger received his medical degree from the University of Paris. Credited with coining the word "nephrology" for the study of kidney disease, Hamburger carried out much of his work as Chief of Nephrology at Necker Hospital in Paris. Hamburger is best known for having performed the first renal transplantation in France. He was the first to describe the various clinical and pathological aspects of acute rejection and suggested the use of cortisone and even non-lethal body irradiation to treat it. Hamburger developed one of the first two artificial kidneys and described several previously unrecognized conditions, including water intoxication, hereditary renal disorders, and diseases involving the filtration system of the kidney. Hamburger was the author of basic research studies on the immunological basis of kidney disease, graft immunology, and auto-immune diseases that advanced the field of renal transplantation.

Hamburger was the founder of the International Society of Nephrology, which established an award in his name. After retiring, Hamburger wrote more than a dozen books on philosophy and literature. Several of these became best sellers in France, and *The Power and the Frailty: The Future of Medicine and the Future of Man* (1973) was published in the United States and translated into multiple languages.

---

## Heimlich, Henry Judah (USA, 1920–)

Born in Wilmington, Delaware, Henry Heimlich received his degree from the Weill Cornell Medical College and specialized in thoracic surgery. In 1963, Heimlich introduced a chest drainage flutter valve (known as the "Heimlich valve"). During the Vietnam War, this simple and inexpensive devise saved the lives of thousands of soldiers shot in the chest. Today, more than 250,000 Heimlich valves are used worldwide each year to treat patients with chest wounds or following surgery.

Heimlich is best known as inventor of the Heimlich maneuver, a technique of abdominal thrusts for stopping choking that was first

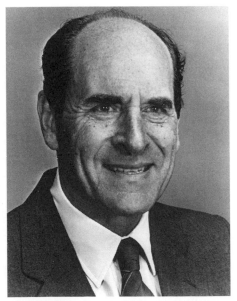

Henry Judah Heimlich. (*Lasker Foundation / Courtesy of Dr. Heimlich's family*)

described in *Emergency Medicine* in 1974. From 1976 to 1985, the choking-rescue guidelines of the American Heart Association and of the American Red Cross taught rescuers to first perform a series of backblows to remove a foreign body obstructing the airway; if these failed, the Heimlich maneuver was recommended. For the next 20 years, backblows were removed from choking-rescue guidelines. However, since 2006, the American Red Cross has returned to its earlier guidelines, recommending that conscious victims receive five backblows; if these fail to remove the airway obstruction, five abdominal thrusts should then be performed (eliminating the phrase "Heimlich maneuver"). Heimlich received the 1984 Lasker Public Service Award for the maneuver bearing his name.

In the early 1980s, Heimlich advocated a controversial treatment called malariotherapy, the deliberate infection of a person with this disease in order to treat ailments such as cancer, Lyme disease, and (more recently) HIV. However, these treatments have not proven successful. Malariotherapy has been attacked as scientifically unsound and dangerous, and the practice has been rejected by the U.S. Food and Drug Administration and Centers for Disease Control and Prevention.

---

### Israel, James Adolf                                    (Germany, 1848–1926)

Born in Berlin, James Israel studied medicine at Friedrich-Wilhelms-Universität in his native city. After serving as a military physician during the Franco-Prussian War, Israel became an assistant surgeon at the Berlin Jewish Hospital. Appointed Deputy Physician-in-Chief of the Department of Surgery in 1875, Israel was promoted to Chief of the Department five years later.

Israel was a pioneer in the development of modern urologic and renal surgery, which developed in the second half of the 19th century in Germany. In addition to being the outstanding renal surgeon of his time, Israel also made major contributions in the field of plastic surgery, particularly in the oral and maxillofacial regions. He also was an early advocate of Joseph Lister's antiseptic practices in the operating room and was credited with designing the mobile hospital railcar (*Lazarett*).

In 1878, Israel gave the first description of actinomycosis in humans, caused by a pathogen that was later given the name *Actinomyces israelii* in his honor.

---

### Jacobson, Ludwig Lewin                                 (Denmark, 1783–1843)

After studying medicine at the Academy of Surgery in his native Copenhagen, Ludwig Jacobson remained there as an assistant surgeon and lecturer on chemistry at the Royal Veterinary and Agricultural College. Turning to comparative anatomy, in 1809 Jacobson published his discovery in mammals of an organ in the nasal cavity that is largely responsible for the sense of smell (later named "Jacobson's organ"). Three other anatomical discoveries are associated with his name, including an instrument that he invented for crushing calculi in the bladder ("Jacobson's lithoclast") which was of great importance to surgery. Both an outstanding scientist and an excellent physician, Jacobson was offered the post of

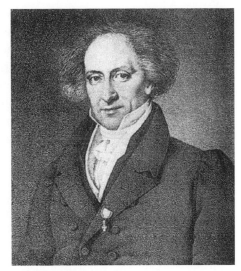

Ludwig Lewin Jacobson. (*NLM / Jerusalem Academy of Medicine*)

Professor of Anatomy at the University of Copenhagen, on the condition that he convert to Christianity, but he refused to abandon his faith. Jacobson also refused to participate in the Scandinavian Naturalists' Congress in Christiania, because Jews were not admitted into Norway at this time.

## Lilienthal, Howard (USA, 1861–1946)

Born in Albany, New York, Howard Lilienthal studied medicine at Harvard University. When the house staff at Mount Sinai Hospital in New York was separated into medical and surgical divisions in 1887, Lilienthal was the first trainee who selected surgery as his primary interest. A pioneer in thoracic surgery, Lilienthal became the first Chief of the Division at Mount Sinai Hospital in 1914, the same year that he performed the first successful pulmonary lobectomy for inflammatory disease of the lung in the United States.

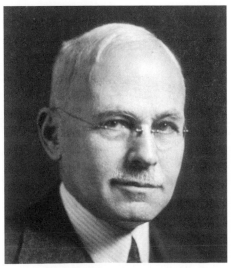

Howard Lilienthal. (*NLM*)

Lilienthal also was the first to perform a thoracotomy (open chest surgery) under intratracheal anesthesia, as well as an extrapleural resection of the thoracic esophagus for carcinoma with the construction of a skin flap to connect the two ends of the remaining mediastinal esophagus (unlike a previous resection in which the esophagus and stomach were connected by an external rubber tube to permit oral nutrition). Lilienthal authored a classic two-volume work *Thoracic Surgery: The Surgical Treatment of Thoracic Disease*, the first textbook in this field written in English.

In addition to his work in thoracic surgery, Lilienthal developed seven new instruments and was among the first surgeons in the Unites States to perform a suprapubic prostatectomy, a colectomy for colitis, and to administrate a citrated blood transfusion (developed by Richard Lewisohn) to a patient.

---

## Lorenz, Adolf                                           (Austria, 1854–1946)

---

Born in Vienna, Adolf Lorenz received his medical degree from the University of Vienna and specialized in surgery. Lorenz remained at the university, but within four years developed a severe allergic skin reaction to the carbolic acid that was routinely used in operating rooms for asepsis. Although the condition prevented him from performing traditional surgical operations, Lorenz continued in the medical profession as a "dry surgeon," treating patients without cutting into skin or tissue and becoming known as the "bloodless surgeon of Vienna."

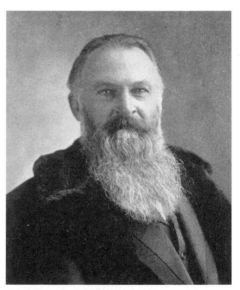

Adolf Lorenz. (*NLM*)

Lorenz developed an international reputation for his manipulative treatment of club feet. He accomplished this by essentially stretching or breaking the tendons, ligaments, and epiphyseal plates until the foot was appropriately aligned, and then applying a cast until the foot healed in that position. Lorenz also developed the use of traction and pulleys to treat scoliosis.

Lorenz also was renowned for his treatment of congenital dislocation of the hip in children. His technique involved putting the patient under light anesthesia, placing the child in a plaster spica cast in abduction, and then using external rotation as the child matured. In addition, Lorenz added a specialized walking frame to give the patient a measure of mobility. In 1903, Philip Armour, a wealthy meatpacking magnate in Chicago, was concerned about his 12-year-old daughter who had a congenital dislocation of the hip. After one attempt at surgical relocation of the hip, Armour invited Lorenz to come to Chicago to treat his daughter. Although reluctant because of the age of the girl and the prior surgery which decreased his chance of achieving a successful reduction, Lorenz finally accepted the invitation and negotiated a huge fee. His successful treatment generated extensive publicity and raised him to the ranks of the most distinguished surgeons in the world, resulting in Lorenz being invited to meet with President Theodore Roosevelt.

## Nissen, Rudolph (Germany, 1896–1981)

Born in Neisse (Silesia) and son of a well-known surgeon, Rudolph Nissen received his medical degree from the University of Breslau. After several years in Munich, Nissen became "professor extraordinary" at the Berlin Charité Hospital, where he performed the first successful pneumonectomy by a Western physician. When the Nazis came to power, Nissen moved to the Ottoman Empire to become Head of Surgery at Istanbul University. In 1938, Nissen immigrated to the United States, where he opened an ambulatory surgical practice in New York and later became Chair of the Surgery at Jewish Hospital and Maimonides Medical Center. In 1951, Nissen ac-

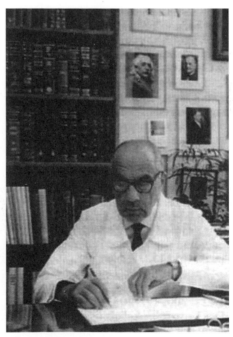

Rudolph Nissen. (*Courtesy of Dr. Nissen's family*)

cepted a professorship in Basel, where he remained until his retirement.

Nissen is best known for fundoplication to treat reflux esophagitis, a surgical procedure that bears his name. When excising an esophageal ulcer, it was necessary to remove a portion of the lower esophagus and join the remaining esophagus to the stomach. To avoid the backflow (reflux) of stomach contents into the patient's esophagus, Nissen wrapped (plicated) folds of the upper stomach (fundus) around the lower esophagus. When the patient recovered, Nissen observed that the patient's symptoms of heartburn had improved after surgery. In 1956, Nissen reported the use of this technique of wrapping the fundus of the stomach around the lower esophagus to successfully treat two patients with reflux esophagitis.

In 1948, Nissen had the distinction of performing an exploratory abdominal operation for pain on Albert Einstein. He discovered a large abdominal aortic aneurysm, which he wrapped anteriorly with cellophane to induce fibrosis. For the next five years, Einstein had only minimal abdominal discomfort until the aneurysm ruptured and he died.

---

## Ravdin, Isidor Schwaner                    (USA, 1894–1972)

A fourth generation physician born in Evansville, Indiana, Isidor Ravdin studied medicine at the University of Pennsylvania, the institution where he would spend the rest of his career. In 1928, Ravdin was appointed to the new Chair of Surgical Research, and in 1945 was named Surgeon-in-Chief at the Hospital of the University of Pennsylvania. Ravdin later served as Vice President for Medical Development, spearheading numerous financial campaigns and building the University of Pennsylvania into one of the finest medical centers at the cutting edge of modern technology. In 1964, the Ravdin Institute was opened, housing 374 beds for inpatients, four operating rooms, and adjacent pathology and

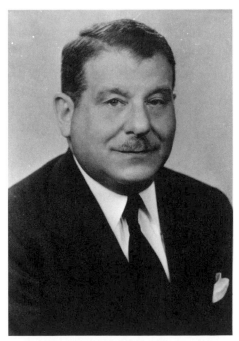

Isidor Schwaner Ravdin. (*Archives of the American College of Surgeons*)

research laboratories. As a recognized expert in the field of surgery with extensive experience with a host of governmental agencies, Ravdin was brought to the White House to treat President Eisenhower as a surgical patient and participated in his emergency operation for ileitis.

Ravdin initially focused his research activities on a systematic study of the gallbladder and then addressed the problem of hypoproteinemia in surgical patients. Immediately before World War II, Ravdin initiated studies on shock, especially the use of blood substitutes to treat war casualties. As a result, he worked with the American Red Cross and the National Research Council, and in 1942 was called on by the government to inspect and treat the casualties of the Pearl Harbor attack. It was there that albumin, a new substance, was used for the first time to treat burn and shock patients. After the war, Ravdin's research concentrated primarily on the study of cancer, and he was a pioneer in anti-cancer chemotherapy.

---

### Stilling, Benedikt (Germany, 1810–1879)

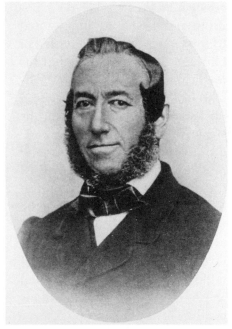

Born in Kirchhain, Benedikt Stilling studied medicine at the University of Marburg. Although prevented by his religion from pursuing an academic career, in 1833 Stilling accepted the position of surgeon to the electoral law courts in Kassel, becoming the first Jewish civil servant in the principality of Hesse-Cassel. When complaints were raised that, as a Jew, he had been elevated to an excessively high position, Stilling was required to transfer to Eiterfeld, a town whose name literally means "Pusfield" and was an apt description. Unwilling to comply, Stilling resigned from this position and for the rest of his life devoted himself to an ever-growing private practice.

Benedikt Stilling, 1901. (*Wikimedia / Pagel: Biographisches Lexikon hervorragender Ärzte des neunzehnten Jahrhunderts. Berlin, Wien 1901, Sp. 1653–1655*)

As a surgeon, Stilling developed a new method for the operative removal of thromboses, improved techniques for surgical treatment of the urinary tract, and was renowned for his expertise in gynecologic surgery. Stilling also made important contributions in the field of neurology, performing research on the structure of the cerebellum and histological studies of the pons. Stilling was the first to discuss the vasomotor nerves that innervate the walls of blood vessels, and also published detailed anatomy of the spinal cord, medulla, and pons based on data from serial sections in three dimensions that he obtained using the microtome he developed. Using this technique, Stilling also described and differentiated almost all the cranial nerve nuclei recognized today and wrote about psychosomatic symptoms, which he attributed to irritation of the spinal cord.

## Thorek, Max                                              (Hungary, 1880–1960)

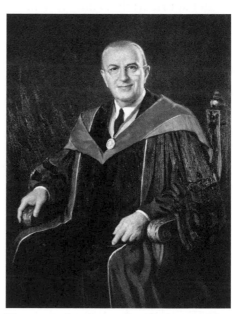

Preparing for university training in Budapest, Max Thorek's studies were interrupted when his younger brother was killed in a pogrom and the family immigrated to the Unites States and settled in Chicago. Thorek completed his medical education at Rush Medical College and specialized in obstetrics and general and reconstructive surgery, developing innovative operative techniques and practices that are still widely used today. Among these was a surgical technique that greatly reduced the mortality rate in gallbladder operations. Together with Solomon Greenspahn, in 1908 Thorek established the American Hospital and was its chief surgeon until his

Photograph of an oil painting of Max Thorek by John Doctoroff, circa 1945. (*Archives of the American College of Surgeons*)

death. This 25-bed hospital was designed primarily to serve members of the performing arts community, and some of its early patients included Mae West, the Marx Brothers, Harry Houdini and Buffalo Bill Cody.

Convinced of the need for an international organization of surgeons dedicated to maintaining the highest possible operative standards while also providing instruction for younger men in the profession, Thorek founded the International College of Surgeons in 1935. In addition to an autobiography entitled *A Surgeon's World* (1943), Thorek wrote *Surgical Errors and Safeguards* (1932) and *Modern Surgical Technique* (1938).

An internationally acclaimed amateur photographer during the pictorialist movement, Thorek authored several books on the subject, including *Creative Camera Art* (1937) and *Camera Art as a Means of Self-Expression* (1947).

## Wolff, Julius (Germany, 1836–1902)

Born in eastern Prussia, Julius Wolff received his medical degree from the Friedrich-Wilhelms University in Berlin and specialized in surgery. Wolff became the first Professor of Orthopaedics at the Charité Hospital and the founder and Director of the First Department of Orthopaedic Surgery in Berlin, effectively establishing orthopaedics as a distinct discipline in medicine.

During decades of research, Wolff, observed that "as a consequence of primary shape variations and continuous loading, or even due to loading alone, bone changes its inner architecture according to mathematical rules and,

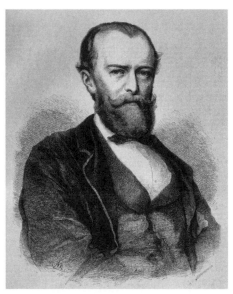

Julius Wolff, 1863. (*Wikimedia / Illustrated Magazine «Die Gartenlaube» (Leipzig-Berlin)*

as a secondary effect and governed by the same mathematical rules, also changes its shape."[57] Simplified, what is generally known as "Wolff's Law" states that the structure and shape of a bone permanently adapts to the amount of loading stress applied to it. If loading on a particular bone increases, the bone will remodel itself over time to become stronger so as to resist that sort of loading. However, if the loading on a bone decreases, the bone will become less dense and weaker due to lack of the stimulus required for continued remodeling.

---

57. Haas NP Duda GN and G. Bergmann, *Founding of the Julius Wolff Institut Charité* – Universitätsmedizin Berlin: Editorial Comment. Clin Orthop Relat Res. 2010 Apr., 468(4): 1050–1051.

## Wölfler, Anton                                    (Austria, 1850–1917)

Born in Bohemia and the son of a doctor who also was a prominent member of the Jewish community, Anton Wölfler received his medical degree from the University of Vienna. A student of Theodor Billroth, Wölfler remained in Vienna for several years as his mentor's assistant before becoming a Professor of Surgery at the University of Graz and later a professor at Charles University in Prague.

Wölfler is best known for his work in gastrointestinal surgery and investigations involving the thyroid gland. In 1881, Wölfler performed the first gastroenterostomy (an anastomosis between the stomach and small intestine) in a patient suffering from narrowing

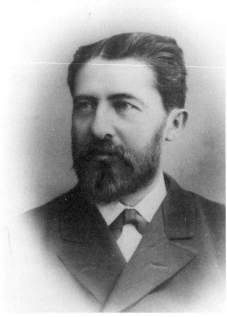

Anton Wölfler. (*Archives of Graz University, Austria*)

of the bowel from an inoperable carcinoma of the pylorus. Wölfler introduced Lister's antiseptic techniques to Vienna. An accessory thyroid gland is named for Wölfler, and he also provided the first detailed description of postoperative tetany related to hypocalcemia, which is secondary to hypoparathyroidism caused by the parathyroid glands being removed or injured during surgical removal of the adjacent thyroid gland.

## VIROLOGY

Blumberg identified the hepatitis B virus, showed that it could cause liver cancer, and developed a prophylactic vaccine against it. Pestka worked on the beneficial antiviral properties of interferon, developing treatments for chronic hepatitis, multiple sclerosis, and cancers. Harry Rubin was a pioneer in the study of how tumor-producing RNS viruses cause the transformation of normal cells into cancer cells, while Gross showed that radiation or a chemical could induce leukemia in an animal by activating a dormant virus. Lwoff studied genetic control of enzyme and virus synthesis, demonstrating that viruses released when the cell is destroyed can then infect new bacteria. Luria investigated the replication method and genetic structure of viruses and showed that bacterial resistance to viruses (phages) is genetically inherited. Isaacs co-discovered interferon, a group of proteins involved in immune regulation and defense against viruses. Salk developed the first injectable vaccine against polio, using formalin-killed viruses, while Sabin developed the first oral vaccine against polio, using live but attenuated viruses. Benjamin Rubin invented the bifurcated vaccination needle, which played an important role in eradicating smallpox.

## Blumberg, Baruch (Barry) Samuel (USA, 1925–2011)

Born in Brooklyn, Barry Blumberg attended the Orthodox Yeshivah of Flatbush for elementary school, studied medicine at Columbia University, and received a doctoral degree in biochemistry at Oxford University.

Blumberg is best known for identifying the hepatitis B virus and showing that it could cause liver cancer. He developed a screening test for the virus to prevent its spread in blood transfusions, as well as a prophylactic vaccine against it. While working at the National Institutes of Health, Blumberg received the 1976 Nobel Prize for Physiology or Medicine (along with D. Carleton Gajdusek)

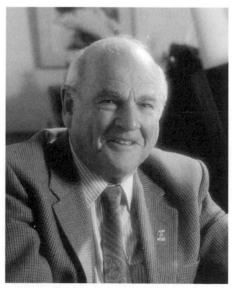

Baruch Samuel Blumberg depicted on a NASA portrait, 1999. (*Wikimedia / Tom Trower*)

for "discoveries concerning new mechanisms for the origin and dissemination of infectious disease."

As described in a press release from the Nobel Committee, Blumberg was trained as a geneticist and studied the variation between certain types of proteins occurring in the blood of different individuals. He discovered a unique protein (Australia antigen) in the serum of a patient with hemophilia who had received several transfusions, observing that it only appeared with (or after) a special type of jaundice that was caused by infectious agents and previously known as "serum" hepatitis. Infection by the hepatitis B virus can lead to a chronic condition, which in some individuals is an important source for further spreading the virus. Today, all blood donors are examined to detect carriers, thus substantially decreasing the frequency of hepatitis due to blood transfusions.

In discussing the factors that shaped him, Blumberg gave credit to the mental discipline of studying Talmud, and he attended weekly Talmud discussion classes whenever possible throughout his life.

---

**Gross, Ludwik**                                              (Poland, 1904–1999)

---

Born in Cracow, where his father was a Jewish member of the Austro-Hungarian Parliament, Ludwik Gross studied medicine at Jagiellonian University in his native city. Specializing in internal medicine, Gross worked at the Pasteur Institute in Paris in the 1930s and wrote medical articles for Poland's largest-circulation newspaper. While on a visit to Cracow in 1939, Germany invaded Poland. As a member of a prominent Jewish family, Gross escaped to Romania just days ahead of the Nazis hunting him. Immigrating to the United States, Gross worked at Jewish and Christ Hospitals in Cincinnati, developing an interest in cancer research. After military service during World War II, Gross became Chief of Cancer Research at the Bronx VA Hospital.

At the time, scientists believed that mouse murine leukemia was a genetic disease and not transmissible. Gross rejected this concept, theorizing that a virus was the agent responsible for the disease. One day, Gross attended a lecture by a scientist working on a different virus, who reported that its harmful effects could be demonstrated by injecting it into suckling mice, but not by introducing it into older mice. This prompted Gross to inject material from leukemic mice into newborn mice of a strain known to be free of this disease, thus isolating a virus. Gross then showed that the virus was passed naturally through successive generations of mice to cause leukemia. Although his claim met with much skepticism and even hostility in the scientific community, this decreased years later when Gross showed that radiation or a chemical could induce leukemia in an animal by activating a dormant virus.

After identifying a second virus causing cancer in mice, Gross hypothesized that viruses also could cause some human cancers. This was later proven by other scientists, who identified two retroviruses (HTLV-1 and HTLV-2) that cause rare types of leukemias and lymphomas – the Epstein-Barr virus, which is linked to Burkitt's lymphoma and to cancer of the nose and mouth; and the hepatitis B virus, which can lead to liver cancer. In 1961, Gross published his encyclopedic textbook, *Oncogenic Viruses*, which is still considered a leading source book for early work in the discovery of viruses causing cancer.

Gross received the 1974 Lasker Award for Basic Medical Research "for his original discovery of leukemia- and cancer-inducing viruses in mammals, and the elucidation of their biology and epidemiology."

As a medical journalist, Gross had many letters published in *The New York Times*. In one, he opposed fluoridation of the water supply to prevent tooth decay, calling fluoride "an insidious poison, harmful, toxic and cumulative in its effect, even when ingested in minimal amounts."[58] In a 1958 letter, Gross urged that smoking be prohibited on airline flights, more than three decades before the industry itself adopted the idea.

## Isaacs, Alick (England, 1921–1967)

Born in Glasgow, Scotland, to immigrant parents who had fled Lithuania in 1880 to escape anti-Semitic persecution, Alick Isaacs studied medicine at the University of Glasgow. Working as a virologist at the National Institute for Medical Research, Isaacs is best known as the co-discoverer (with Swiss virologist Jean Lindenmann) of interferon in 1957. Considered a major breakthrough of the 1950s, this discovery fundamentally influenced subsequent research in immunology and virology. Interferon, a group of proteins involved in immune regulation and defense against viruses, is now used to treat such varied conditions as hepatitis C, multiple sclerosis, and some cancers.

## Luria, Salvador Edward (Italy, 1912–1991)

Born in Turin to a Sephardic family, Salvador Luria graduated from medical school at the University of Turin. Introduced to the theories of Max Delbrück on the gene as a molecule, Luria began to formulate methods for using bacteriophages (viruses that infect bacteria) to test genetic theory. In 1938, Luria received a fellowship to study with Delbrück in the United States, but was prevented from using the funds because of a decree by the fascist regime of Benito Mussolini banning Jews from academic re-

---

58. http://www.wellthychoices.net/2013/02/03/fluorine-is-an-insidious-poison-harmful-toxic-and-cumulative-in-its-effects/.

search fellowships. Lacking a funding source for work in the United States or Italy, Luria moved to Paris to become a researcher at the Institute of Radium. However, when the German army invaded France two years later, Luria fled on bicycle to Marseilles, where he received an immigration visa to the United States and settled in New York City.

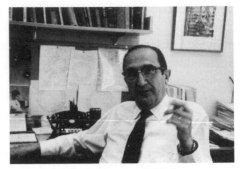

Salvador Edward Luria. (*NLM*)

In 1943, Luria collaborated with Delbrück in a statistical study demonstrating that inheritance in bacteria must follow Darwinian rather than Lamarckian principles, and that mutant bacteria occurring randomly can transmit viral resistance even in the absence of the virus.

Luria shared (with Max Delbrück and Alfred Hershey) the 1969 Nobel Prize in Physiology or Medicine "for their discoveries concerning the replication mechanism and genetic structure of viruses" – that bacterial resistance to viruses (phages) is genetically inherited. The concept was later extended to explain how bacteria develop resistance to antibiotics.

## Lwoff, André Michel                                      (France, 1902–1994)

Born in Ainay-le-Château (Allier) in Auvergne, André Lwoff graduated with a science degree from the University of Paris and joined the Pasteur Institute while still a teenager. In the 1930s, Lwoff studied in Heidelberg and Cambridge, earning both a medical degree and doctorate. He was named department head at the Pasteur Institute in Paris in 1938, remaining in this positon until being appointed as Professor of Microbiology at the Sorbonne in 1959.

Lwoff focused much of his research efforts on the phenomenon of lysogeny, in which the nucleic

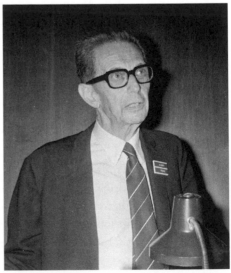

Andre Lwoff, 1971. (*Wikimedia / Dutch National Archives and Spaarnestad Photo*)

acid of a bacteriophage (bacteria-infecting virus) is integrated into the genome of the host bacterium, which continues to live and reproduce normally. However, at each cell division, the genetic material of the bacteriophage is transmitted to succeeding generations in a non-infective form (prophage). Lwoff showed that under certain conditions, such as in response to ultraviolet radiation or the presence of certain chemicals, the prophage gives rise to an infective form that causes lysis (disintegration) of the bacterial cell. Viruses released when the cell is destroyed can then infect new bacteria. For this work, Lwoff shared (with François Jacob and Jacques Monod) the 1965 Nobel Prize in Physiology or Medicine for "their discoveries concerning genetic control of enzyme and virus synthesis."

---

**Pestka, Sidney** (Poland, 1936–2016)

Born in Drobin, Sidney Pestka immigrated to the United States before age 2. Pestka received his medical degree from the University of Pennsylvania and joined the National Institutes of Health, working in the Nirenberg Laboratory on the genetic code, protein synthesis, and ribosome function. Moving to the Roche Institute of Molecular Biology in Nutley, New Jersey, Pestka worked on the beneficial antiviral properties of interferon, developing antiviral treatments for chronic hepatitis B and C, multiple sclerosis, and cancers. He especially contributed to the development of producing clinically relevant quantities of interferon at reasonable cost.

From 1986–2011, Pestka served as Professor and Chairman of the Department of Molecular Genetics, Microbiology and Immunology at the UMDNJ-Robert Wood Johnson Medical School in Piscataway, New Jersey. Pestka received the US National Medal of Technology in 2001.

---

**Rubin, Benjamin** (USA, 1917–2010)

Born in New York City, Benjamin Rubin was a microbiologist working at the Wyeth Laboratory. He is best known as the inventor of the bifurcated vaccination needle, which played an important role in eradicating smallpox. Although a smallpox vaccine had been developed in the 18th century, when in 1965 Rubin began working on a method for providing rapid smallpox vaccinations, this highly contagious viral disease was killing more than 2 million people per year. At the time, the standard method of delivery was the multiple insertion method. Needles were dipped into the vaccine vial and then jabbed into the patient's arm multiple times. Although this process was effective, it was both painful and time consuming. To simplify the technique, Rubin's solution was grinding off the end of a sewing machine needle, which opened the thread hole (the eyelet) and resulted in a needle that was divided into two branches, like a fork. Rubin found that his new needle would hold just enough vaccine within the small space between the two sections to vaccinate a person with just a few pokes. The needle could easily be replicated in areas that were less developed, and since his bifurcated needle used less of the vaccine, more people could be vaccinated in areas where the supply of serum was short. By 1980, the World Health Organization declared that smallpox had been eradicated.

## Rubin, Harry                                                 (USA, 1926–)

Born in New York City, Harry Rubin received a doctorate in veterinary medicine from Cornell University and specialized in virology and cell biology. After stints at the Virus Laboratory of the United States Public Health Service and the California Institute of Technology, Rubin joined the faculty at the University of California, Berkeley, where he was appointed Professor of Virology and later Professor of Molecular and Cell Biology.

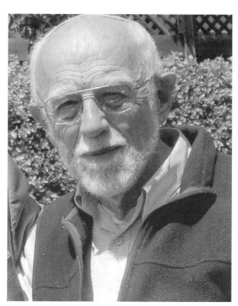

Rubin pioneered the study of how tumor-producing RNA viruses cause the transformation of normal cells into cancer cells.

Harry Rubin. (*Courtesy of Dr. Rubin's family*)

Working in the laboratory of Renato Dulbecco, Rubin developed a method for the study of the tumoral transformation of cultured chick cells by the Rous sarcoma virus (RSV). He found that this RNA virus actually consists of two viruses. When separated, the RSV alone caused the malignant transformation, but the transformed cells contained no infectious virus even after many passages. The other virus, known to cause chicken leukosis, did not cause malignant transformation although it multiplied in all cells. When leukosis virus was added to the cells transformed into cancer cells from the RSV alone, the cells produced not only the leukosis virus but also RSV. This proved that the virus could not mature without the help of a second virus, called a helper virus, which provides its protein coat to the RSV.

Rubin (and Dulbecco) received the 1964 Lasker Award in Basic Medical Research for their discovery that cells can carry for many generations a foreign nucleic acid, whether RNA or DNA, that is responsible for the malignant properties of these cells.

## Sabin, Albert Bruce (Poland, 1906–1993)

Born Albert Krugman Saperstein in Białystok, the family immigrated to the United States in 1921. After graduation from the New York University Medical School, Albert Sabin immediately began research on the nature and cause of polio, a viral infection of worldwide epidemic proportion that could cause paralysis or death. Sabin joined the staff of the Rockefeller Institute in New York and then the Children's Hospital Research Foundation in Cincinnati. There Sabin proved that polio viruses not only grew in nerve tissue, as was generally assumed, but that they also lived in the small intestine. This discovery indicated that polio might be vulnerable to an oral vaccine.

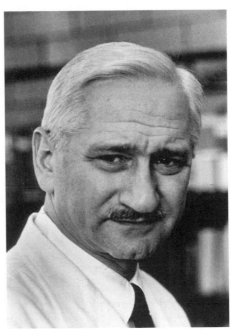

Albert Bruce Sabin. (*NLM / Lasker Award Archives*)

During World War II, Sabin served in the U.S. Army Medical Corps, where he developed vaccines against mosquito-borne encephalitis and dengue fever. After the war, Sabin returned to Cincinnati and isolated a mutant form of poliovirus that was incapable of producing the disease. This virus could be grown in culture and introduced into the intestine, where it would reproduce rapidly and overwhelm the virulent forms of the virus, thus protecting the human host from disease. Sabin and his research laboratory associates tested the vaccine on themselves and hundreds of prisoner-volunteers with no harmful effects.

Although ready for large-scale tests, Sabin could not carry them out in the United States because a rival polio vaccine, using a killed form of the virus and developed by Jonas Salk, was already being tested among American school children. However, the Salk vaccine had some drawbacks – it had to be injected into the body and was only effective for a relatively short time, thus requiring periodic booster injections. Moreover, Salk's vaccine had been accidentally contaminated with some live virulent polio

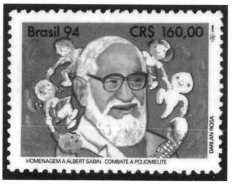

Albert Bruce Sabin depicted on a Brazil stamp for the campaign against polio. 1994. (*Author's private collection*)

viruses, causing death or severe illness in several hundred school children. In contrast, Sabin's vaccine was free of dangerous viruses, easily administered orally, and effective over a long period of time.

Some foreign virologists, especially those from the Soviet Union, were convinced of the superiority of the Sabin vaccine. From 1955 to 1957, the oral vaccine was tested on millions of children and adults in Russia and other Eastern Bloc nations. Finally, in 1960 Sabin's vaccine was safely tested on large numbers of children in Cincinnati. Ultimately, it was a live oral vaccine that was used in the United States and the rest of the world to eliminate polio.

Sabin received the 1965 Lasker Award in Clinical Medical Research for his oral polio vaccine.

---

## Salk, Jonas Edward                                               (USA, 1914–1995)

---

Born in New York City, the son of Russian-Jewish immigrants, Jonas Salk graduated from the New York University School of Medicine. He decided to pursue a career in medical research rather than becoming a practicing physician.

In the mid-20th century, polio was a crippling and killing disease that affected millions of people throughout the world annually and was a frightening public health

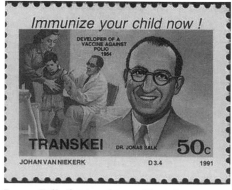

Jonas Salk depicted on a Transkei stamp, 1991. (*Author's private collection*)

scourge in post-war United States. In 1947, Salk joined the faculty at the University of Pittsburgh Medical School to lead a project funded by the March of Dimes (National Foundation for Infantile Paralysis) to determine the number of different types of polio virus. He detected three distinct types and assembled a research team to develop a vaccine against the disease, working intensively on this project for the next seven years. By 1953, Salk had injected 600 people with a formalin-inactivated vaccine, which was shown to be safe. In one of the largest field trials ever undertaken, during the next year more than a million children (as

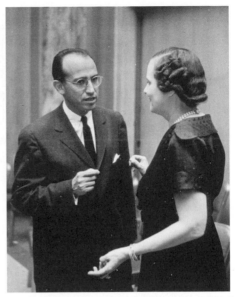

Jonas Salk talking with Mary Lasker. (*NLM / Lasker Award Archives*)

well as Salk and his family) received three injections for the three types of viruses. The new vaccine proved to be the first answer in combating polio, but it had the drawback of requiring periodic booster injections.

News of the success of the vaccine was made public in 1955, and Salk was hailed as a miracle worker. Huge immunization campaigns were instituted throughout the world. Salk had no interest in personal profit and refused to patent the vaccine, stating: "Could you patent the sun?[59]" Salk received the 1965 Lasker Award in Clinical Medical Research for his polio vaccine.

In 1960, he founded the Salk Institute for Biological Studies in La Jolla, California, which today is a center for medical and scientific research. Salk's final years were spent searching for a vaccine against HIV.

---

59. https://www.awesomestories.com/asset/view/Jonas-Salk-Could-You-Patent-the-Sun-.

# PHYSICIANS AND MEDICINE
## IN THE STATE OF ISRAEL

∽: ∾

ZIONISM is the modern political movement for the return of the Jewish people to Zion, the prophetic and poetic biblical name for the city of Jerusalem, which includes the walled city and the Temple Mount. Deemed the capital of this world and the future messianic city of God, the term Zion became a symbol for the ingathering of the Jewish people to their ancient homeland and the restoration of Jewish sovereignty in the Land of Israel.

Ever since the destruction of Jerusalem by the Romans in 70 C.E. and the exile of the Jewish people from their ancient homeland, Jews clung passionately to the hope for a return to Zion. Despite extreme poverty and physical dangers that threatened their very survival, Jews turned in prayer toward Zion three times each day. With the rise of nationalism in Europe during the 19th century, Jews slowly became convinced that the time was ripe for them to develop an independent state in their own land. The Zionist political movement they developed had largely secular leadership, but deep religious and historical roots. A major political victory was achieved with the issuance of the Balfour Declaration, a letter from Arthur James Balfour, British Foreign Secretary, to Lord Lionel Walter Rothschild, president of the Zionist Federation of England, sent on November 2, 1917. The Balfour Declaration included the famous sentence: "His Majesty's government view with favor the establishment in Palestine of a national home for the Jewish people." Five years later, the League of Nations authorized Great Britain to create the political, administrative, and economic conditions that would enable the establishment of a Jewish homeland in the British Mandate of Palestine. To appease budding Arab nationalism, Britain removed two thirds of Mandatory Palestine to create the separate Arab territory of Transjordan. A series of White Papers were issued to curtail Jewish immigration into Mandatory Palestine, despite the increasing persecution of German Jews under the Nazi regime. Following World War II, Jewish military resistance to British rule grew steadily, as the Jewish community in Mandatory Palestine sought to bring the survivors of the Holocaust to the Land of Israel. Underground extremists carried out sabotage operations and direct attacks on British military and government installations. Jews and Arabs engaged in armed clashes. Eventually, the British grew weary of the challenge of the Mandate, and on May 14, 1948, it ceased to operate. After the British withdrawal, the Declaration of Independence proclaimed the State of Israel as the fulfillment of the Zionist dream.

A concept of the Labor Zionists was the "New Jew," a polar opposite to the traditional ghetto Jew who was scorned as downtrodden and weak as a result of centuries in exile. This "New Jew," like the ancient Maccabees, would be strong, brave, active, and rooted in nature rather than alienated from it. Instead of a slave to the *halachah*, the rabbis, and rabbinic Judaism, the "New Jew" would be free, relying on innate abilities and strengths to construct a new secular Jewish society. Unlike the "Old Jew," who did not fight for his self-defense, the "New Jew" fought in Jewish resistance movements, such as the Palmach, and proudly served in the Israel Defense Forces (IDF) after the founding of the State.

## Adler, Saul Aaron (Russia, 1895–1966)

Born in Russia, Saul Adler was taken to England at age 5. After medical studies at the University of Leeds and the Liverpool School of Tropical Medicine, Adler served as a doctor with the British army in the Middle East during World War I. He made *aliyah* to the Land of Israel in 1924, settling in Jerusalem. Four years later, Adler was appointed Director of the Parasitological Institute of the Hebrew University Medical School. Adler

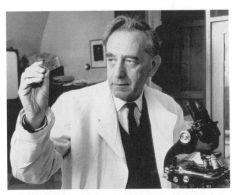

Photograph of Saul Aaron Adler by Harris. (*Wikimedia / Wellcome Collection*)

earned an international reputation for his pioneering research into leishmaniasis and its carrier, the sandfly. In addition to making important contributions to the study of such disorders as malaria, leprosy, and kala-azar, Adler translated Charles Darwin's *Origin of Species* into Hebrew, thus convincingly demonstrating that the language could be used for modern scientific expression.

### Kligler, Israel Jacob                                    (Austria-Hungary, 1888–1944)

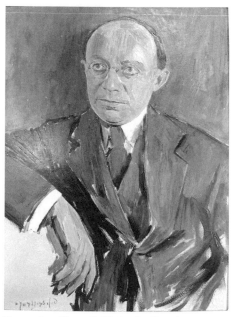

Born in what is now the Ukraine, at age 8 Israel Kligler's family moved to New York City, where he received a doctorate in bacteriology, pathology, and biochemistry at Columbia University. An ardent Zionist since his youth, Kligler made *aliyah* in 1921 and became manager of the laboratories of the Hadassah Hospital in Jerusalem. Four years later, Kligler was one of the first four professors of the Hebrew University and the founder of its Department of Hygiene and Bacteriology, which he headed till his death.

A pioneer in public health, Kligler's greatest achievement was the planning and organization of the complete eradication of ma-

Portrait of Israel Kligler by Pinchas Litvinovsky. (*Wikipedia*)

laria in the Land of Israel, which was fully achieved after his untimely death. An active member of associations that promoted physical activity among the youth of the *Yishuv* and a founder of the Anti-Tuberculosis League, Kligler led faculty researchers in conducting the first survey of nutrition in the country. This demonstrated the poor nutritional status of schoolchildren and resulted in a plan to provide a daily glass of milk to schoolchildren. For ten years after its establishment in 1929, Kligler was head of the Nathan and Lina Straus Health Center in Jerusalem (now part of Hadassah Medical Center), which under his leadership gained a strong reputation as a leader in developing public health programs. He also developed Kligler Iron Agar, a culture medium still used for the isolation and the identification of intestinal bacteria.

## Mazie, Aaron (Belarus, 1858–1930)

Aaron Mazie settled in the Land of Israel in 1888, and from 1902 served as Head of the Department of Internal Medicine at Bikur Holim Hospital. He was the central figure in writing the first and largest Hebrew Dictionary of Medicine and Science. Editor of the medical journal *ha-Refu'ah*, a publication of the Hebrew Physicians' Association of Palestine, Mazie's *The Book of Medical and Scientific Terms* was the culmination of 40 years of gathering material and consisted of 790 double-sided pages. The work was completed and edited by famed poet and pediatrician Shaul Tchernichovky, who published it in Jerusalem in 1934, four years after Mazie's death.

## Nordau, Max (Hungary, 1849–1923)

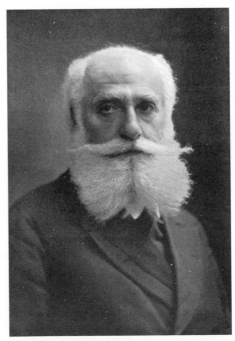

Portrait of Max Nordau. (*Wikimedia*)

Born Simon Maximilian Südfeld in Budapest, then part of the Austrian Empire and now in Hungary, Max Nordau received a medical degree from the University of Budapest and specialized in neurology. After changing his name and traveling for six years throughout Europe, Nordau spent two years practicing medicine in Budapest. In 1880, he moved to Paris as a correspondent for *Die Neue Freie Presse*. Although born into an Orthodox family, Nordau became an agnostic, fully assimilated, and acculturated European Jew. As with Theodor Herzl, the Dreyfus Affair and its evidence of the universality of anti-Semitism triggered Nordau's conversion to Zionism. With Herzl, Nordau was a co-founder of the World Zionist Organization. At the 1898 Zionist Congress, Nordau coined the term "muscular Judaism" to describe his ideal vision of a Jewish culture and religion that would result in a stronger, more physically assured Jew rather than the stereotype of one who was weak and intellectual.

## Pinsker, Leon (Judah Leib)                                        (Poland, 1821–1891)

Born in Poland, Leon Pinsker was one of the first Jews to attend Odessa University, where he studied law. However, after discovering that as a Jew he had no chance of becoming a lawyer, he switched to medicine. Pinsker was one of the founders of the first Russian Jewish weekly, *Razsvet* (Dawn), which attempted to acquaint the Jewish population with Russian culture, encourage them to speak the language, and thus become assimilated into Russian society. However, Pinsker and other enlightened Jews were shattered by the pogroms of 1881, which began in Odessa, and the undisguised anti-Semitism of the government. The following year, Pinsker published his famous work, *Autoemancipation*, in which he analyzed the psychological and social roots of anti-Semitism. Terming it a "disease" caused by fear of the alien, stateless Jew, Pinsker called for the establishment of a Jewish national center. Initially, Pinsker believed that a Jewish homeland could be established anywhere. However, after contact with the *Hibbat Zion* (Lover of Zion) movement, he became convinced that the Land of Israel should be the Zionist goal.

## Rachmilewitz, Moshe                                              (Russia, 1899–1985)

Born in what is now Belarus, Moshe Rachmilewitz studied medicine at the University of Berlin. Rachmilewitz immigrated to Mandatory Palestine in 1926 and became Head of Hadassah Hospital on Mount Scopus. One of the founders of the Hebrew University-Hadassah Medical School in 1949, Rachmilewitz served as Dean of the Faculty from 1958–1961. An expert in internal medicine and hematology, Rachmilewitz was the personal physician of many of Israel's leaders. He was awarded the Israel Prize for Medicine in 1964 and named a Yakir Yerushalayim (Worthy of Jerusalem) in 1970.

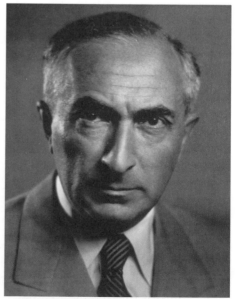

Photograph of Moshe Rachmilewitz by Ganan. (*Wellcome Collection*)

## Saliternick, Zvi (Ukraine, 1897–1993)

Born in Proskurov, Zvi Saliternick studied medicine in Kiev before emigrating to Mandatory Palestine in 1920, working in an anti-malarial program. After several years, Saliternick studied biology at the Hebrew University in Jerusalem and earned a doctorate in entomology. Saliternick focused his research on combatting malaria, serving as director of the anti-malaria department at the Ministry of Health from 1949–1962, where his efforts led to the eradication of the disease in Israel. Saliternick also directed the program leading to the elimination of the parasitic disease schistosomiasis from the country, and he was awarded the 1962 Israel Prize for medicine.

## Sheba, Chaim (Austria-Hungary, 1908–1971)

Born Chaim Scheiber in what is now Frasin, Romania, and a descendant of the famous Hasidic house of Ruzhin, Chaim Sheba began medical studies in Cernăuți and received his degree in Vienna. Immigrating to Mandatory Palestine in 1933, he practiced as a rural doctor for several years before joining the staff at Beilinson Hospital in Tel Aviv. A member of the Jewish Brigade and later the Haganah, after the War of Independence Sheba commanded the Medical Corps of the Israel Defense Forces for two years before leaving to become Director General of the Ministry of Health. Sheba then became Director of Tel Hashomer Hospital, which was later renamed the Chaim Sheba Medical Center in his honor.

A Professor of Medicine at the Hebrew University of Jerusalem, Sheba was one of the founders of

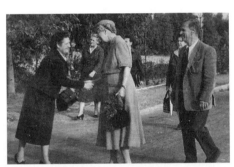

Chaim Sheba (right) escorts Eleanor Roosevelt during her visit to Sheba Medical Center, 1952. (*Wikimedia / Pikiwikisrael*)

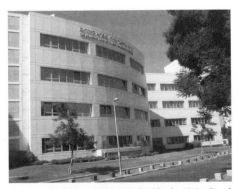

Safra Children Hospital, Sheba Medical Center, 2007. (*Wikimedia / David Shay*)

the Tel Aviv University Medical School and helped to establish medical schools in Jerusalem and Haifa.

## Sherman, Moshe                                    (Russia, 1881–1969)

Born in Nikolayev, Moshe Sherman studied medicine in Odessa and Berlin before graduating from the University of Dorpat (Estonia) and pursuing postgraduate studies in otolaryngology at Moscow University. In 1911, Sherman settled in Jaffa as the first otolaryngologist in the Land of Israel, setting up a private practice and soon becoming a famous specialist. Sherman volunteered at Sha'ar Zion, the Jewish hospital in Jaffa, and twice a year spent several weeks in Jerusalem seeing patients and performing small operations. In 1912, Sherman joined five other physicians to lay the foundation for the first doctors' organization in Israel. Long a consultant at Hadassah Hospital in Tel Aviv, in 1932 Sherman directed the newly established department for ear, nose and throat diseases. A prolific writer of articles in his specialty and on the history of Jewish organizations in the country, Sherman served as Editor-in-Chief of *Harefu'ah*, the official journal of the Israel Medical Association.

## Szold, Henrietta                                    (USA, 1860–1945)

Born in Baltimore about a year after her parents arrived in the U.S. from their native Hungary, Szold became a teacher at an elegant female academy and conducted classes for children and adults at the Conservative congregation where her father was the rabbi. The massive influx of Russian Jews after 1881 prompted Szold to at-

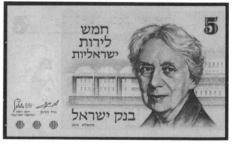

Henrietta Szold featured on a 5-lira Israel bank note, 1973. (*Author's private collection*)

tempt an experiment in practical education – a night school for immigrants – that she directed from 1888–1893. By the time the school was taken over by the city five years later, it had instructed more than 5,000 pupils (Christians as well as Jews) and had become the model for what later became the predominant pattern of Americanization of immigrants. This experience made Szold a confirmed Zionist, and in 1909 she made her first visit to the Holy Land. She was as impressed by the beauty and desirability of the land as by the misery and disease among its people. In 1912, invitations were issued for an organizational meeting of women interested in "the promotion of Jewish institutions and enterprises in Palestine,"[60] and 38 women constituted themselves as the Hadassah Chapter of Daughters of Zion. At the first convention of the young organization in 1914, the name was changed to Hadassah and Szold was elected the first president. Under her leadership, Hadassah (also known as the Women's Zionist Organization of American) established schools, hospitals, children's clinics, and welfare stations throughout the Land of Israel, where Szold resided after 1920. Seven years later, Szold was elected one of the three members of the Palestine Executive Committee of the World Zionist Organization, the first woman ever to serve in this capacity. Her portfolios were education and health. In 1930, Szold was elected to serve on the *Va'ad Leumi* (National Council of Jews in Palestine), which entrusted her with the responsibility for social welfare.

At age 73, Szold wanted to return to America and retire from public life. However, the advent of Nazi rule accelerated German immigration to the Land of Israel and brought about the implementation of a plan to send German adolescents there to complete their education. Consequently, the always-vigorous Szold undertook a new challenge, becoming director of a new agency (Youth Aliyah) set up for this purpose. In October 1934, Szold laid the cornerstone of the new Rothschild-Hadassah-University Hospital on Mount Scopus.

---

## Tchernichovky, Shaul (Russia, 1875–1943)

Born in the Ukraine, Shaul Tchernichovsky was raised in a religious home that was open to the ideas of the Enlightenment and Zionism. Failing to gain admission to a Russian university, Tchernichovsky studied medicine at the University of Heidelberg before receiving his degree in Lausanne. From then on, he combined his activities as a pediatrician with his increasing fame as a poet. In 1931, Tchernichovsky was commissioned to edit *The Book of Medical and Scientific Terms* (in Hebrew, Latin, and English) of the late Aaron Mazie, which enabled him to settle in the Land of Israel. Upon completion of this work in 1934, four years after the death of its primary author, Tchernichovsky was appointed physician of the municipal schools of Tel Aviv.

Heavily influenced by Greek and Roman literature, Tchernichovsky

---

60. http://www.jewishvirtuallibrary.org/hadassah-organization.

translated many classic foreign works into Hebrew. His poetry, considered among the masterpieces of modern Hebrew literature, reflected the wholesome and happier phases of traditional life in Eastern Europe and was distinguished by a vigorous sense of beauty and closeness to nature. Committed to the idea of a national and cultural revival of the Jewish people, Tchernichovsky's poems often deal with the Land of Israel landscape and provide a glimpse into the historical saga of Zionist aspirations of the preceding decades. Twice awarded Israel's coveted Bialik Prize, Tchernichovsky is one of four poets whose portrait appears on Israeli currency.

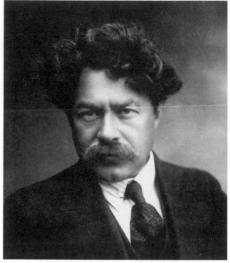

Portrait of Shaul Tchernichovsky by Š. Bajeris (Laisvės Al. 58, Kaunas), 1927. (*Wikimedia / Israel National Photo Collection*)

## Theilhaber, Felix A.                            (Germany, 1887–1956)

Born in Bamberg and the son of a doctor of obstetrics and gynecology, Felix Theilhaber's family moved to Munich when he was one year old and he studied medicine in Berlin and Munich. As a teenager, Theilhaber had become a member of the local Zionist chapter and made his first trip to the Land of Israel in 1906. Recognizing the trend of German Jews mi-

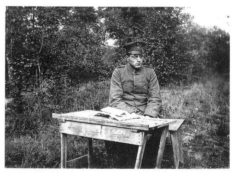

Felix Theilhaber. (*National Library of Israel*)

grating from the countryside to the big cities and having high rates of mixed marriages and a birth rate of less than one child per family, Theilhaber concluded that only Zionism could rejuvenate the Jewish people in the Diaspora, with the establishment of a Jewish homeland the only possibility for stopping the demise of the Jewish people.

After serving in a field hospital during World War I, Theilhaber settled in Berlin and specialized in skin and venereal diseases. A pioneer sexologist, he campaigned for birth control and against the criminalization of abortion and homosexuality, and was cofounder and sexologic adviser of one of the first birth control and sex advisory clinics in Berlin. The author of 20 books, in 1933 Thielhaber was imprisoned for two months when the Nazis took control of Germany and his medical license was revoked. Two years later, Thielhaber moved to Mandatory Palestine and, with other doctors of German origin, established the Maccabi Sick Fund as a private health insurance with free choice of doctor (and promoting awareness of the importance of physical activity) as an alternative to the system developed under the socialist workers' union. Today, the Maccabi Sick Fund remains one of the largest health maintenance organizations in Israel.

## Ticho, Abraham (Moravia, 1883–1960)

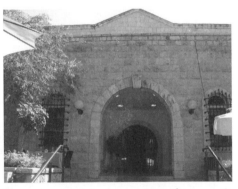

Trained in ophthalmology, Abraham Ticho immigrated to Jerusalem in 1912, devoting his professional career to fighting trachoma and other endemic eye diseases that caused thousands of cases of blindness among the local population. He founded and headed Jerusalem's first ophthalmic hospital, working tirelessly to save the eyesight of all who approached him. Among his patients was Emir Abdullah, later the king of Jordan.

Entrance to Ticho house, Jerusalem, 2008. (*Wikipedia*)

During the 1929 riots, Ticho was stabbed and seriously wounded outside his eye clinic near the Damascus Gate. Thousands of residents in the Jewish, Christian, and Muslim communities prayed for Ticho, and he eventually recovered from his injuries. Ticho then established his new eye clinic in the first floor of a 19th-century mansion in downtown Jerusalem, one of the first homes built outside the Old City walls, which he and his artist wife Anna had purchased several years previously. The Ticho House became a meeting place for local and British government officials, artists, writers, academics, and intellectuals. Anna willed their historic home, including her husband's Judaica collections and library, to the city of Jerusalem. It is now part of the Israel Museum and includes a restaurant and cultural center.

Fascinated by Chanukah menorahs, sometimes even accepting exotic ones in exchange for treatment, Ticho donated his remarkable collection to the Israel Museum.

## Zollschan, Ignaz                                          (Austria, 1877–1948)

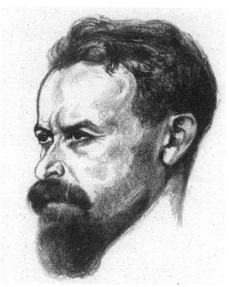

Born in Vienna, Ignaz Zollschan studied medicine at the University of Vienna. He specialized in radiology and established a private practice in Carlsbad. During a visit to the Middle East in 1928, Zollschan served as Chief of the X-ray Department of the Hadassah Medical Organization in Mandatory Palestine and gave a series of lectures at the Hebrew University in Jerusalem, but was unsuccessful in attempting to secure an academic position and returned to Carlsbad.

Also an anthropologist and later a vocal critic of Nazism, Zollschan was a prolific writer on the "Jewish racial question." Recognizing

Portrait of Ignaz Zollschan by Hermann Struck. (*Leo Baeck Institute Art and Objects Collection*)

the rise of racial anti-Semitism in his native Austria, he argued that Jews should be united by their racial origin rather than religion. Concluding that it was critical to preserve the Jewish race, Zollschan maintained that this quest was doomed in the Diaspora and could only be achieved through Zionism. Consequently, he strongly supported *Binyan ha-Aretz* (Building of the Land), a German Zionist organization that urged the immediate establishment of Jewish farms, businesses, and towns in Mandatory Palestine. When the Nazis occupied Austria, Zollschan fled to England.

# Bibliography

Burger, Natalia (ed). *Jews and Medicine: Religion, Culture, Science*. Philadelphia: The Jewish Publication Society, 1997.

Efron, John M. *Medicine and the German Jews: A History*. New Haven: Yale University Press, 2001.

Friedenwald, Harry. *The Jews and Medicine*. Baltimore: Johns Hopkins Press, 1944.

Friedenwald, Harry. *Jewish Luminaries in Medical History*. Johns Hopkins Press, 1946.

Heynick, Frank. *Jews and Medicine: An Epic Saga*. Hoboken (NJ): KTAV, 2002.

Isaacs, Ronald L. *Jews, Medicine, and Healing*. Norwalk (NJ): Jason Aronson, 1998.

Mann, Vivian B. *Gardens and Ghettos: The Art of Jewish Life in Italy*. New York, Jewish Museum.

Ruderman David B. *Jewish Thought and Scientific Discovery in Early Modern Europe*. New Haven: Yale University Press.

Ruderman, David B. *Kabbalah, Magic and Science: The Cultural Universe of a Sixteenth-Century Jewish Physician*. Cambridge, Harvard University Press, 1988.

Shatzmiller, Joseph. *Jews, Medicine, and Medieval Society*. Berkeley: University of California Press, 1995.

Whaley, Leigh. *Women and the Practice of Medical Care in Early Modern Europe, 1400–1800*. New York: Palgrave MacMillan, 2011.

# Alphabetical Index of Names